The NaProTECHNOLOGY *Revolution*

Unleashing the Power in a Woman's Cycle

THOMAS W. HILGERS, MD

BEAUFORT BOOKS
New York

What every woman has a right to know about her body...her health...her future!

Library of Congress Cataloging-in-Publication Data

Hilgers, Thomas W., 1943–
The naprotechnology revolution : unleashing the power in a woman's cycle /
Thomas W. Hilgers.
    p. cm.
Includes bibliographical references and index.
ISBN 978-0-8253-0626-6 (alk. paper)
1. Natural family planning. I. Title.
RG136.5.H552 2010
613.9'4—dc22
2010018419

10 9 8 7 6 5 4 3 2

Design and layout: Erik E. Baumgart, BFA
Layout editing: Victoria L. Sage, BSc
Cover design: Victoria L. Sage, BSc

Printed in China

Published by:
Beaufort Books
New York, New York
www.beaufortbooks.com

* The term **"NaProTECHNOLOGY"** has been registered in the U.S. Patent
and Trademark Office by the Pope Paul VI Institute for the Study of Human
Reproduction. It can be used freely by any person or entity as long as its use
reflects the medical concepts and values presented in the textbook,
"The Medical & Surgical Practice of NaProTECHNOLOGY,"
Pope Paul VI Institute Press, Omaha, Nebraska, 2004.

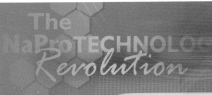

Tips On How to Use This Book

OU SHOULD APPROACH this book in a way that will allow it to be the most help to you. Here are a few tips for letting that happen.

First of all, by reading the *author's introduction,* you will get a sense of the feel, emotion and capability of the new women's health science, **NaProTECHNOLOGY** (Natural Procreative Technology).

The first four chapters of the book are important reading because they give you a good background on why **NaProTECHNOLOGY** and the **CREIGHTON MODEL Fertility*Care*™ System** were developed, what the motivating forces have been and a contrast between two different approaches to reproductive medicine. These first four chapters are a **must read** for everyone.

Chapters 5, 6 and 7 give the reader a review of basic anatomy and physiology, the various hormones of the menstrual and fertility cycle, how they interact and how they work. It also will introduce the reader to a variety of different myths, areas of ignorance and various insults that have been leveled at this work over the years. This, too, should be considered a **must read**.

The next series of chapters, Chapter 8 through Chapter 14, introduce the reader to a number of areas of *new understanding* that both the **CREIGHTON MODEL System** and **NaProTECHNOLOGY** introduce to the medical framework for the evaluation and treatment of a variety of conditions from which women of reproductive age suffer. It will introduce the reader to the **CREIGHTON MODEL**, how it can be used to date the beginning of a pregnancy, and how it can be used to target the cycle correctly for the proper and adequate evaluation of certain hormones that are produced during the course of the menstrual and fertility cycles. In addition to that, these chapters will introduce the reader to various aspects of normal and abnormal ovarian function, the difference between hormones that are produced normally in the body and artificial chemicals that are currently used day-in and day-out for the treatment of various conditions (in this book these are called *artimones*, artificial substitutes for hormones). It will introduce the reader to the use of progesterone support during the course of pregnancy and also the surgical aspects of **NaProTECHNOLOGY**. Perhaps the most important is the basic description of the charting system of the **CREIGHTON MODEL**. A little study of this chapter will help you immensely to understand the ensuing chapters.

Ultimately, **NaProTECHNOLOGY** has components that are medical, surgical and pregnancy-related. Once the first 14 chapters have been read, then the remaining portions of the book *can be read in any order*. This will undoubtedly be related to what your interest might be or what your own personal medical problem might be. Of course, we think that all of the chapters are important and you might wish to read about all of them, but definitely begin with those chapters that are most pertinent to your own situation.

Most of these chapters are not complex in their reading. However, a few of them are more technical, particularly from a medical point of view. Even though they have been written in a fashion that is strictly not overly medical, the lay reader may still find some of it technical. Thus, for your individual use, we have placed, at the conclusion of this book, a *"Glossary of Terms"* that you can use to better understand some of the more technical chapters.

Concepts presented in this book are heavily documented. The complete reference list, for those who might be interested, can be downloaded from the Internet Appendix for this book (*www.unleashingthepower.info*). There are additional resources at this website that can also be downloaded (at no charge).

Throughout the book, there are patient testimonials and comments that re-enforce the medical and educational substance of the content.

At the conclusion of a number of the chapters, there are "Action Items" and more technical details for physicians under "For the Doctor."

At the conclusion of the book, there are chapters that deal with the cost-effectiveness of **NaProTECHNOLOGY**, the need for insurance reform, and other important elements to the future of this new science and to your health. These chapters also should be read to give you the complete breadth of what this work challenges us to do.

Thomas W. Hilgers, MD, Dip. ABOG, ABLS, SRS, CFCMC

Director of the **Pope Paul VI Institute for the Study of Human Reproduction** in Omaha, Nebraska, he began his first research in the natural regulation of human fertility in 1968 as a senior medical student. Working at St. Louis University and Creighton University Schools of Medicine, he and his co-workers developed the **CREIGHTON MODEL Fertility***Care*™ **System**. Those intrinsically involved in the development of this system for the last 34 years, along with Dr. Hilgers, are K. Diane Daly, RN, CFCE; Susan K. Hilgers, BA, CFCE; and Ann M. Prebil, RN, BSN, CFCE.

Dr. Hilgers is currently a senior medical consultant in obstetrics, gynecology, reproductive medicine and surgery at the Pope Paul VI Institute and is a Clinical Professor in the Department of Obstetrics and Gynecology at Creighton University School of Medicine. He is director of the Institute's Education Programs and its National Center for Women's Health. He is board certified in Obstetrics and Gynecology, Gynecologic Laser Surgery and he is a member of the Society of Reproductive Surgeons. Furthermore, he is certified by the American Academy of Fertility*Care* Professionals (AAFCP) as a **Fertility***Care*™ Medical Consultant (CFCMC). In 1994, Dr. Hilgers, along with his wife, Susan, was named by Pope John Paul II to a five-year term to the Pontifical Council for the Family, and he also was appointed an active member of the Pontifical Academy for Life.

FOR FURTHER INFORMATION,
CONSULT THE FOLLOWING WEB SITES:

www.naprotechnology.com
Provides additional information on the new
woman's health science of **NaProTECHNOLOGY**
including an exhaustive listing of medical references.
The medical textbook,
"The Medical & Surgical Practice of **NaProTECHNOLOGY**",
can be ordered on this site.

www.creightonmodel.com
Provides some additional information on the
CREIGHTON MODEL Fertility*Care*™ System.

www.popepaulvi.com
The website of the Pope Paul VI Institute and how to seek
assistance from the Physicians at the Institute
and its National Center for Women's Health

www.fertilitycare.org
The website of **Fertility*Care*™ Centers of America** and listing of
CREIGHTON MODEL teachers and medical consultants.

www.DrHilgers.com
Dr. Thomas W. Hilgers' website for
"straight talk on women's health care"

www.aafcp.org
The official website of the
American Academy of Fertility*Care* Professionals.

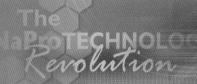

Table of Contents

Tips On How to Use This Book   v

About the Author   ix

Table of Patient Testimonials and *For the Doctor*   xiii

Introduction   xv

Acknowledgments   xxv

An Important Cautionary Note   xxvi

A. The State of Modern Reproductive Medicine

   Chapter 1:   Dissent and Discovery   3

   Chapter 2:   The Medical and Social Consequences   15

   Chapter 3:   Women Healed: **NaProTECHNOLOGY**   25

   Chapter 4:   Two Approaches to Reproductive Medicine   31

B. How the Reproductive System Works

   Chapter 5:   Basic Anatomy and Physiology   43

   Chapter 6:   The Cycle of Hormones   53

   Chapter 7:   Myths, Ignorance and Insults   61

C. A New Understanding

   Chapter 8:   **CREIGHTON MODEL** and its Charting System   73

   Chapter 9:   Dating the Beginning of Pregnancy   97

   Chapter 10: Targeted Hormone Evaluation and Treatment   103

   Chapter 11: Abnormal Ovarian Function   115

   Chapter 12: Hormones vs. Artimones   127

   Chapter 13: Progesterone Support During Pregnancy   137

   Chapter 14: Surgical **NaProTECHNOLOGY**: Surgery of the Heart   157

D. Conditions, Diseases, and **NaProTECHNOLOGY**

Chapter 15: Effects of Stress   169

Chapter 16: Recurrent Ovarian Cysts   175

Chapter 17: Premenstrual Syndrome   181

Chapter 18: Postpartum Depression   199

Chapter 19: Infertility: What Progress Over 50 Years   207

Chapter 20: **NaProTECHNOLOGY** and Infertility   227

Chapter 21: Recurrent Miscarriage   259

Chapter 22: Endometriosis   275

Chapter 23: Polycystic Ovarian Disease   285

Chapter 24: Absence of Menstrual Periods   299

Chapter 25: Male Infertility   303

Chapter 26: Menstrual Cramps and Pelvic Pain   313

Chapter 27: Chronic Vaginal Discharges   321

Chapter 28: Unusual Bleeding   331

Chapter 29: Prevention of Preterm Birth   351

E. The Future

Chapter 30: Costs and Insurance Reform   377

Chapter 31: New Insights from Current Research   387

Appendices

Internet Appendix: www.unleashingthepower.info   399

    1. Complete List of References for this Book

    2. Introduction to the CrMS

    3. Scientific Foundation of the Creighton Model System

    4. Medical Risks of Infertility

    For a Teacher or Medical Consultant: www.fertilitycare.org

Glossary of Terms

Glossary of Terms   403

Index

Index   423

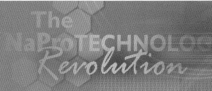

The NaProTECHNOLOGY Revolution

Table of Patient Testimonials and *For the Doctor*

Patient Testimonials

Debra: Hormonal depression — 182

Susan: Premenstrual syndrome — 196

Five patients: Abandoned by the medical profession — 225

Jeanine: Infertility, miscarriage, and pelvic pain — 257

Marcia: Recurrent miscarriage — 270

A young woman: Endometriosis — 275

A nurse: Mainstream treatment of fertility-related issues — 285

Kathy: Unusual bleeding — 346

Jeanine: Prevention of preterm birth — 373

For the Doctor

Targeted hormone evaluation and treatment — 111

Abnormal ovarian function — 122

Progesterone support during pregnancy — 150

Recurrent miscarriage — 180

Premenstrual syndrome — 194

Postpartum depression — 205

Recurrent miscarriage — 273

Polycystic ovarian disease — 297

Absence of Menstrual Periods — 302

Chronic vaginal discharge — 329

Unusual bleeding — 348

ARE YOU A WOMAN of reproductive age (12 to 50 years)? Are you a woman in this age group who has been to your obstetrician/gynecologist with *recurrent ovarian cysts, menstrual cramps, long and irregular cycles, irregular bleeding* and/or other conditions related to the menstrual and fertility cycles? Has your doctor given you birth control pills to treat your symptoms? Have you felt *frustrated* after that because the doctor did not actually do any testing to find out what the cause of the problem was? Did you feel like you had only received a Band-Aid?

Are you a woman who has experienced an *infertility problem?* Have you gone to your obstetrician-gynecologist with the idea in mind of finding out why it is you are having difficulty achieving a pregnancy? Did your doctor give you Clomid (an ovulation inducing medication) for a few cycles and then refer you to an *in vitro* fertilization (IVF—test tube baby) clinic without ever looking into the underlying causes? Did you go to the IVF clinic only to find out that they were not interested in what was wrong with you? *Was this frustrating?* Or maybe you are a woman who has experienced infertility and has been afraid to go to an infertility specialist because you know that you will be exposed to a whole variety of approaches to reproductive health that you, quite frankly, don't believe in.

Are you a woman who experiences significant *mood swings, premenstrual syndrome* or just a feeling that your hormones are *"all wacked out?"* Have you been to your doctor for these symptoms? Did they automatically prescribe either birth control pills, antidepressants or anti-anxiety medications without evaluating your hormones or doing anything to find out what was wrong? Maybe you have suffered from *postpartum depression* only to be treated with antidepressants that are slow to work, make you feel drugged and never return you to normal. And yet, you are never told about a simple hormone therapy that can bring about rapid relief in nearly 95 percent of cases.

Have you been a *pregnant woman,* where during the course of your pregnancy, you experienced pelvic pressure, the uterus knotting up like a ball, low backache, vaginal discharge and so forth? When you told your obstetrician about this did he or she have a blank stare or offer the only treatment as bedrest and "drink lots of fluids"? Or was the obstetrician just patronizing and reassuring that everything is going to be okay? If this was your situation, did you deliver your baby *prematurely,* in spite of what your doctor prescribed for you? Were you somewhat frustrated by the lack of attention given to your symptoms?

If you have found yourself in any of the above situations, and also found yourself either *dissatisfied* or *frustrated* or even *abandoned,*then you are not alone! In my experience, over the last 30 years, you are a member of a growing number of women who are deeply dissatisfied with today's approach to reproductive health care. Health care that is neither reproductive (usually) nor healthy (often).

Are you aware, for example, that severe menstrual cramps are often caused by endometriosis and that treating the endometriosis surgically can be of great long-term benefit to you in reducing the pain that you experience? In fact, for adolescents, who are often placed on birth control pills for severe menstrual cramps, in our experience, the incidence of endometriosis in that population is 100 percent.

Did you know that long and irregular cycles are often associated with *polycystic ovarian disease* and that this is also the cause of much of the irregular bleeding that a woman experiences in such circumstances? Indeed, polycystic ovarian disease is a multifaceted disease condition which increases a woman's risk of uterine cancer, breast cancer, heart abnormalities, abnormalities with one's lipid profile (including cholesterol and triglycerides) and so forth.

Do you have *premenstrual spotting?* Do you have *brown bleeding at the end of your menstrual flow?* Have you told your doctor about these without much response except, "I think the birth control pill will help." These are all symptoms of what are associated with either *abnormal hormone function* or possibly even *chronic infection or inflammation* within the lining of the uterus.

Did you know that infertility has many different causes, and that, in fact, these causes are often present all at the same time? In fact, infertility has many facets to it. Many women have endometriosis, others have pelvic adhesions, others still have polycystic ovaries. Associated with these, there may be underlying *hormonal abnormalities* and *ovulation-related defects* that cannot be diagnosed with basal body temperature, the urinary ovulation test kits, or even a serum progesterone level on Day 21 of the cycle. Many of these women have *defects in the production of cervical mucus* which can be readily identified. Furthermore, did you know that these are easily identified and tracked? Did you also know that the profession of obstetrics and gynecology has **completely disregarded and ignored such tracking?**

Did you know that the *prematurity rate has nearly doubled in the last 40 years?* Did you know that the treatment protocols recommend, before a patient is given progesterone, a hormone that has been proven to help reduce the prematurity rate, that *she should first experience at least one premature birth?* Why would they subject **any** pregnancy to the risk of preterm birth? Why, in this era of modern medicine, has the prematurity rate nearly doubled over these years?

Did you know that it is possible to cut your prematurity risk nearly in half with a treatment approach *available to all physicians* in the United States and the Western world? Did you know that by reducing prematurity, you could also protect your baby from the very real threats that a preterm birth poses? Did you know further that the increase in prematurity is, at least in part, due to physician-related causes? In other words, some treatments that physicians implement can cause premature birth. Women who achieve a pregnancy with the artificial reproductive technologies (such as IVF) have an increased risk of multiple birth and these multiple pregnancies are, in turn, associated with a prematurity rate of 50 to 100 percent.

It is hard to believe that during these last 40 to 50 years, we, as a culture, have accepted this standard for the practice of reproductive medicine. In effect, *it is an approach to medical care which is based on treating symptoms, but not the disease.* It does not discover the underlying problem, and whatever control of symptoms it provides, it is nearly always temporary with the symptoms returning once the treatment has been discontinued, and this is because the disease or cause has not been treated.

While there have been, over these many years, large volumes of published research in the field of reproductive medicine especially as it relates to contraception and IVF, *there is one huge blank space!* It is as if the research stopped! Relatively few studies have been done to better understand a woman's menstrual and fertility cycles and, of those studies in this area that have been published, they have been largely *ignored.* These major physiologic events that affect greater than 50 percent of our population during the reproductive years, have been almost ***completely ignored by the medical profession.*** Furthermore, the patients who do not wish to use artificial contraceptives, be sterilized, have an abortion or select *in vitro* fertilization, have been largely *abandoned.*

This trend in reproductive health care began in 1960 when the oral contraceptive was placed on the market. This birth control pill suppressed the pituitary gland, stopped ovulation (for the most part), and gave to a woman an artificial bleed on a monthly basis, which was not her menstruation, but a withdrawal bleed from the chemicals in the birth control pill. This birth control pill (with many variations to come in the next 40 to 50 years) was quickly adopted as a treatment approach for any number of menstrual cycle irregularities suffered by many women in the reproductive years. *But, in fact, it has cured none of them.* It is an artificial suppressant of the reproductive system, which gives symptomatic relief (along with a long litany of side effects) and provides for the doctor the camouflage that he or she was providing a treatment and, for the woman, the thought that this was the best and only treatment available.

In the late 1960s and early 1970s, abortion became widely available in the United States and women who had high-risk pregnancies were told, in many cases, that the only treatment for their condition was to abort the pregnancy.

In 1978, the first baby was born by *in vitro* fertilization performed by a group of doctors in England. The main reason given for performing this test-tube baby procedure was the scar tissue and blockage of the fallopian tubes experienced by this woman and in the future for other women. That was the only indication in 1978. Now it is used and promoted for almost all aspects of infertility treatment. Like its predecessors, the birth control pill and abortion, the woman is not investigated for determining what the underlying causes are.

So that basically brings us up to date. We have now developed a dominant profession in obstetrics and gynecology that has accepted, as an approach to the evaluation and treatment of women with reproductive problems, programs that *either suppress their fertility or destroy it.* There is the thought that a woman cannot handle a diagnosis. It reminds me of the days prior to telling patients they had cancer when the doctor would keep this information to themselves.

We are now exposed to a way of thinking in reproductive medicine which is basically different from any other area of medicine. The search for a diagnosis of what's causing the problem is often not made and the woman is placed on a treatment which provides only symptomatic relief masquerading itself as a form of real cure.

It is easy, in some ways, to see how this has happened. But in order to understand it, you must understand that it is *a way of thinking* that is at the foundation of these last 40 to 50 years in reproductive medicine. *The major professional organizations of the dominant culture in obstetrics and gynecology have adopted, promoted, established as policy, and for the most part, sanctified this approach.* They have promoted it to the physicians who practice in this field, made it the framework upon which new medical students and young obstetricians and gynecologists are trained and have been the foundation upon which third party reimbursement agencies (both health insurance companies and government insurance programs) have established their reimbursement policies. In other words, the entire profession and all that supports it has pushed forward with a philosophy of reproductive medicine that often *does not establish a diagnosis, does not treat the underlying diseases and supports cheap programs of treatment which carry with them various risks that ultimately make it more expensive.* Indeed, this has all happened in a very seductive way while nobody has been able to challenge it.

This has led to a whole host of problems that go unmet. These are the things that I have great concern about:

- The millions of women who suffer from infertility without ever knowing the reason (the diagnosis) for the infertility and without it being properly treated.
- The hundreds of thousands of miscarriages that occur each year because of inadequate evaluation and treatment.
- The thousands of women who have unnecessary hysterectomies each year and needless surgery for functional ovarian cysts.
- The hundreds of thousands of women who suffer from complications of pregnancy that could be prevented with adequate progesterone support. Perhaps even worse is the lack of good and adequate research in these areas.

- The thousands of babies that are born prematurely in the United States, many of them unnecessary and preventable.

- The needless cerebral palsy, mental and motor retardation and other physical and mental effects that come as the result of the incredibly poor record that has been established in the United States for the prevention of preterm birth.

- The hundreds of thousands of women who suffer needlessly from postpartum depression after having a baby, a miscarriage, an ectopic pregnancy, or an induced abortion.

- The millions of women who suffer needlessly from premenstrual syndrome.

- The millions of women who suffer needlessly from menstrual cramps, pelvic pain, and pain with intercourse because of poorly and inadequately treated endometriosis and pelvic adhesive disease.

- The thousands of women who suffer from the long-term ill effects of long and irregular cycles.

- The millions of women who subject themselves needlessly to the contraceptive and abortion practices of this culture.

- A dominant profession in obstetrics and gynecology that has been controlled financially by the contraception-abortion corporate complex (CACC) – both private and public (including a third party reimbursement system that rewards this approach to reproductive medicine).

- The scarcity of research that is being done to reduce these concerns.

I have asked several of my patients if they would write a short description of their experiences in receiving reproductive health care at the Pope Paul VI Institute and then to contrast that with the care they have received through other clinics. I wanted them to describe the contrasts because it is such a recurring story that I wanted it to be highlighted. Specifically, however, I asked them not to mention any physicians' names. The types of stories that are integrated into the various chapters of this book found in Section D are so incredibly common in our experience that to name the physician involved would be non-productive. Physicians' attitudes towards the various conditions outlined here are often very negative and this has become the predominant care pattern. But these are real people who have real problems and they deserve better.

If medicine does not have a solution that can be approved by a professional organization, it is still the *physician's responsibility* to attempt to implement medical strategies that potentially can be of help. In order to do this effectively, however, one needs to know what the underlying problems are and one needs to choose treatment approaches, which by themselves should not threaten the patient's health. So there is *a science* and *an art of medicine*. The science of medicine has often been usurped by the various professional organizations (but still is the responsibility of the individual physician). At times, this science is deeply biased by a philosophical relativism that is often prejudicial, antagonistic, and discriminatory. The *art of medicine is fully the responsibility of the individual physician* and how he or she interacts with and cares about and for the patient. The professional organizations aren't able to take over this responsibility. The patients I asked to write about this accepted my invitation without hesitation and they have often put their name to it.

While testimonials of and by themselves are not scientific proof of the effectiveness of a particular treatment strategy, they still are important, especially in this work in reproductive medicine because the contemporary approaches tend to be cold and lack heart. They tend to be opinionated without an adequate understanding of the science and, if the patient believes in certain principles that are different from the physician's beliefs, then pray for that patient because she will not get the help that she desires and needs.

In this book, I have the honor of presenting a new women's health science. The research and scientific foundations for this new science have come a long way and have already been published in detail in a 1,244-page medical textbook written for doctors (Hilgers, TW: The Medical & Surgical Practice of **NaProTECHNOLOGY**. Pope Paul VI Institute Press, Omaha, Nebraska 2004. See *www.naprotechnology.com*). This book is written for the lay public so that they may also have access to this new approach.

NaProTECHNOLOGY refers to *natural procreative technology*. In **NaProTECHNOLOGY**, we study the basic concepts of the normal menstrual and fertility cycle. We look at a way of tracking the cycle that is *objective* and *standardized*. With this we can begin to describe and understand what is normal and what is not normal or what is diseased. By taking this approach, we can also find and look for the underlying causes which then allow us to effectively treat it for long-term health. Indeed, **NaProTECHNOLOGY** uses the **CREIGHTON MODEL Fertility*Care*™ System** and its biological markers which are gained through education to guide its medical and technological resources so that it can be used *cooperatively* with the woman's cycle. This is key to the new science of **NaProTECHNOLOGY**. It is a new women's health science that has been built through the process of *listening to women*. It is not one which suppresses or destroys, but rather one that works cooperatively with the woman's cycle. It is this that allows this new science to *unleash the power that exists in a woman's cycle.* This power is one of *knowledge, understanding* and *medical application.*

This is the story of one physician's resistance to a dominant profession that has chosen approaches that are largely suppressive and destructive. Approaches that have, as their very foundation, a way of thinking which too often doesn't care about the underlying diseases. It is the story of how a new women's health science was conceived, born and raised within a dominant profession that thinks differently. It approaches problem solving by looking for the underlying problem. *It approaches patients by listening to them!* It approaches treatment by working toward eliminating the cause or the disease which is causing the symptoms. To accomplish this, an orderly and thorough study of *both* the *menstrual* and *fertility cycles* had to be conducted. In many ways this would seem to be a "no-brainer." But the dominant profession throughout the decades of its existence has done very little of this and what has been done, for the most part, has been ignored or ridiculed. This process has been like solving a puzzle, by putting all of the pieces in the right place. To do this, we have had to work toward *unraveling the mysteries of a woman's cycle.*

If you are one of the many women who have not been able to get satisfactory answers to the problems you have experienced with your menstrual cycle, your fertility or any number of related problems, you may have adopted the attitude that finding the cause or the remedy is truly hopeless. I am here to tell you that it is HOPELESS NO MORE! **NaProTECHNOLOGY** is an approach to a woman's reproductive health that works toward identifying the root cause and treating it effectively.

Experience over the years has revealed the amazing fact that most women **do not know the basics** about how their **body** works and functions. In some ways, the profession has "hidden" important aspects of this. The basic principles of how this information can be integrated so that a woman's **health** can be monitored, maintained and improved is also not known to most women and to their health care providers. Because there are any number of ill effects associated with the way reproductive medicine is practiced in today's world (and these may affect both the woman and her child), this can, in turn, profoundly and adversely affect her **future.** This book introduces you to another way of approaching this. **NaProTECHNOLOGY** teaches a woman about how **her body works,** how this information can be used constructively to improve her health and how *all of this impacts in a positive way her future* and *the future of those around her.* This book introduces you to the new women's health science of **NaProTECHNOLOGY**. It presents vital information that a woman has a **right to know** about **her body…** **her health…** and **her future!** It is truly a **bold new way of thinking,** **approaching** and **healing** in women's health!

In 2004, an international conference "Introducing **NaProTECHNOLOGY** to the World" was held at the Qwest Center in Omaha, Nebraska. The new medical textbook "The Medical & Surgical Practice of **NaProTECHNOLOGY**" (Pope Paul VI Institute Press, Omaha, Nebr., 2004) was formally presented. It detailed the nearly 30 years of scientific research that went into this approach. What has happened since then has been something that I would never have imagined to occur in my lifetime. Lay and medical professionals have come from six continents to be trained as providers of the **CREIGHTON MODEL** **System** and **NaProTECHNOLOGY**. These services have since expanded to a number of additional European nations (Poland, Switzerland, Italy, France, Croatia, Slovakia, Ukraine), Nigeria, Australia, Taiwan, Singapore, and Japan. They have merged with countries where these services were already available including the United States, Canada, Mexico, Ireland, United Kingdom, the Netherlands, and Germany. The ultimate list is nearly endless! There has been brewing a revolution—"the **NaProTECHNOLOGY** revolution"! This is happening because of the research that decoded the mysteries of the menstrual and fertility cycles— "unleashing the power in a woman's cycle"!

I hope that this book will serve as an introduction to the lay public of this remarkable approach. It is my honor and privilege to present it to you.

Thomas W. Hilgers, MD

Thomas W. Hilgers, MD
Senior Medical Consultant
Obstetrics, Gynecology, Reproductive Medicine and Surgery
Clinical Professor
Department of Obstetrics and Gynecology
Creighton University School of Medicine
Director
Pope Paul VI Institute for the Study of Human Reproduction

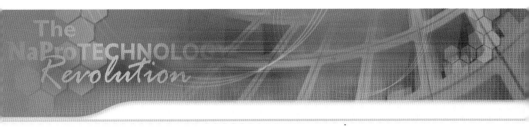

The author wishes to acknowledge with gratitude the invaluable role that a number of people have played in seeing this project come to completion.

First and foremost are those research assistants who have provided invaluable aid to its completion. These people include: Pamela Yaksich, BS; Jeremy Kalamarides; Paula Maslonka, BS; and Christy Schoen, BS. Additional research assistance also was provided by Jennifer Davis, Kristina Garnett, Stephen Hilgers, Michael Hilgers, Paul Houser, Amanda Mafilika Austin, Anh Nguyen, Rae Nguyen, Jennifer Pavela, Teresa Sobie, Brian Tullius, and Patrick Yeung. In addition, Nelson Fong, PhD, assisted with some of our biostatistical analyses and John Vasiliades, PhD, served as a consultant in biochemistry. Ken Oyer, librarian at the Dr. John Hartigan Medical Library at Bergan Mercy Medical Center, and the librarians at Creighton University and University of Nebraska Schools of Medicine are also acknowledged for their professional support.

The invaluable, expert layout and design services of Erik Baumgart, BFA, along with the secretarial assistance of Terri Green and the graphic design work of Victoria Sage, BSc, are gratefully acknowledged.

The work could not have been accomplished without the development of the **CREIGHTON MODEL Fertility*Care*™ System** and the great assistance of its co-developers, K. Diane Daly, RN, CFCE; Susan Hilgers, BS, CFCE; and Ann Prebil, RN, BSN, CFCE.

The medical technicians in the National Hormone Laboratory of the Pope Paul VI Institute also have provided invaluable assistance: Barbara Gentrup, Deborah Frahm, and Janice McAlpine. Our ultrasonographers, Jeanine Johnson and Sandra Keck, also are gratefully acknowledged.

Our nursing staff headed by Linda Cady, RN, along with Barbara Schimerdla, RN; Marlene Beckman, RN; Teresa Kenney, APRN; Cheryl Dorman, Tanya Land, Cathy Broderson, and the assistance of the directors of the **FertilityCare™ Centers of Omaha**, Kathy Cherovsky, CFCS, and Jeanice Vinduska, CFCP, CFCE, also are gratefully acknowledged.

The author wishes to thank Mary Pat Wilson for her artistic skills in assisting with the production of the **CREIGHTON MODEL FertilityCare™** charts that are included in this book. In addition, Stacee Milan, computer graphics assistant at Creighton University's Biocommunications Center, is acknowledged for assisting in the production of many of the graphs presented in this book.

The author also recognizes the American Academy of FertilityCare Professionals who, over the last 27 years, have given a forum to the presentation of the ideas presented in this book so that they could be publicly presented, discussed and implemented. Their collegial support has been deeply appreciated and the development of **NaProTECHNOLOGY** could not have occurred without their assistance.

I also thank Lisa Maxson for her expert editing and proofreading assistance. In addition, I am grateful for the proofreading of Kirsten Lillegard. I also thank Deborah Colloton for her expert guidance in the creation of this book.

Finally, this work also could not have been accomplished without the financial support of those who have so deeply believed in this work. This includes many individual and institutional donors who have been extraordinarily generous in supporting this effort.

A special note of appreciation, too, to L. Paul Comeau for his support and friendship and to the entire staff of the Pope Paul VI Institute.

A very special appreciation goes also to my dear wife Susan and our entire family (Paul, Stephen, Michael, Teresa, and Matthew) for their support. I will tell you that this work could not have been accomplished without Susan's tremendous love and support.

For all of the above, the author expresses his deep and sincere appreciation and gratefully acknowledges their assistance and support.

The **CREIGHTON MODEL Fertility***Care*™ **System** (CrMS) is a new and unique model of advanced procreative education. It allows for the first time the opportunity to network family planning with women's health and it accomplishes this in a way that is *completely natural and cooperative* with a woman's menstrual and fertility cycles.

This book *does not replace adequate instruction in this system.* The system is designed to be learned through an adequate instructional experience provided by a properly trained **CREIGHTON MODEL Fertility***Care*™ **Practitioner** (FCP) or **Fertility***Care*™ **Instructor** (FCI) who has a thorough grasp of the principles outlined in this book and its associated teaching materials. Such a provider can be found at *www.fertilitycare.org.*

Medicine is an ever-changing field. Standard safety precautions must be followed but, as new research and clinical experience broaden our knowledge, changes in treatment and drug therapy become necessary or appropriate. Readers are advised to check the product information currently provided by the manufacturer of each drug to be administered to verify the recommended dose, the method and duration of administration, and the contraindications. It is the responsibility of the treating physician, relying on experience and knowledge of the patient, to determine dosages and the best treatment for the patient. Neither the publisher nor the author assume any responsibility for any injury and/or damage to persons or property.

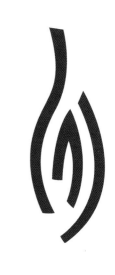

The State of
Modern Reproductive
Medicine

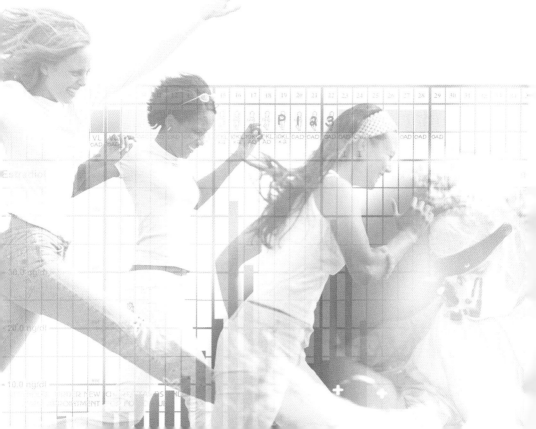

Dissent and Discovery

I<small>N</small> 1960, after a number of years of experimentation on poor women in Puerto Rico, the Food and Drug Administration approved for commercial application the first birth control pill. It was used instantly by many women. The only thing that was needed for its widespread distribution was a medical degree, a license to practice medicine and a prescription pad. There were, of course, hundreds of thousands of such doctors worldwide and "The Pill" has been used extensively ever since.

The oral contraceptives are generally made up of a combination of a synthetic orally-active estrogen-like chemical and a synthetic orally-active progesterone-like chemical. The estrogen-like *chemical* present in the oral contraceptive is *not human identical.* It is thus not natural to the human body, but it does absorb orally and it has some estrogen-like properties. The same is true for the progesterone-like *chemical.* It also is *not human identical.* It is an artificial progesterone-like substitute that metabolizes, at least in part, to male androgenic hormones. The chemicals in the birth control pill can be referred to as *artimones* (artificial hormones that are not human identical – see Chapter 12).

While the oral contraceptive was released as a contraceptive agent (to be used for birth control), it soon became a drug that was prescribed by physicians for nearly *any type of female health problem* in women of reproductive age. Some of the health problems include the following: *irregular menstrual cycles, abnormal bleeding, recurrent ovarian cysts, severe menstrual cramps, endometriosis, premenstrual syndrome, and*

3

almost any other condition that affects the menstrual cycle. In other words, it was released as a contraceptive agent, but then was phased in for the treatment of a variety of women's health problems. Nearly all of its uses for health problems, with the exception of acne, are *"off label" uses.* This means that the Food and Drug Administration has not approved the labeling of the contraceptive agent for these purposes.

Between the years 1968 and 1973, there was a gradual legalization of abortion that occurred in the United States culminating in the Supreme Court decision of January 22, 1973, *Roe v. Wade.* This legalized abortion for almost all reasons throughout the course of the entire pregnancy. It is, one can argue, the most extreme abortion policy of any country in the world (perhaps with the exception of China).

The first baby born through *in vitro* fertilization (test-tube baby) was born July 25, 1978. This was hailed as a new treatment for infertility and it was a treatment that initially was thought to apply only to women who had blocked fallopian tubes. Today, however, it is used for almost any infertility problem that exists.

Each of these *three major developments* in the field of reproductive medicine—the release of the birth control pill, the legalization of abortion, and the introduction of *in vitro* fertilization—has had a major impact on the practice of obstetrics and gynecology and the health care of women.

In the case of the birth control pill when it is prescribed for various abnormalities of the menstrual cycle, it is a *symptomatic form of treatment only.* In other words, when the doctor prescribes the oral contraceptive for a medical reason, he or she does so without actually knowing what the underlying problem is. The doctor may know the symptoms because the patient has conveyed those symptoms to the doctor, but when the physician prescribes the birth control pill, he or she almost always does not look for the underlying cause and is only treating symptoms and not the disease.

In the case of abortion, it initially had been promoted for the solution of various social problems within society. It can be argued that none of these social problems have been adequately treated as a result of abortion. In fact, they have been almost all made worse (see Chapter 2). For the purposes of this book, however, it is important for the reader to recognize that when a high-risk problem occurs in pregnancy, it is not unusual for abortion to be recommended, even when the condition can be treated successfully without using abortion as a "treatment."

In vitro fertilization (IVF) has become the main approach to the treatment of infertility, and yet, it does so with very little knowledge of what the causes of the infertility problem might be. In fact, many doctors who recommend IVF do so specifically with the idea in mind that they *do not need to know what the underlying diseases are* that are causing the infertility problem. So if one is treated with IVF, she will continue to have the underlying diseases that are causing the infertility problem to begin with.

These three major developments have had a marked impact on how physicians approach problem-solving in women's health care. They have dominated the treatment approaches of the obstetrician-gynecologist and specialists in reproductive medicine over the last 45 to 50 years.

Dissent

One might wonder why an obstetrician-gynecologist from Omaha, Nebraska, would be so bold as to say that he has developed a new insight into the evaluation and the treatment of many women's health problems, when, in fact, it goes so contrary to the general approaches taken by the dominant profession. This is a legitimate question and it deserves a fair response.

I am a Roman Catholic and when I was in medical school there was a great debate within the Catholic Church as to whether or not the Church would approve various methods of contraception, including the new birth control pill. I followed that controversy closely thinking actually that the Church was going to change its long-held position of being opposed to contraception. Then, on July 25, 1968, Pope Paul VI issued a papal letter (formally referred to as an encyclical letter) called *Humanae Vitae* (Of Human Life). This letter was addressed not only to Catholics, but also to "all men of good will." It described the Catholic Church's position on contraception and it reiterated its centuries-old position of opposition.

The encyclical letter was met with an *instant and well-organized dissent* from Catholic theologians and philosophers all throughout the United States and in other countries. This had the effect of pulling the rug out from underneath the teaching and leading Catholics in the direction of contraception so that today, there is virtually no difference within the population as to the percentage of Catholics who use contraceptive measures.

At the time, I thought it would be a good idea to read this encyclical letter. I already had understood that the coverage of such an issue by the main print and television outlets was certain to be strongly biased against the teaching. I went to the Newman Club (Catholic) chaplain at the University of Minnesota (where I was attending medical school) and I asked him where I could get a copy of it. He looked at me with some degree of surprise and said, "What do you want to read that kind of trash for?" I wasn't really expecting that response, but in spite of it, I was able to finally obtain a copy of the encyclical letter and it had a major impact on the rest of my personal, as well as professional life. It is worth our while to reflect a bit on what this letter had to say.

First of all, it described the characteristic marks and demands of conjugal love and the supreme importance of having an exact idea of what these are. Primarily, this love is *"fully human,"* … and "this love is *total,"* … *"it is faithful and exclusive until death,"* and … "this love is *fecund."* In that regard, it taught that "Marriage and conjugal love are by their nature ordained toward the begetting and educating of children. Children are really *the supreme gift of marriage* and contribute very substantially to the welfare of the parents"[1] (emphasis applied). The encyclical letter went on to say:

> "The teaching, often set forth by the Magisterium, is founded upon the inseparable connection, willed by God and unable to be broken by man on his own initiative, between the two meanings of the conjugal act: the unitive meaning and the procreative meaning. Indeed, by its intimate structure, the conjugal act, while most closely uniting husband and wife, capacitates them for the generation of new lives, according to two laws inscribed in the very being of man and of woman. By safeguarding both these essential aspects, the unitive and the procreative, the conjugal act preserves in its fullness the sense of true mutual love and its ordination toward man's most high calling to parenthood. We believe that the men of our day are particularly capable of seizing the deeply reasonable and human character of this fundamental principle."[2]

After reading these paragraphs from *Humanae Vitae*, it became clear to me that the Church wished to preserve the connections between *love and life* and that Her ultimate decision had to be a rejection of contraception, sterilization and abortion. To see that this was accomplished, Pope Paul VI issued what I have often referred to as the "challenges of *Humanae Vitae.*" These were presented in Part III of this encyclical, the *Pastoral Directives*. Two of the challenges seemed to be addressed to me:

To men of science

"We wish now to express our encouragement to men of science who 'can considerably advance the welfare of marriage and the family, along with peace of conscience, if by pooling their efforts, they labor to explain more thoroughly the various conditions favoring a proper regulation of births.'… In this way, scientists, and especially Catholic scientists, will clearly demonstrate in actual fact, that, as the Church teaches, 'a true contradiction cannot exist between the divine laws pertaining to the transmission of life and those pertaining to the fostering of authentic conjugal love.'"[3]

To doctors and medical personnel

"We hold those physicians and medical personnel in the highest esteem who, in the exercise of their profession, value above every human interest, the superior demands of their Christian vocation. Let them persevere, therefore, in promoting on every occasion, the discovery of solutions inspired by faith and right reason. Let them strive to arouse this conviction and this respect in their associates. Let them also consider as their proper professional duty, the task of acquiring all of the knowledge needed in this delicate sector, so as to be able to give to those married persons who consult them wise counsel and healthy direction, such as they have a right to expect."[4]

When I read these "challenges of *Humanae Vitae*" I felt the Church was speaking directly to me, although I fully realize the Church was speaking to all of us. By December 1968, I began my very first research project trying to better understand the natural methods of family planning. Working with six female medical students, I evaluated the salivary albumin concentration as it fluctuated in the menstrual and fertility cycles. While it was an interesting research project, it was not very productive.

Faith and Reason

There has, over the years, developed in Western society, the thought that religion and science are in irrevocable conflict. On September 14, 1998, Pope John Paul II issued an important response in his encyclical letter, *Fides et Ratio* (Faith and Reason).[5] For those who may hold some of these views, it is important to understand that Pope John Paul II was clearly one of the greatest intellects of the 20th and the newly formed 21st century. He was a trained philosopher in the tradition of St.

Thomas Aquinas. He wrote extensively, continuing the longstanding 2000-year tradition in the Catholic Church of intellectual discipline. It is worth reciting some of what he has written in *Fides et Ratio*, for he addresses a number of the important questions that have existed in the faith versus reason conflict. It is not possible for me to be able to consolidate all of what the Holy Father addressed in this 57-page encyclical letter, but I would like to share a few excerpts so that perhaps we can all learn from it.

With regard to the thought of St. Thomas Aquinas, the Holy Father said:

"Both the light of reason and the light of faith come from God, he (St. Thomas Aquinas) argued; hence there can be no contradiction between them. More radically, St. Thomas recognized that nature, philosophy's proper concern, could contribute to the understanding of divine revelation. Faith, therefore, has no fear of reason, but seeks it out and has trust in it. Just as grace builds on nature and builds it to fulfillment, so faith builds upon and perfects reason… human reason is neither annulled nor debased in assenting to contents of faith, which are, in any case, attained by way of free and informed choice."[6]

Pope John Paul II went on to say that:

"It is not too much to claim that the development of a good part of modern philosophy has seen it move further and further away from Christian revelation, to the point of setting itself quite explicitly in opposition… As the result of the crisis of rationalism, what has appeared finally is nihilism. As a *philosophy of nothingness* it has a certain attraction for people of our time. Its adherents claimed that the search is an end in itself, without any hope or possibility of ever attaining the goal of truth. In the nihilist interpretation, life is no more than an occasion of sensations and experiences, in which the ephemeral has pride of place. Nihilism is at the root of the widespread mentality, which claims that a definitive commitment should no longer be made because everything is fleeting and provisional"[7] (emphasis applied).

It is this question of faith being viewed as "myth or superstition" as I have heard some people say, right up there next to "witchcraft", which troubles much of modern society. There is the thought, for example, that human reason can find the answers to all things and that faith is not necessary. *The work contained in this book, however, is the result of questions that have been asked because of faith.*

The nature of research is to ask questions. It is the question that forms the foundation of the investigation. The questions that are asked are the result of the values that the investigator holds. No matter what type of research is being conducted, it always emanates from the values that the investigator(s) holds. In fact, research becomes very boring and empty if it is not stimulated by values.

Discovery

In 1976, as an assistant professor in the Department of Obstetrics and Gynecology at St. Louis University School of Medicine, I recruited a team to begin an independent investigation of the Billings Ovulation Method. This was a new method of natural fertility regulation that had been developed in Melbourne, Australia. Our work, supported by a grant from the Missouri Division of Health and the National Institutes for Child Health and Human Development, began to thoroughly investigate this system. Out of those investigations came the *standardization of the mucus observations* and the subsequent development of what is now known as the **CREIGHTON MODEL FertilityCare™ System**.

This work moved to the Department of Obstetrics and Gynecology at Creighton University School of Medicine in July 1977 and a special research center was developed within that department that continued to work on and further develop this system. I continued our professional relationship with the team in St. Louis. In 1978, we began the first class of Natural Family Planning Practitioners (teachers of natural family planning) in a 13-month Allied Health Education Program. This was developed through the education and research efforts of our program at Creighton University School of Medicine. This program has been ongoing since that time. Our teachers are now called **FertilityCare™** *Practitioners, Educators and Supervisors.* The physicians trained in this system and in the new women's health science of **NaProTECHNOLOGY** (Natural Procreative Technology) are eligible to be certified as **FertilityCare™** *Medical Consultants.* This was the first and continues to be the only training program in natural family planning that is fully designed to meet the academic demands of an Allied Health Professional Education Program. We also train *nurse practitioners, physician assistants, nurse midwives and pharmacists.*

On August 6, 1978, the Feast of the Transfiguration, Pope Paul VI died. My wife and I, going to a late Mass on that Sunday afternoon, heard of his death through an extraordinary tear-filled eulogy given by our parish priest. On our way home that evening, we turned to each other and said, "We must build a lasting memorial to Pope Paul VI and his encyclical letter, *Humanae Vitae,* and to his call to men of science and to doctors and medical personnel. We will call this the Pope Paul VI Institute for the Study of Human Reproduction."

Several years went by before we were able to open the doors of this new Institute. This Institute, which opened in 1985, was dedicated to scientific and educational research in the field of human reproduction, but would ask questions from a uniquely Catholic perspective. By this time, contraception, sterilization, abortion and the artificial reproductive technologies (ART) had completely taken hold in the profession of obstetrics and gynecology. In fact, this monolithic view has continued up to the present day among professionals in obstetrics, gynecology and reproductive medicine, and it supports their approach to the health care of women. The only exception is in the area of abortion where there still are a group of obstetrician-gynecologists who are able to express their opposition.

This answers, at least in part, the question of how a doctor from Omaha, Nebraska, might be able to provide new insight into the evaluation and treatment of women's health issues. As one of only a handful of physicians who pursued "the road less travelled," new insights were bound to be observed.

When it comes to contraception, sterilization or the artificial reproductive technologies such as *in vitro* fertilization (IVF), there has developed within this profession one view and one view only. In fact, many obstetrician-gynecologists have said over the years that you cannot even practice this profession without prescribing oral contraceptives, doing sterilizations or referring people for the artificial reproductive technologies, such as IVF or artificial insemination. During these years, our research with the **CREIGHTON MODEL System** has shown that *this was 100 percent incorrect.* In fact, services can be provided to women that are completely consistent with the highest of ethical and moral principles and, in fact, these services can be provided with a very high level of medical expertise and with excellent success.

In 1991, I wrote a small textbook called "The Medical Applications of Natural Family Planning".[8] The subtitle of this book was "A Physician's Guide to **NaProTECHNOLOGY**." This was, in effect, the official birth of a new women's health science. I have been amazed by how this little textbook was able to reach out to so many physicians throughout this country and several foreign countries. We have been able to observe, through training programs that we have conducted over these years, the development of these physicians toward a practice of medicine that is completely consistent with their values and the values of their patients. They have often done this, I might point out, in the face of significant ridicule, prejudice and discrimination by their colleagues and peers. But, they have observed the disturbing trends in the health care of women, children and families (see Chapter 2 – The Medical and Social Consequences), and they are deeply concerned about them. They do not wish to continue being a contributor to the role that either they have played or the medical profession as a whole has played in the cultivation of these trends. They have, in effect, decided not to be a part of that portion of medicine that cultivates these negative outcomes.

In this book, I will introduce the new women's health science of **NaProTECHNOLOGY**. When we first started our work in 1976 as simply an independent investigation of a natural method of family planning, we had no idea it would lead to this. The system we were working with was a system that involved the study of certain types of vaginal discharges, including menstrual bleeding, and the mucus flow around the time of fertility. Once this system was *standardized* and then became known as the **CREIGHTON MODEL FertilityCare™ System**, we began to have women of reproductive age chart their cycles regardless of what type of symptom or medical problem they might have. *This charting system led to an observation of a variety of abnormalities that raised new questions for research*—new questions that could *only be seen* because of this charting system. These new questions then led to new approaches to treatment.

Now with the **CREIGHTON MODEL System** as its foundational family planning system, the new women's health science of **NaProTECHNOLOGY** offers great hope to women of reproductive age. *It looks for the underlying cause, it treats the diseases and it allows for a foundation to be laid for continued exploration of the causes of these abnormalities so that new treatments can be developed further.*

This system, which is an *extremely reliable family planning system*, also is especially good in evaluating and eventually treating women who have *infertility, recurrent miscarriages, recurrent ovarian cysts, premenstrual syndrome, postpartum depression, menstrual cramps and a whole variety of other conditions.* Even for those women who achieve a pregnancy, research born out of **NaProTECHNOLOGY** has resulted in a significant decrease in the prematurity rate.

NaProTECHNOLOGY is *not* ineffective. There is no question that this approach to medical care is effective in those areas to which its promises are made. A summary of its effectiveness can be seen in Tables 1-1 and 1-2.

As our research progressed, more than 8,000 individual patients contributed in some way to the knowledge of the **CREIGHTON MODEL System** and **NaProTECHNOLOGY**. There have been over 36,000 patient research contacts and over 200,000 individual research observations that have been made in putting together this approach. Indeed, the results of these observations now have been published extensively in a 1,244-page medical textbook titled "The Medical & Surgical Practice of **NaProTECHNOLOGY**" (Pope Paul VI Institute Press, Omaha, Nebraska, 2004). With **NaProTECHNOLOGY**, we have undertaken *extraordinary research evaluations, verified them and*

Table 1-1: An Effectiveness Summary: NaProTECHNOLOGY vs. Artificial Reproductive Technologies

NaProTECHNOLOGY Success rates (in percent)		Artificial Reproductive Technologies Success rates (in percent)	
To Avoid Pregnancy		**To Avoid Pregnancy**	
Creighton Model Fertility*Care* System[1]		Birth control pills	
Perfect Use	99.5	Perfect Use	99.5
Typical Use	96.8	Typical Use	90-96
Infertility Treatment		**Infertility Treatment**	
Surgical NaProTechnology associated with:		Traditional surgical approach	
Endometriosis	56.7-76.4[2]	Endometriosis	57.0[2]
Polycystic ovarian disease	62.5-80.0[2]	Polycystic ovarian disease	41.8[2]
NaProTechnology		*In vitro* fertilization	
Endometriosis	56.7-76.4[3]	Endometriosis	21.2[3]
Polycystic ovaries	62.5-80.0[3]	Polycystic ovaries	25.6[3]
Tubal occlusion	34.4[3]	Tubal occlusion	27.2[3]
Diagnosis of Luteal Phase		**Diagnosis of Luteal Phase**	
NaProTechnology		Current medical approach	
Detect by properly targeting hormone evaluation	98.2[4]	Not available (n/a)	n/a
Premenstrual Dysphoric Disorder (PMS)		**Premenstrual Dysphoric Disorder (PMS)**	
NaProTechnology	95.2[5]	Current Treatment	43.0
Postpartum Depression		**Postpartum Depression**	
NaProTechnology	92.4-96.7[6]	Antidepressants	Slow improvements over 6-12 months
Generally within 1-10 days			

1. Completely comparable to oral contraceptives.
2. Measured by survival curve analysis at 36 months and compared to published results from Johns Hopkins University Medical Center.
3. A range of effectiveness acquired from different study designs.
4. Using the Creighton Model Fertility*Care*™ System to target evaluation of the post-ovulatory hormone phase of the cycle.
5. With the use of targeted HCG hormonal support and oral naltrexone.
6. With the use of IM progesterone therapy.

published them prior to writing this book, which is specifically designed for the lay person and introduces **NaProTECHNOLOGY** to the general public.

NaProTECHNOLOGY reveals success rates that, in many cases, exceed those of contemporary obstetrics, gynecology and reproductive medicine. The treatment of infertility and recurrent miscarriage, for example, exceeds what is currently available in contemporary medical practice. With **NaProTECHNOLOGY** approaches to the pregnant woman, we have been able to reduce the preterm birth rate from twleve percent down to seven percent. *This is an extraordinary accomplishment* given the fact that over the last 35 years the prematurity rate in the United States has nearly doubled.

There will be some who will reject this work because of its close association with Catholic philosophical concepts. They will say that the Church has no platform on which to speak because of past and certainly present sexual abuses. For my part, I can understand that. Those within the Church have definitely not practiced all of what the

Table 1-2: An Effectiveness Summary: NaProTECHNOLOGY vs. Artificial Reproductive Technologies

NaProTECHNOLOGY Success rates (in percent)		Artificial Reproductive Technologies Success rates (in percent)	
Prematurity & Severe Prematurity Rate		**Prematurity & Severe Prematurity Rate**	
NaProTechnology		Traditional treatment	
Prematurity rate	7.0[1]	Prematurity rate	12.1
Severe prematurity rate	1.3[1]	Severe prematurity rate	3.9
Recurrent Spontaneous Abortion		**Recurrent Spontaneous Abortion**	
NaProTechnology	79.0	Current medical approach	Lower
Dating the Beginning of Pregnancy		**Dating the Beginning of Pregnancy**	
Creighton Model System	100.0[2]	Using date of last menstrual period	86.0[2]
Chronic Pelvic Pain		**Chronic Pelvic Pain**	
Surgical NaProTechnology		Current medical approach	
Hysterectomy rate	11.5	Hysterectomy rate	40.0
Cost-effectiveness		**Cost-effectiveness**	
Creighton Model System	$494[3]	Birth Control Pills	$1,866[3]
Infertility	$322[4]	IVF	$9,226[4]
Prematurity	$16,795[5]	Current medical approach	$28,556[5]
PMS evaluation and treatment	$3,218[6]	Current medical approach	$5,104[6]

1. Using the Prematurity Prevention Protocol of the Pope Paul VI Institute.
2. Within 10 days.
3. Based on five years of use.
4. Based on costs per cycle of treatment.
5. Based on cost savings generated by decrease in prematurity rate to 7.0 percent.
6. Includes cost savings due to improved productivity.

Church preaches. Unfortunately, the Church, like all other earthly groups, is administered by human beings who are frail and imperfect. As Vicki Thorn, co-founder of "Project Rachel," has often said, "The Church is not a hotel for saints, but, rather, it is a hospital for sinners." We need to keep these things in perspective and not let it prejudice our observations. Indeed, while it is the result of research that has been stimulated by Catholic philosophical insights, the approaches taken here are "for all men of good will" and not just for Catholics. The medical principles outlined in this book can potentially help all women of reproductive age regardless of religious background.

If we have been created "in His image and likeness,"[9] then an individual human person can grow closer to God and better understand Him by understanding and listening to how the body works, by understanding the language of the body. The **CREIGHTON MODEL FertilityCare™ System** is "an authentic language of a woman's health and fertility." We have been called to build a *civilization of love.*[10] As a physician, there is no reason on earth that we should not respond to this call.

So, as I started this work in 1976, it began under a cloud of rejection, which has, for the most part, persisted until the present day. Even my patients very often experience antagonism from other physicians because of the approaches I have chosen to utilize. This is to be expected since these approaches seriously challenge the current medical paradigm in obstetrics, gynecology, and reproductive medicine. These approaches, however, *offer more hope to women* in many areas than the contemporary approaches currently in use. It is not meant to be a threat to other physicians, only an approach developed out of a very sincere and disciplined approach to scientific investigation in areas that have been *nearly completely ignored* by the medical establishment.

The Medical and Social Consequences

VER THE LAST 45 YEARS, there has been a *well-documented* disintegration of the family and with it a *well-documented* increase in adverse medical and social reproductive outcomes. There is evidence to suggest that this is, at least in part, related to the widespread availability of contraceptive agents, which have clearly increased sexual promiscuity. Some of this is related to the increased use of abortion and still others to the increased use of IVF. Some *truly disturbing trends* have been observed in the health care of women, children and families. It is vital that these trends be examined and reflected upon so that actions can be taken to reverse them.

In the United States, beginning in the early 1960s, a significant increase in *the divorce rate* and in *the number of children involved in divorce* was observed. Divorce adversely affects adult relationships and it also has a generally negative impact on the physical, emotional and economic well-being of the children involved.[1]

In the past, there have been some variations of the divorce rate in the United States. There was a short episode of variation, for example, during the Great Depression, and somewhat sharp increases following World Wars I and II.[2] Each of these increases were followed by a decline (although the overall trend continued to increase slowly). These changes in patterns for divorce are small in comparison to the *exponential increase* that occurred beginning in the early 1960s. It is legitimate to ask why such a trend occurred.

Professor R. T. Michael[2] of the University of Chicago reported a sizeable and robust statistical analysis of the various potential causes of this increase in divorce. He found that the standard potential causes, such as a change in the divorce laws, unemployment, involvement in the military or public assistance variables, were not major forces in this increase. Even such things as income variables or variables in age composition between the spouses contributed only moderately. *The major variable that accounted for the increase in divorce was the introduction on a widespread scale of the various contraceptive technologies,* which included mostly the oral contraceptive and intrauterine device and then female and male sterilization.

The rise in the divorce rate since the 1960s parallels the increase in the use of technological contraceptives suggesting a close association between the two.[1, 3-7] While some have argued that the change in the divorce laws in the early 1960s led to the increase in the divorce rate, evidence suggests that the changes in the laws followed and codified social change instead of preceding and causing these social changes.[2]

This rise in the divorce rate has had an enormous impact on the *living arrangements* of the children affected by divorce. The *number of children living with both biological parents has significantly decreased,* while the *number of children living with their mother only has significantly increased* during this same period of time. This breakup of the family was bound to have a significant sociologic impact. For example, it is well recognized that children have the best chance for psychological, physical and economic success if they are raised in families where both parents are present and have shown affirmation and love to the children.

In the late 1960s, with changes in abortion legislation in various states, the number of abortions began to increase. There was *a major increase in the number of abortions performed* following the implementation of the *1973 Supreme Court decision, Roe v. Wade.*[9-11] There was *a parallel increase* in the use of contraceptives, which occurred in *advance* of the rise in induced abortion.[12] While there has been a tendency over the last 10 to 15 years to look at small declines in the abortion rate and view it positively, when looking at abortion rates one should view the data in perspective by going back to the early 1960s. At that time, there were very few abortions performed. *Since then, the increase in abortion has been monumental!*

Some would say that prior to the legalization of abortion, there were large numbers of illegal abortions performed in the United States with a large number of women dying. I spent six months working at Cook

County Hospital in Chicago prior to the Supreme Court decision. This was one of the largest obstetrical units in the United States and the population was nearly all at or below the poverty line. During my experience there, completely in obstetrics, the number of illegal abortions observed was low. Furthermore, those who argue that we need contraception in order to reduce the number of abortions *simply have no evidence* that this occurs and, in fact, the evidence is to the contrary. The introduction of widespread technological contraception *positively* influenced the number of abortions being performed in the United States.[3-7, 9-12] The explosion of *contraceptive availability* and use *has had only one impact,* that is to *increase the number of abortions.* It also is well recognized that those organizations that are most supportive of contraception also are in support of abortion.

There has been a six- to seven-fold *increase* in *the number of unmarried women who have given birth* in the last 40 years.[13] While the widespread availability of contraception and abortion promised to reduce this trend, it is noteworthy that the only impact observed has been to *increase the number of births to unmarried women.* In fact, the *pregnancy rate* (which differs from the birth rate) among teenage women age 15 to 19 *also has increased significantly* during this same period of time.[14, 15]

Child abuse and neglect figures are difficult to obtain because over the years there has not been an organized effort to collect this data in a universally acceptable form. Nonetheless, it seems quite clear from data that is available that *the number of children who are involved in both child abuse and neglect situations has increased* along with the increased divorce rate, the increase of children born to unmarried women, the increased use of contraceptives and the increase in abortion.[15, 16]

During this same period of time, the estimated *violent crime rate also has increased* dramatically[16] along with the percentage of juveniles who have been taken into police custody and referred to either a criminal or adult court. Concomitant with these increases has been the increase in drug use among teenagers.[17, 18]

The *suicide rates* for young people age 15 to 19 *also have increased significantly.* Suicide is now *the third leading cause of death among teenagers* in the United States.[19, 20] The increase in the suicide rate has been significantly higher for teenage boys than it has for teenage girls.[17] Depression is well-recognized as the major cause of suicide. With the extraordinary sociologic changes that have occurred over the last 40 years with the disintegration of the family and the fragmentation of parental support, it is not difficult to see why depression is now more prevalent.

Depression and sexual activity also have been evaluated in teenage boys and girls. Sexually-active teenagers describe themselves as "depressed sometimes," "depressed a lot," or "depressed most/all the time" more frequently than teenagers who are not sexually active.[21] This finding is stronger among teenage girls. In fact, when surveyed, the majority of sexually-active teens indicated that they wished they had waited longer before beginning their sexual activity. This finding is, again, more prominent among teenage girls than it is in teenage boys.[21]

Planned Parenthood's call is that teenagers "are going to have sex anyway no matter what we do" so contraceptives should be widely available to them. Data, however, suggests this is inaccurate. There is a distinct relationship between sexual values and the sexual activity rates. The sexual activity rate was nearly 10 times less (7.8 percent) for those who strongly agreed with the statement, "It is against my values for me to have sex while I am an unmarried teen" than those who strongly disagreed with that statement (72.4 percent).[22] This type of data suggests that if teenagers are adequately trained in a value formation setting that will allow them to understand the potential harm that can come from sexual activity at that age, they will see to it that their sexual activity significantly decreases. Furthermore, it has been shown that the recidivism rate, following the use of contraceptives (with regard to subsequent pregnancy) is very high. The same is true for young women who have abortions. They often have what is referred to as an "atonement pregnancy" following the abortion (usually within the next year).

There is a striking relationship between the use of alcohol and subsequent sexual activity rates as well. For those teenagers who have used alcohol recently, there is a greater than six-fold increase in the percent engaging in sexual activity.[22] Although television advertisements speak strongly against the use of drugs and alcohol, few, if any, have made the connection to their association with premature sexual activity.

There has been *a near doubling* in the *prematurity rate* (births at less than 37 weeks gestation) in the United States since 1967 and *the prematurity rate continues to increase*.[23-26] This is extraordinary given the relatively widespread availability of perinatologists (specialists in high-risk pregnancy). Their presence has made *no identifiable impact* on the prematurity rate in the United States. The *high prematurity rate is a national tragedy* and is linked to a variety of different problems that have been discussed (including the increased rate of teenage pregnancies and, as will be pointed out later, the increased use of artificial reproductive technologies – IVF – with their increase in multiple pregnancy and the increase in sexually-transmitted diseases). The *increasing number of babies born* with what is considered *low birth weight* (less than 2500 grams) and those born with *very low birth weight* (less than 1500 grams) also has *increased* over the last 30 to 40 years. This increase significantly threatens the health of these newborns.[27]

There has been a large increase in the number of multiple pregnancies over the last 30 years. The number of triplets and other high-order multiples *has increased more than four-fold* during this period of time. This is related to the number of artificial reproductive technology cycles that have been started for the treatment of infertility.[28-30] These approaches to treatment are associated with very high rates of multiple pregnancy ranging from 25 to 50 percent.

This is tragic! The infant mortality rate for triplets of all gestational ages is 10.9 times greater than for singleton live births. Babies from high-order multiple pregnancies are born at a much lower birth weight.[31] What is not reflected here is a significant *increase in neonatal morbidity* among those babies who survive their prematurity. It is well recognized that such morbidity is significantly increased and thus the health of these children is compromised.

It seems clear that the number of women who have experienced both childlessness and infertility also has increased during this same time interval. These increases in the infertility rates have been well documented at this point in time. It is estimated that there are 9.5 million women in the United States who have impaired fecundity[32] (this includes not only infertility, but also previous abnormal reproductive outcomes, such as miscarriage, ectopic pregnancy and stillbirth). At the same time, modern medicine offers these women the artificial reproductive technologies, such as *in vitro* fertilization. In 2006, about 41,000 women had a baby as a result of IVF.[32] Thus, *these most "technologically-advanced" programs assist only 0.44 percent of all women in the United States who have impaired fecundity.* These programs also are associated with multiple pregnancies, frozen embryos, surrogacy programs, postmenopausal motherhood, embryo experimentation and so forth.

The occurrence of *sexually-transmitted diseases also has increased significantly.* While the reported rates of gonorrhea have decreased over the last 30 years (preceded by a marked increase),[33] there has been a significant increase in *human papilloma virus* (genital warts and cervical cancer)[33] and *Chlamydia infection* (especially among women).[33] In addition, the number of ectopic pregnancies in the United States as measured by both inpatient and outpatient estimates also has increased significantly.[34, 35] These increases are directly attributable to the sexual promiscuity that has accompanied the epidemic increase in these diseases that often cause impairment of tubal function.

It has been estimated that there are more than *15 million new cases* of sexually-transmitted diseases (STDs) in the United States each year. Furthermore, there are well over *50 million total cases of viral STDs in the United States*. The direct medical cost for caring for this epidemic is *$8.4 billion per year!*[36]

Women who have used oral contraceptives are now shown to be *at an increased risk of invasive cervical cancer.*[37] This is related to the epidemic in human papilloma virus infection of the cervix, which is a sexually-transmitted disease.

Some have argued that there are health benefits to the use of oral contraceptives because, at least in part, the ovarian and endometrial cancer rates have been shown to decrease with their use. The increase in cervical cancer and also the increased risk of breast cancer in women who have long-term oral contraceptive use seems to be incontrovertible at this point in time.[38-40] There also is a well-recognized association between induced abortion and the development of breast cancer.

The issues related to cancer and contraception also point out the shift that has occurred in medicine over the last few decades from one whose focus was on the individual patient to one whose focus is more general. This is illustrated by a recent review of the net effect of oral contraceptive use on the risk of cancer in women in the United States. After recognizing the net increase in the number of breast, cervical and liver cancer victims amongst oral contraceptive users and a net decrease in endometrial and ovarian cancer victims in similar users, the conclusion is reached that, *"from a population perspective,* there are only small cancer-related risks and benefits associated with oral contraceptive use, and, on balance, the net effect *is negligible"*[41] (emphasis applied). This approach *depersonalizes health care* and places it only in aggregate terms. *Medicine should be at the service of the human person!* For the woman who has fallen victim to a breast, cervical or liver cancer as a result of her use of oral contraceptives, the effect on her health is not well served by being described as "negligible."

The AIDS virus also has increased significantly. While some of these infections are related to blood transfusions and unclean needle use, the overwhelming majority are related to sexual promiscuity in both men and women. Acquired immune deficiency syndrome is a fatal illness and the increased mortality rate for both men and women has been well documented.[42, 43] The number and percentage of AIDS cases in women greater than 13 years of age has continued to increase significantly over the years. Condom distribution is usually proposed to eventually decrease the spread of the AIDS virus. Data now suggests that there is a *parallel increase in condom distribution and the spread of the HIV/AIDS virus.*[44]

Many people also have argued that while these trends have occurred, they can be reversed by increasing the dollars that are spent both on research and distribution of technological contraceptive services and abortion. There has been a significant increase in the federal dollars given to support AIDS research and also a significant increase in the federal funding of Planned Parenthood over this same period of time.[45] The incidence and prevalence of all of the conditions mentioned have increased significantly in spite of the increase in the number of dollars spent for programs that largely continue to support sexual promiscuity, the use of contraceptive agents, sterilization, abortion and the artificial approaches to reproduction.

This chapter has not addressed the influence of pornographic literature or the widespread availability of sexually-alluring content of television programs, movies, the Internet and so forth. Beginning in 1956, there was a well-documented increase in the sexual explicitness of that literature.[46] It has been said that this was the beginning of the sexual revolution. Few can deny that it was the beginning of a shift in sexual behavior. While some would call it revolutionary, *in reality the "sexual revolution" has stifled human growth and development, trivialized sex and produced an epidemic of victims.* Instead of it being sexually revolutionizing, it has been *sexually retarding.*

The health of women, children and families distinctly has been harmed by these changes over the last 45 years. Some have suggested that these are victimless trends. And yet, the data shown in this chapter of well-documented demographic analyses clearly indicate the opposite. The tragedy is that this is a revolution whose major victims have been innocent children, although adult men and women also have been significantly victimized.

There is evidence to suggest and a strong trend analysis to show that the increase in divorce, which leads to an increase in children being affected by divorce and no longer living in a family unit, is connected to *the increase in sexual promiscuity,* which has been fueled by the widespread infusion of technologically-oriented contraception and ultimately the increase in abortion rates. Contrary to what many have suggested, *there is simply no data to support the use of contraception as an answer to abortion.* In fact, the data clearly shows the close correlation between *the rise in technological forms of contraception and the subsequent rise in abortion.* Furthermore, it is becoming clear that perinidational abortion has become an emphasis. Oral contraceptives are, to some extent, *abortifacient.*[47] Intrauterine devices are also *abortifacient* (at times). Embryo experimentation, the frozen embryos that are stored in freezers throughout the United States and in other foreign countries, the push towards cloning and other forms of experimentation are the fallout from this same "revolution."

A woman with a problem of infertility, vulnerable in the position she finds herself, goes to her physician to seek care for that problem and is offered artificial reproductive technologies. She does not expect to be delivering triplets, quadruplets or quintuplets. Superficially, it may even be enticing. And yet, the data is clear that these pregnancies and the children resulting from them suffer enormously. Those who promote contraception and abortion have an abortive solution to the multiple pregnancy problem. It is referred to as "selective reduction." In this procedure, one or two or more of the babies are aborted so that the pregnancy is "reduced" to one or two fetuses, thus reducing some of these risks. And yet, this is an ethical and service principle *that is based on the development or protection of life through its destruction.* In a society that generally prides itself on respect for life, this is ultimately incompatible.

There are several reasons why prematurity rates and the occurrence of low-birth weight infants have increased. As will be discussed later in this book, on the prevention of prematurity, there is a strong suggestion that there is an infection-related explanation for many of the premature births that occur. This also may be related to the fallout from the widespread sexual promiscuity that has occurred in this nation and much of the Western culture.

The widespread increase in sexually-transmitted diseases affects mostly women. Men are often not affected (with the exceptions of AIDS). While men are often infected, usually it is not symptomatic and causes little harm. Women need to become more sexually savvy. That is to say, *they need to become more assertive with regard to the protection of their own sexuality, their own bodies and their own self-respect.* To continue submitting themselves to the harm of abortion, sexually-transmitted diseases, multiple births, premature birth, delivery of a low-birth weight infant and the risk of marriage dissolution is foolhardy. This needs to be reversed and women must take the lead in seeing that this is accomplished!

They do not need to do this out of resentment, although their resentment would be very understandable. Women should approach it by challenging society to respect them as human persons who have dignity and integrity; to respect their bodies as the nurturers of life and to respect the offspring that may be created in the union between man and woman. While I do not believe, in any way, that men are "hopeless" in this endeavor, in my more than 30 years of work with both men and women I have seen that women have a far more sensitive, intuitive and palpable connection to these events. Men often are concerned with other issues. That does not make them bad by nature. They can be educated and they often will respond positively. In fact, one of the reasons I have been involved in this work over so many years is because of the positive and liberating impact it can have on men.

The major story in health care over the past 45 years or more has been the epidemic *increase in family violence* that has been brought with us from the 20th to the 21st century. *The very way in which medicine is practiced has endangered the health of women, children and families.* The evidence cited here is from nationally-recognized data collection systems. It tells a story of *a society that has lost its fundamental moorings by sacrificing its most important resources.* Our priorities have undergone a seismic shift and, with it, left a trail of victims (see Table 2-1). One would need to be incredibly insensitive to not see these connections.

This book does not promote the notion of going backwards to the 1950s. There also has been a good deal of positive progress that has been made over these same 45 years. But, at the same time, the data shows that it is our current culture and its priorities and behaviors that have created these dangers. The data also shows that family violence, to this great extent, need not exist.

TABLE 2-1: THE LITANY OF SOCIOLOGIC AND MEDICAL TRENDS THAT HAVE SIGNIFICANTLY INCREASED[1] OVER THE LAST 45 YEARS[12]

↑	Divorce rate	↑	Sexually-transmitted diseases
↑	Children affected by divorce	↑	Multiple pregnancies
↑	Abortions	↑	Prematurity rate
↑	Teenage pregnancy rate	↑	Low-birth-weight babies
↑	Out-of-wedlock births	↑	Very low-birth-weight babies
↑	Child abuse and neglect	↑	Neonatal morbidity
↑	Violent crime rate	↑	Invasive cancer of cervix
↑	Drug use among teenagers	↑	Breast cancer
↑	Suicide rates among teens	↑	Liver tumors
↑	Teenage sexual activity	↑	Ectopic pregnancy
↑	Infertility	↑	AIDS

1. In each of these situations, the increase has been very significant and often very dramatic.

Ultimately, *there needs to be another response.* The portion of that response being proposed in this book is a new women's health science referred to as **NaProTECHNOLOGY**. This is described in the chapters ahead. *It is truly 180 degrees different from the current artificial, suppressive and destructive approach of the artificial reproductive technologies that have been used over the last 40 to 50 years.* What has been happening over the last 40 years is a national, and to some extent, international tragedy. It now must be taken seriously and programs must be developed to reverse these trends. *I believe that it must begin now!*

Women Healed: NaProTECHNOLOGY

*N*APROTECHNOLOGY (Natural Procreative Technology) can be defined as a new women's health science that is designed to *cooperate* with the menstrual and fertility cycles. It has as its spectrum of application the reproductive-age woman during her months or even years that may exist prior to her conceiving a new pregnancy. It continues to be applicable around the time of conception and then during the entire course of pregnancy through the birth of the child and the immediate and even long-term postpartum period (Figure 3-1). It has *medical, surgical and perinatal applications.*

NaProTECHNOLOGY is the *first system* to fully network *family planning* with *procreative* and *gynecologic-health monitoring and maintenance.* Its use has applications in *family planning,* the evaluation

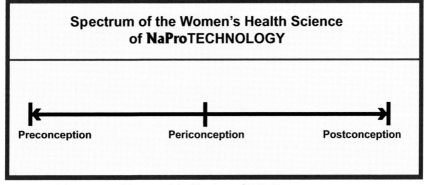

Spectrum of the Women's Health Science of NaProTECHNOLOGY

Preconception — Periconception — Postconception

Figure 3-1: The spectrum of the women's health science of NaProTECHNOLOGY.

and treatment of *infertility* and other reproductive disorders, such as *recurrent miscarriage, abnormal bleeding,* various *abnormal hormone conditions* of the menstrual cycle including *premenstrual syndrome and recurrent ovarian cysts,* the *dating of the beginning of pregnancy,* the *prevention of preterm birth* and *postpartum depression* (among others).

NaProTECHNOLOGY is a medical science that has *the education of the patient* as its foundation *integrated with good medical practice.* Specifically, it educates women in the objective parameters of their menstrual and fertility cycles in such a way that *they can develop a partnership with the properly-trained physician* in the evaluation and eventual treatment of whatever gynecologic or reproductive problem they may encounter.

This *education is standardized* so that it can be used throughout the United States and in other foreign countries. Because of its standardization, it also is *objective.* Because it is objective, it is *reproducible.* The information that the women gather can be interpreted and used for both medical evaluation and treatment purposes.

All of the above features of **NaProTECHNOLOGY** are *unique* at this point in the history of obstetrics, gynecology and reproductive medicine. They are incredibly important to being able to identify the underlying cause(s) of a particular medical problem(s), and then establish a form of treatment. While education is one of its foundations, **NaProTECHNOLOGY** also relies on developments in *medical technology.* This is best exemplified by its use of *targeted hormone surveys, expert ultrasound evaluation and various surgical approaches* that utilize *laser technology, microsurgical applications and anti-adhesion strategies.* **NaProTECHNOLOGY** allows for therapeutic approaches to be taken that are different from the ones currently in use. Because of this, *it can solve many problems that we have not been able to solve in the past!* These treatments hold great promise, and they are all used within a respect for a woman's health and the health of a woman's baby.

The research that has led to the development of **NaProTECHNOLOGY** began in 1976 when I recruited a research team to begin an independent investigation of one of the newest methods being used to naturally regulate fertility. At the beginning of this research, I had no idea that this would progress to become an entirely new women's health science. In fact, our only goal was to see whether or not the claims made with regard to this newest method of natural fertility regulation were scientifically correct. Indeed, we were able to substantiate those claims while advancing this methodology on a very wide scale.

The system that we were investigating was the Billings Ovulation Method. This was developed by Drs. John and Lyn Billings, a husband and wife medical team from Melbourne, Australia. The Billings Method was brought to the United States by Dr. John Billings in 1971.[1] As with all new advances in science, there was a need for this methodology to be independently reviewed, investigated and verified. That was really our only goal at the beginning.

This system is based upon a *woman's observations* of a variety of different vaginal discharges that occur during the course of the menstrual and fertility cycle. It is a system of making the observations, recording them and interpreting them. The Billings Method was *subjective* in the approach it took in teaching women how to make these observations and the language used to describe them. Within the first year of our work, I was able to recognize that these various discharge patterns would lend themselves nicely to *an objective, common language.* The development of this language along with a basic routine for observing the various discharges led to *the single most important discovery* in what later would become **NaProTECHNOLOGY**. This discovery was the *standardization of the system.* By 1980, with this standardization in place and a number of new education tools that were designed to standardize the teaching of the women and men who were to use this system, it became officially known as the **CREIGHTON MODEL** Natural Family Planning System. Later, because the term "natural family planning" no longer applied to this work, it became known as the **CREIGHTON MODEL Fertility***Care***™ System** (see Chapter 8).

As an obstetrician and gynecologist (Dr. John Billings was a neurologist and Dr. Lyn Billings a pediatrician), I had a natural interest in the application of this system to reproductive-age women. I began to have these women chart their cycles using the **CREIGHTON MODEL System**. Over a period of 15 years, I began to see various reproducible signs in the charts that reflected ongoing abnormalities in the woman's reproductive system. During this period of time, we extensively used *hormone measurements, ultrasound testing and diagnostic laparoscopy* (a minor surgical procedure where a scope is placed into the abdominal cavity and the uterus, tubes and ovaries are evaluated for the presence or absence of any organic disease). With these various diagnostic tools and hours upon hours of research investigation, we began to identify some of the underlying causes of these problems. These all will be discussed as you read this book.

In 1991, the term **NaProTECHNOLOGY** was first used in a small textbook I wrote titled "The Medical Applications of Natural Family Planning: A Physician's Guide to **NaProTECHNOLOGY**."[2] This book began to attract other physicians to this work and our training programs, which began in 1978, were now expanding.

The research that began in 1976 has continued ever since. The basic research team is still intact and continues to work on improving the system. The textbook that was published in 1991 was not a definitive description of the new science of **NaProTECHNOLOGY**. That would occur in 2004 when "The Medical and Surgical Practice of **NaProTECHNOLOGY**" was published – all 1,244 pages of it. This book was the first definitive presentation of this new women's health science. With **NaProTECHNOLOGY**, we have undertaken an extraordinary research evaluation, verified the results and published them prior to writing this book, which is specifically designed for the lay person and introduces **NaProTECHNOLOGY** to the general public.

This approach to reproductive health care is clearly *counter-cultural.* By that, I mean it represents a *significant paradigm shift* in the delivery of health care services to reproductive-age women. It is definitely not a breech in the "standard of care." The Code of Professional Ethics of The American College of Obstetricians and Gynecologists[3] makes this clear. It says that "… maintenance of medical competence through study, application and enhancement of medical knowledge and skills is an obligation of practicing physicians." It goes on to state that "The patient-physician relationship is the central focus of all ethical concerns, and the welfare of the patient should form the basis of all medical judgments." Furthermore, it says that "The obstetrician-gynecologist should serve as the patient's advocate and exercise all reasonable means to ensure that the most appropriate care is provided to the patient." It goes on to say that "The patient-physician relationship… is built on confidentiality, trust and honesty." In addition, "In emerging areas of medical treatment where recognized medical guidelines do not exist, the obstetrician-gynecologist should exercise careful judgment and take appropriate precautions to protect patient welfare." And, with regard to informed consent, "The obstetrician-gynecologist has an obligation to obtain the informed consent of each patient."

Indeed, in all of these areas, the research that has been conducted to substantiate and validate this new women's health science of **NaProTECHNOLOGY** meets these guidelines and responses to "standard of care." In fact, much of what **NaProTECHNOLOGY** is comprised of, from a scientific point of view, is bolstered by the over 2,000 peer-reviewed scientific papers that are cited in the **NaProTECHNOLOGY** textbook (see *www.naprotechnology.com*).

In spite of this, the principles in **NaProTECHNOLOGY** are practiced only by a small group of physicians nationwide at the time of the publication of this book. It is a growing number of physicians and I do anticipate that it will grow significantly in the next several years. There are reasons why many physicians do not practice in this fashion at this time. This includes the enormous financial support provided to the medical profession by the pharmaceutical industry by way of advertisements in medical journals, support of professional educational meetings and the ability of pharmaceutical representatives to speak directly to the physicians themselves. In addition, young obstetricians and gynecologists receive very uneven surgical training in their residency programs and are not adequately equipped to venture into the surgical **NaProTECHNOLOGY** arena.

In addition to the above, the number of published scientific papers on a worldwide basis over one year or over a few years is truly staggering. No individual physician can legitimately keep up with all that is published. Recognizing this, professional medical societies often resort to the publication of committee "opinions," which have the tendency to dictate the practice of medicine within that profession. This is particularly true in the field of obstetrics and gynecology where The American College of Obstetricians and Gynecologists (ACOG) is constantly publishing such "opinions." And yet, it is clear that a significant portion of funding of ACOG activities comes from the pharmaceutical industry that supports contraception, sterilization, abortifacient medications and *in vitro* fertilization, and many of their "opinions" clearly reflect that support. Are their opinions obstructed by a "conflict of interest?" It appears so. In fact, the ACOG is so dominant in its support of contraception, sterilization, abortion and ART that it appears to have *abandoned* the medical needs of those patients who do not share their anti-life perspective. *Patient abandonment is a very serious issue* and it needs to be corrected.

In spite of this, **NaProTECHNOLOGY** has continued to grow over the last several years. When women become more knowledgeable about the ignorance that has been fostered, I believe they will become more and more interested in **NaProTECHNOLOGY** where they can have *the* *root cause of their problem identified and treated,* they can be *a true partner* in their own health care and they *can be educated* with the principles of how their body works. Many of the medical, surgical and perinatal applications of **NaProTECHNOLOGY** will be presented as this book unfolds. They can be compared to other approaches and they will do very well in such a comparison.

Two Approaches to Reproductive Medicine

ITH THE DEVELOPMENT of **NaProTECHNOLOGY**, there are now legitimately two approaches to medicine in women of reproductive age. There is the current "giant," the artificial reproductive technologies and the current "David," **NaProTECHNOLOGY**. The artificial reproductive technologies include all methods of contraception, sterilization, abortion (and abortifacient medications) and *in vitro* fertilization and its various approaches. These artificial approaches have dominated the approach to reproductive medicine over the last 45 years and because of that, we have lost valuable time in our ability to both evaluate the root causes of various reproductive abnormalities or abnormalities in the menstrual and fertility cycle and the various treatments that might be successful for them.

When the birth control pill was approved by the Food and Drug Administration for use as a contraceptive agent, a whole new concept was introduced into the practice of medicine. Up until this time (1960), the basic premise was *"First, do no harm."* With the introduction of the oral contraceptive and the ability to suppress a sensitive and sophisticated hormonal system between the hypothalamus, pituitary gland and the reproductive organs, it became ethically appropriate *to do harm*, so long as it appeared that there was some good that would come from it.

The use of oral contraceptives for the treatment of a whole variety of gynecologic conditions comes from a profession that found it easy and pragmatic to prescribe the oral contraceptive, not only for contraceptive purposes, but also for a variety of medical conditions to which they had no other solution. What has been so disturbing has been the medical profession's disinterest in looking at the underlying causes. It is almost as if the profession, as a whole, developed a defeatist attitude with regard to what the underlying causes might be. They have accepted this *"Band-Aid"* approach and not moved on. This premise has truly infected the practice of obstetrics and gynecology and specialists in reproductive medicine.

In the field of infertility, we have been made to think that the single best treatment for infertility involves the use of the various artificial reproductive technologies. This includes techniques such as *in vitro* fertilization and ICSI (intracytoplasmic sperm injection). *What you have not been told* is that the *"per-woman" success rate* for the treatment of infertility has *substantially declined* over the last 40 or 50 years. What you have not been told is that success rates in the treatment of infertility were actually better for some conditions in 1950 and for others in the early 1970's than they are today. There has been a well-documented decrease in the effectiveness of medical treatment for women who have suffered from infertility over this period of time.

It might be interesting for you to read what the husband of one of my patients wrote to me about their experiences in going to a reproductive specialist:

> "… We have never experienced a group of doctors who have assigned as much divinity to themselves as they have. Our first experience was with a reproductive specialist who flat out stated there was little hope and asked if we contemplated using donor eggs! Needless to say, he never heard back from us. We are sure none of this comes as a surprise to you. It was quite a revelation to us. Revelation, from the perspective of how impersonal and dehumanizing the entire process is. At every stage in this process, we have been together; from every doctor's appointment, to every blood test, to every ultrasound, to administering the medication. During the overwhelming majority of times, my wife and I have been the only couple in the doctor's office. We couldn't help but notice how many women did not bring their spouses along. What was a striking discovery for us in doing our homework on infertility was the "business" aspect to their practices. Forgive us, but more had to do with financial matters than the true health and wellbeing of their patient."[1]

I cannot tell you how often I've heard something similar to this from patients who have come to see me. These are approaches to reproductive medicine that specifically *do not look for the underlying causes.* For a patient who wants to know "What's wrong with me?" – which I suspect represents a significant percentage of patients – they cannot understand the approach of a specialist who does not concern himself with these issues.

Sterilization in a variety of different ways for both women and men also has become a mainstay in the contraceptive culture. For many women and some men, they never knew an alternative existed. In the 30 years that we have been providing **CREIGHTON MODEL** services in the Omaha metropolitan community, I can count on one hand the number of referrals we have received from local physicians. Our scientific papers have been published in peer-reviewed medical journals as early as 1978. And yet, this information has been kept from patients.

More and more, abortion has become institutionalized in the practice of reproductive medicine and in the practice of perinatology (high-risk obstetrics). If a woman carries a child that has a genetic defect such as Down syndrome, she is offered abortion. She is, however, often not offered supportive medical and social services. If you are age 35 or greater, some states *mandate* that testing be done to search out a Down syndrome child or other types of abnormalities. The expectation is that that woman also will be referred for abortion. If a woman ruptures her membranes early in pregnancy, she may be told that the only method of treatment is to "terminate" the pregnancy even though the baby will die. Abortion, too, has become one of the mainstays of the current practice of mainstream reproductive medicine. If one of their treatments results in a high order multiple pregnancy (triplets or greater), the patient is referred to the perinatologist for "selective" reduction. This is an abortion procedure that is *not* selective but does reduce the pregnancy to twins or a singleton pregnancy. At some clinics, patients have to sign a consent form for such an abortion prior to beginning treatment if they find themselves in this position.

One of the obstacles in the current approaches dominating obstetrics, gynecology and reproductive medicine over the last 40 to 50 years is the view that *women are tarnished* by the presence of their procreative abilities. In some ways, the menstrual cycle is still viewed as a "curse"[2] and the fertility cycle is viewed as a burden and an obstacle to be suppressed or destroyed. In addition, many in the profession view fertility and pregnancy as a "disease."[3] These mindsets have so ingrained themselves within the profession that when one approaches obstetrics, gynecology, and reproductive medicine from a different perspective or point of view, it raises significant antagonisms.

In **NaProTECHNOLOGY**, however, *fertility is not considered a disease.* The menstrual flow and the fertility cycle are thought of as normal biologic and physiologic processes, which can, of course, become dysfunctional and abnormal. Nonetheless, the cyclic physiologic process of menstruation and fertility is a normal process. A pregnancy that results from that physiologic event also is normal. While abnormalities of pregnancy can occur and result from certain diseases, the fundamental process of pregnancy, childbirth and delivery is considered normal.

Approaching women with the educational principles of their menstrual and fertility cycles and helping women to *discover the power that exists within their cycle* (this power is *knowledge* and *understanding*) allows the physician to approach women as *total human persons. This* (**NaProTECHNOLOGY**) *is a medical science that is at the service of the human person.* It not only encourages the female patient to become a partner in the evaluation and treatment of her reproductive health, but such participation is an actual component of the approach.

The achievement of pregnancy is not considered a "sexually-transmitted disease" as some have expressed it in the past.[3] Achieving a pregnancy is not considered a violation of the demographic ecology, but rather an event that calls all of us to support and care. The developing child within the mother's womb is neither viewed as a parasite nor as a potential human being. *Rather, the unborn child is viewed as a human being with potential!*

In modern reproductive medicine, the approach to family planning is one ultimately of either *suppression* or *destruction*. There are no current contraceptive systems that work cooperatively with the reproductive system. Oral contraceptives, for example, suppress the function of the pituitary gland so as to suppress ovulation. When an ovulation is not suppressed and a pregnancy develops, then the contraceptive works by destroying the newly-developing embryo at the time of implantation.[4]

In current approaches to contraception, sterilization has become one of the major technologies. One of the principles behind sterilization is that it requires no motivation. Sterilization relies on the principle that human beings are unable to develop any level of self-mastery when it comes to their expression of genital sexuality. In **NaProTECHNOLOGY** and with the **CREIGHTON MODEL System**, the patients and clients are accepted as individuals who are quite capable of living in a positive way with the normal function of fertility.

Sexual Freedom v. Sexual License

Over the past 45 years, there has been a movement sometimes referred to as the "sexual revolution." The clarion call of this movement has been "sexual freedom." But, as we have now looked at this over the past four decades, it is hard to support the notion that what has occurred is the result of an authentically-developed freedom.

The people who *are sexually free* are able to say both "yes and no" to the genital expression. With a natural means to regulate fertility, this expression of sexual freedom is in-built within the system. However, the modern contraceptive culture allows people to say "yes" while only giving token expression to their ability to say "no."

The "sexual freedom" of the contraceptive movement has harmed many people over its existence (see Chapter 2). It clearly has not been victimless. It is difficult to appreciate a concept of freedom where so many people have been harmed and so much pain and agony has been created while at the same time, so many people have ignored the pain and suffering.

This "sexual freedom" has fostered a significant disruption in human relationships over the four to five decades of its existence. It is difficult to believe that true freedom would generate such disruption. This "sexual freedom" has been physically violent as well. This "sexual freedom" has specifically harmed countless numbers of women under the guise of their liberation. One could hardly consider that having a woman seek an abortion and having the embryo or fetus dismembered by surgical instruments is the product of true freedom. It is difficult to believe that true freedom would be so destructive.

A more appropriate term for this "revolution" would be *sexual license.* This license is different from true freedom. It is self-centered and not other-oriented. It is pleasure-seeking rather than joy-and-fulfillment seeking. It is not nearly so concerned about others as its proponents would make one think. Indeed this "sexual freedom" is not freedom at all, but rather it has produced a kind of *tyranny* in which people are often trapped. This is because it results from sexual license and not true freedom.

In the **CREIGHTON MODEL Fertility*Care*™ System** and in other natural methods of family planning, legitimate choices are made relative to the achievement or avoidance of pregnancy, communication exists between the spouses, and the virtue of chastity is respected. This promotes a deep and profound respect, not only for the individual person who holds these principles, but also towards those individuals with whom they are shared. There is a willingness to reach out to others and truly care for them and with them. It is neither self-centered nor pleasure-seeking as its primary objective. Rather, it is mutual. It promotes growth over a period of time and not instant gratification. It is not an arrested, adolescent approach, but a full, mature and loving approach that respects *the value and dignity of each and every human life, the dignity of women and the integrity of marriage.* This can be argued to be an *authentic sexual freedom* and carries with it the possibility of establishing a legitimate sexual revolution.

Prospective v. Retrospective Data Collection

As a new medical science, **NaProTECHNOLOGY** relies on the *prospective* accumulation of objective and standardized data on the menstrual and fertility cycles. *In reproductive medicine, this has never occurred before.* It is easy to see that reproductive medicine has been entrenched for at least a century in the retrospective collection of data. A survey of textbooks in obstetrics, gynecology and reproductive medicine from 1915 until the present time shows clearly that the emphasis has been on the relatively unreliable retrospective collection of data on the menstrual and fertility cycles.[5-36]

The **CREIGHTON MODEL System** changes all of this. For the first time, women are instructed in the function of the menstrual and fertility cycle and the observation of its various parameters. These parameters are often referred to as *biomarkers* (biological markers). The research that has been done over the last 30+ years shows that these biomarkers allow the woman and the physician to make proper evaluations and find the eventual treatment. Furthermore, abnormalities in these biomarkers are closely associated with underlying pathophysiologic abnormalities. *Since these biologic markers have mostly been ignored over the last century, many important insights into reproductive medicine have been missed.* It is well recognized that the prospective collection of data is *far superior* to its retrospective collection. Specialists in reproductive medicine and obstetrics and gynecology have accepted without question the inferior form of retrospective data collection, even in spite of the presence of an objective, standardized means of collecting the data in a prospective fashion (the **CREIGHTON MODEL System**).

Band-Aid Approaches v. Getting to the Underlying Causes

In reproductive medicine, the current approach to problem solving is what could easily be called a "Band-Aid" approach. A woman comes to the physician with *menstrual cramps* and she is placed on birth control pills rather than finding out why she has the cramps. A woman comes with *irregular cycles*, and, instead of finding out why she has irregular cycles, she is placed on the birth control pill. A woman comes to the physician because of *irregular bleeding* and she is placed again on birth control pills so that she can artificially bleed regularly often without looking for the underlying causes. A woman who is being investigated for *recurrent ovarian cysts*, instead of being investigated for the underlying causes, is placed on oral contraceptives. A woman has *an infertility problem* and the doctor places her on medication to stimulate ovulation without looking for the cause of her infertility. If she does not get pregnant in one to three cycles, she is often referred to the artificial reproductive technologist. Those doctors have not been interested in looking for the underlying causes.

In **NaProTECHNOLOGY**, the focus is on looking for the underlying pathophysiologic event or events that allow for a rational approach to treatment. It is a philosophical approach, a concept used in most other medical specialities, but is absent from reproductive medicine. This approach allows for the physician to look for and investigate those underlying causes and then develop or implement effective treatments for these conditions.

Cooperative Approaches v. Suppresive and Destructive Approaches

A fundamental principle in **NaProTECHNOLOGY** is to work *cooperatively* with both the menstrual cycles and the fertility cycles. **NaProTECHNOLOGY** solves many problems that we have not been able to solve in the past and allows for approaches to be taken that are different than current approaches. At the same time, it allows for the implementation of treatments that hold great promise. On the other hand, modern reproductive technology's fundamental principle is to overcome the menstrual and fertility cycle by either suppressing or destroying it. These two approaches, the artificial reproductive technologies and **NaProTECHNOLOGY**, are at polar extremes.

The work presented in this book was originally supported by the Missouri Division of Health and with that, the St. Louis University Natural Family Planning Center was established at St. Louis University School of Medicine. Additional funding was provided by the National Institutes of Child Health and Human Development for a project, which allowed us to investigate the correlation of various biological markers with the hormonal events that stimulate them. This is the beginning of what started out as an opportunity to do an independent investigation of a new natural method for the regulation of fertility.

The program eventually moved to Creighton University School of Medicine in the Department of Obstetrics and Gynecology. The Creighton University Natural Family Planning Education and Research Center was developed and was functional as a full division within that department for eight years. The projects that previously had been funded had been completed and were published in major peer-reviewed medical journals.[37-40] For the most part, the work went unnoticed and ignored.

The **CREIGHTON MODEL System**, which is the fundamental family planning system that is necessary to implement **NaProTECHNOLOGY**, is a system that focuses on both the naturally-occurring phases of infertility and fertility and it has something very unique to offer. Since it was *standardized*, it allowed for very specific and reproducible observations to be made and it was this development that eventually led to **NaProTECHNOLOGY**. In fact, its special focus on human fertility, specifically, has provided insights that simply have not been available before this time. Because this work has been so completely ignored by the dominant profession, they have missed the focus of it. Many of the biomarkers that are present in the **CREIGHTON MODEL System** can be observed in no other way than by charting the menstrual and fertility cycle using the concept of the **CREIGHTON MODEL System**.

In 1978, the first Allied Health Education Program for Natural Family Planning Practitioners (now called **FertilityCare™ Practitioners**) was started. These programs have been conducted in affiliation with Creighton University School of Medicine ever since. By 1981, physicians were being trained and the program continued to grow and develop.

In September 1985, the Pope Paul VI Institute for the Study of Human Reproduction was opened. This institution allowed the natural regulation of fertility to be placed at the highest level of administrative priorities. As a part of the Institute, its Division of Reproductive Ultrasound was established. This division is nationally accredited by the Ultrasound Practice Accreditation Commission of the American Institute of Ultrasound in Medicine. This Institute also has a National Hormone Laboratory. This laboratory specializes in the accurate measurement of various reproductive hormones. It is Medicaid, Medicare and CLIA approved; it is inspected every two years by the State of Nebraska Department of Health; and it participates in a number of major quality control programs. It is a laboratory that is established to run at the highest level.

Most recently, a one-year, *full-time Fellowship* in Medical and Surgical **NaProTECHNOLOGY** has been established at the Institute in affiliation with Creighton University School of Medicine. This program will train young obstetrician-gynecologists in the various principles involved in the medical and surgical aspects of this practice. In this way, we should be able to expand the programs to more and more people (see our web site at *www.popepaulvi.com* and *www.fertilitycare.org*).

So, indeed, there are now two approaches to reproductive medicine. Over the years, women have endured a highly negative form of evaluation and treatment that often suppresses and destroys and does not get to the root causes. These women never knew of any alternative. But now there is a medically authentic alternative. In the months and years ahead, it will be of great interest to see how many women choose this new alternative.

*How the
Reproductive System
Works*

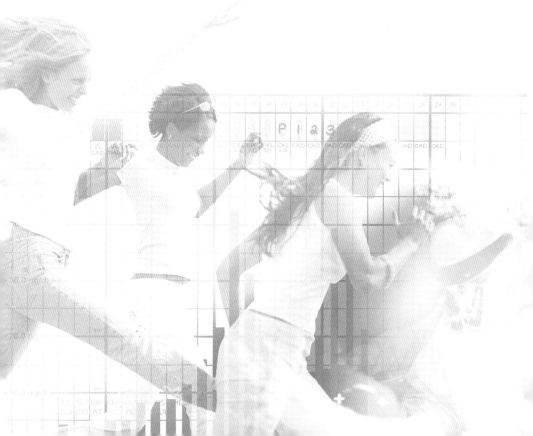

T IS IMPORTANT FOR those who want to learn about the **CREIGHTON MODEL System** (CrMS) and **NaProTECHNOLOGY** to have a basic understanding of how their bodies work and function. This chapter reviews the basic anatomy and physiology of the human reproductive system and allows the individual an opportunity to better understand this system and how it works. If these basic concepts are understood, it will be easier to understand the basic principles of the **CrMS** and also the new women's health science of **NaProTECHNOLOGY**.

One of the most simple of all principles is the fact that *men are always fertile*. A man's fertility will begin at the age of 12 or 13 (the age of puberty) and continue for the remainder of his life. This is an important realization for men in order to appreciate the nature of their own fertility. In addition, men must understand their role in the fertility process if the **CrMS** is to be used successfully.

The cell of human reproduction that is contributed by the male is called the *sperm* or *spermatozoa* (Figure 5-1). The genetic material for procreation is contained in the head of the sperm and the ability of the sperm to move from one place to the next comes predominantly from the motion of its tail.

The sperm are produced in two glands called the *testes* or the *testicles* (Figure 5-2). The testicles are located on the outside of the man's body. They are located there primarily because the sperm are highly sensitive to heat and if the testes were located inside the body,

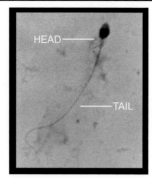

Figure 5-1: A photo micrograph of a spermatozoa showing its head and its tail.

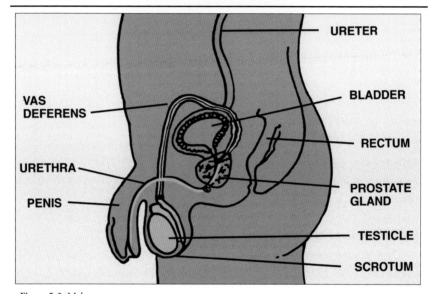

Figure 5-2: Male anatomy

the increased temperature would destroy or inactivate some of the sperm. On occasion, that may be a cause of male infertility.

After the sperm are produced in the testicles, they are transported along a tube called the *vas deferens*. From the vas deferens, the sperm go through the *prostate gland* into the *urethra* and are transported to the outside of the man's body. The urethra is the channel that normally connects the bladder to the outside of the body.

While men are always fertile, *women are, for the most part, infertile.* Women are fertile for only a short period of time during each menstrual cycle. Of course, it is not at all correct to talk about the man's fertility and the woman's fertility separately. The only meaningful point of discussion is the *combined fertility* of the couple. Since women are, for the most part, infertile, this means that the couple is, for the most part, infertile. Since men are always fertile and women are, for the most part, infertile, the understanding of the *couple's fertility* is focused by necessity upon the cyclic variations of fertility and infertility that occur in the woman.

This cyclic variation of a woman's fertility is one of the most marvelously sophisticated events in all of nature. It is a *finely-tuned, well-balanced, ecologically-sensitive* system. The events are outwardly visible by the regular occurrence of menstruation, the characteristic flow of cervical mucus and the absence of any discharge.

The reproductive organs of the woman lie within the protection of her pelvic cavity. In Figure 5-3, the location of the reproductive organs, the uterus, tubes and ovaries are shown as they exist in the woman's pelvis. Unlike the man, the reproductive organs of the woman are located inside of the body.

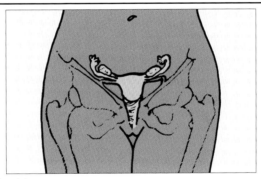

Figure 5-3: Female pelvic organs

The internal reproductive organs of the woman, the uterus, tubes and ovaries, are shown in the diagram in Figure 5-4. The ovaries are almond-shaped organs located on each side of the uterus, which is basically a muscle that is pear-shaped. There is a cavity within the uterus and at its opening there is an organ called the *cervix*. Lining the canal of the cervix are the *cervical crypts*. These are out-pouchings that come off of the *cervical canal. The cervical mucus is produced within these cervical crypts.* The mucus is discharged as a cervical fluid to the outside of the woman's body where all of the observations of the **CrMS** are made. There are no internal examinations involved in the use of the system. The location at the opening of the cervix where a Pap smear (Papanicolaou smear) is taken also is shown in Figure 5-4.

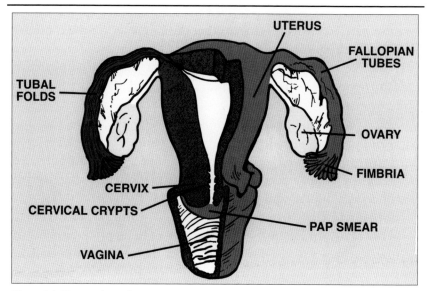

Figure 5-4: Uterus, tubes and ovaries

The *menstrual cycle* begins with the first day of menstrual bleeding and ends with the last day prior to the beginning of the next menstrual period. The length of this cycle tends to be somewhat irregular. While the average length of the menstrual cycle is around 28 days, most women will experience menstrual cycles from 21 through 38 days in duration during their reproductive life. Many people wonder why one menstrual cycle may be short while another may be more regular in length and still another may be long in duration. In Figure 5-5, the different phases of the menstrual cycle are shown. There are basically two phases that are important: The *preovulatory phase* and the *postovulatory phase.* The preovulatory phase of the cycle is counted from the first day of menstrual bleeding until the day of ovulation. The postovulatory phase of the cycle is counted from the day after ovulation until the day before the beginning of the next menstrual period.

It is the *preovulatory phase* of the cycle that is *highly variable.* The *postovulatory phase* is *quite stable* in its length. From the time of ovulation until the beginning of the next menstrual period averages about 13 days, although a range of nine to 17 days can be expected in a population of women.[1] In the individual woman, there is great consistency in the length of the postovulatory phase of the cycle. It is the variable length of the preovulatory phase that ultimately determines whether a cycle will be short or long.

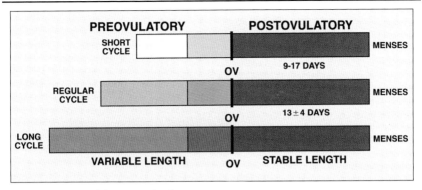

Figure 5-5: Phases of the menstrual cycle

During the course of the menstrual cycle, there is an event occurring within the ovary that is called the *"ovulation cycle"* (Figure 5-6). The menstrual cycle and its accompanying ovulation cycle are the result of the close interaction of several hormones. The pituitary gland (the master gland of the body) produces two hormones that are very important to the smooth functioning of these cycles. These hormones are FSH (follicle-stimulating hormone) and LH (luteinizing hormone). The FSH stimulates the development of an egg within the ovary. The LH actually stimulates the release of the egg from the ovary (ovulation—see Chapter 6).

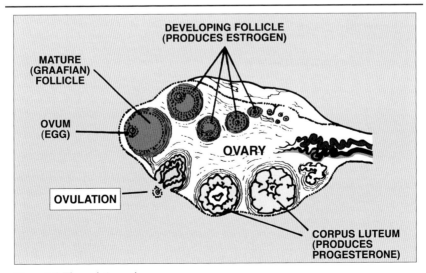

Figure 5-6: The ovulation cycle

There are several hundred thousand individual, undeveloped eggs in the ovary. Early in the menstrual cycle, one or two of these eggs is selected to develop toward ovulation. These eggs develop within a *follicle*. A follicle is a small cyst-like structure. The follicle begins to grow and develop, and just prior to ovulation, is about 1-inch in diameter. At that time, it is called a *mature follicle*. With the rupture of this follicle, the egg is released from the ovary in a process called *ovulation*. The same ovarian tissue that was the mature follicle now becomes what is called a *corpus luteum*.

The changes that occur in the lining of the uterus during the course of the menstrual cycle are shown in Figure 5-7. It is the lining cells of the uterus (the endometrial cells) that slough at the time of *menstruation* (Figure 5-8). The *ovulation cycle* also is shown in Figure 5-7 to assist the reader in coordinating the events of the ovulation cycle with the events occurring within the lining of the uterus. The phase of follicular development in the ovary coincides with the *proliferative phase* in the lining of the uterus and the formation of the corpus luteum with the *secretory phase*.

Once ovulation occurs, the egg lives for only 12-24 hours if it is not fertilized. If anything, the lifespan of the egg is closer to 12 hours than it is to 24 hours. This lifespan of the egg is so short that if our fertility depended upon this fact alone, few women would become pregnant

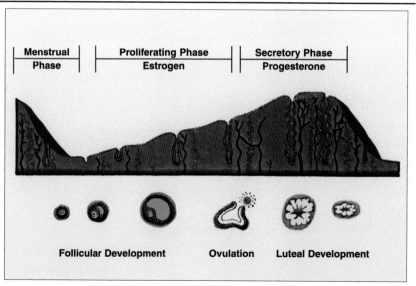

Figure 5-7: Changes in the lining of the uterus. The ovulation cycle is shown at the bottom.

during their entire reproductive life. The length of the fertility cycle is extended by another vital factor. *That vital factor is the cervical fluid.* It is the cervical fluid that allows the sperm to survive long enough to become available when an egg is released, and, of course, it is the cervical fluid that is involved in learning and understanding one's fertility through the use of the **CrMS**.

The sperm need cervical mucus to survive. Sperm, in the absence of good mucus, will die literally within hours or even minutes when placed into the vagina. This is because the vagina is very acidic and hostile to the sperm. In the presence of good cervical mucus, however, the sperm may live for three to five days. This is because the cervical mucus is alkaline and neutralizes the acids of the vagina. *Sperm survival* is directly dependent upon the presence of good cervical mucus.

The *estrogen* hormone rises to a very high level, a peak, just prior to the time of ovulation. It is this rise in the estrogen hormone that stimulates the production of cervical mucus. After ovulation, the predominant hormone is *progesterone.* The progesterone hormone inhibits the effects of estrogen on the production of cervical mucus. The mucus that had been stimulated to be produced by the estrogen hormone is halted in its production by progesterone. It also helps to prepare the lining cells within the uterus, as mentioned earlier, for the implantation of a new human life (see Chapter 6).

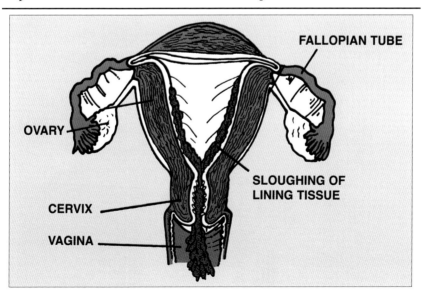

Figure 5-8: Menstruation: the sloughing of the lining of the uterus.

Human life begins at the time when the egg and sperm unite. This begins the process—a process we have all gone through—that allows the new baby to grow and develop within the mother's womb. Some would like to call this a "potential human being," but it is rather a "human being with potential" (see Figures 5-9 through 5-12).

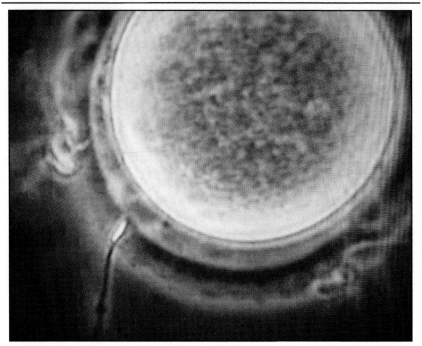

Figure 5-9: Sperm surrounding the egg just prior to its penetration into the egg resulting in a new conception.

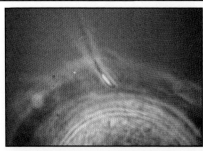

Figure 5-10: A sperm entering the the zona pellucida of the egg.

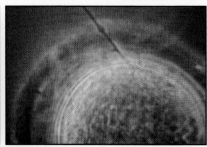

Figure 5-11: A sperm, after entering the zona pellucida, all the way inside the ovum and now without its nucleus.

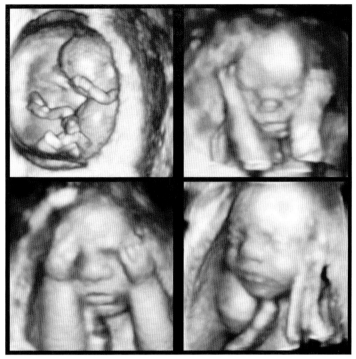

Figure 5-12: Ultrasound pictures from four-dimensional ultrasound videos of human babies at (top left to right) 11 weeks and 19 of pregnancy and at (bottom) 27 weeks of pregnancy (from Pope Paul VI Institute Reproductive Ultrasound Center).

A very important function of the cervical mucus in human fertility is shown in Figure 5-13. On the left side of the diagram is an illustration of a very characteristic type of cervical mucus that is only produced when the estrogen levels are rising or are very high. This type of mucus arranges itself in parallel strands, literally forming swimming channels for the sperm so that they can penetrate through the cervix and go up to the fallopian tubes where conception will occur. This type of cervical mucus is referred to as *Type E mucus*. On the right side of the diagram is the type of mucus that is produced when the estrogen levels are very low or when the progesterone levels are rising or are elevated. This type of mucus is called *Type G mucus* and is very thick and dense and, in fact, acts as a barrier to sperm penetration.

These two types of cervical mucus act, in effect, like a *biological valve*. The valve is open, allowing sperm to penetrate through the cervix, when the Type E or estrogen-stimulated mucus is present. The valve is closed to sperm penetration when the mucus is Type G. This biological valve is essential to human fertility and assures that fresh sperm and fresh eggs are available at the time of conception.

In the **CREIGHTON MODEL System** the couple is taught how to determine, in effect, when the biological valve is open (a time of fertility) and when it is closed (a time of infertility). The system will give *reliable information* on these events with *external observations* that women are taught when they learn the system. These observations are easy to do and require very little time (Figure 5-14), but you do need to work with a trained **Fertility*Care*™ Practitioner** (FCP) so that you learn all of the principles properly *(www.fertilitycare.org)*.

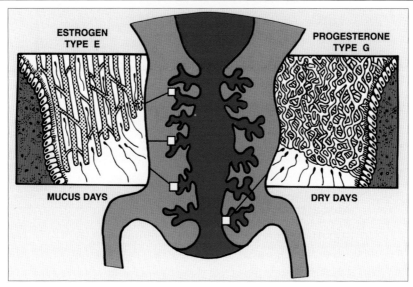

Figure 5-13: The cervical canal showing the production of Type E and Type G cervical mucus (see text) that functions as a biologic valve.

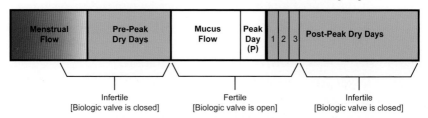

Figure 5-14: The basic pattern of a woman's menstrual and fertility cycle (see text).

The Cycle of Hormones

HERE ARE TWO HORMONES that are especially important in the regulation of the menstrual and fertility cycles. They are produced in the *pituitary gland*. These two hormones are *follicle-stimulating hormone* (FSH) and *luteinizing hormone* (LH). They regulate the function of the ovary as it proceeds towards ovulation and then again after ovulation. The *ovary* produces *two additional hormones* called *estrogen* and *progesterone*. As ovulation approaches, it begins to produce estrogen, *the dominant preovulatory hormone*. It is the estrogen hormone that stimulates the cervix to increase its production of cervical mucus and to change the qualities of that mucus so that it will be receptive to both the survival and penetrability of the sperm. The estrogen hormone also stimulates the lining of the uterus so that it regenerates after it has been shed at the time of menstruation.

Once the egg is released (*ovulation*), the follicle becomes a *corpus luteum* (the Latin words for "yellow body"). In fact, the corpus luteum does have a yellowish appearance to it when observed in its real form. The corpus luteum is a gland that produces *both* progesterone and estrogen, but *the dominant hormone at this stage of the cycle (the post ovulation phase) is progesterone*. Progesterone has the effect of sharply decreasing the production of cervical mucus that was formerly stimulated by the estrogen hormone. It is the production of the progesterone hormone that accounts for the woman's observation of the *Peak Day* (see Chapter 8). It also is progesterone that increases the body temperature (the basal body temperature). This is referred to as the *thermogenic* action of progesterone. The relationship of the estrogen and progesterone hormones along with FSH and LH as they occur during the course of the menstrual and fertility cycles is shown in Figure 6-1.

The production of estrogen prior to ovulation has an effect on the lining of the uterus (the endometrium). With the rising levels of estrogen being produced by the developing *follicle* (the small cyst on the ovary that contains the egg), the endometrium undergoes a proliferation (a regrowth after it has been shed at the time of menstruation). The *proliferative* phase of the menstrual cycle regenerates the endometrium. When ovulation occurs, the endometrium develops the ability to secrete a nutritious fluid that is important to the early days of the survival of the blastocyst (the early developing human being). This is called the *secretory phase* of the menstrual cycle.

The endometrium sheds when the corpus luteum discontinues its production of both progesterone

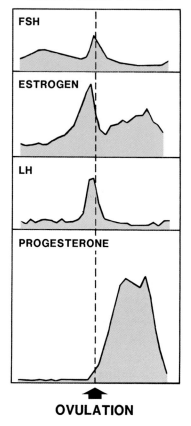

HORMONES OF THE MENSTRUAL CYCLE

FSH

ESTROGEN

LH

PROGESTERONE

OVULATION

Figure 6-1: The hormones of the menstrual cycle, including FSH, estrogen, LH, and progesterone.

and estrogen. This hormonal change occurs over a period of four to five days prior to the actual onset of the menstrual bleed. Without the hormonal support of both progesterone and estrogen (but primarily progesterone), the endometrium is designed to shed. This process is referred to as *menstruation* (Figure 6-2). Once menstruation occurs, then the whole sequence within the ovary and the endometrium (along with its associated changes in the cervix) start all over again and repeat the occurrence of the *ovulation cycle* and the *menstrual cycle* respectively.

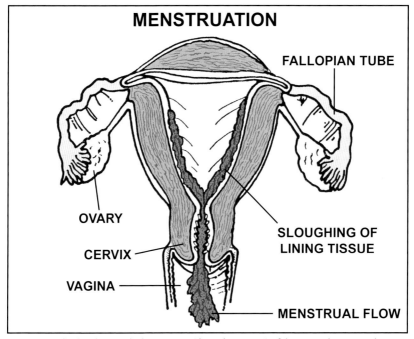

Figure 6-2: The sloughing in the lining tissue (the endometrium) of the uterus that occurs during menstruation.

The Fertility Pacemaker

It has been known since 1932 that a central command for the control of the various hormones that regulate both the ovulation and the menstrual cycles might be located within the brain.[1] It has taken many years of intensive scientific research to further investigate and understand the very complex hormonal interactions that are ultimately responsible for these cyclic functions.

The *hypothalamus* is a small gland weighing only 10 grams and is located just behind the pituitary gland. The hypothalamus produces a hormone called *gonadotropin-releasing hormone (GnRH)*. This hormone is produced in a *pulsatile fashion*, and, with each pulse, it stimulates the pituitary gland to produce both FSH and LH in pulses that correspond to the GnRH pulses (see Figure 6-3).

GnRH is produced in pulses that vary during the course of the menstrual and ovulation cycles. During the *first week* of the cycle, the pulses are of lower amplitude, but occur more frequently. They occur approximately 60 minutes apart. During the *second week* of the cycle (or the week prior to the timing of ovulation), the pulse frequency is approximately 90 minutes. There is some evidence to suggest that the pulse frequency increases some just prior to ovulation. *Following ovulation,* however, the pulse frequency slows significantly to 120-180 minutes while the amplitude increases. These pulses of gonadotropin-releasing hormone are sometimes referred to as the "Fertility Pacemaker" or "Mission Control" of the reproductive system.

The following summary traces the events of the menstrual and ovulation cycles relative to the hormones that actually regulate it:

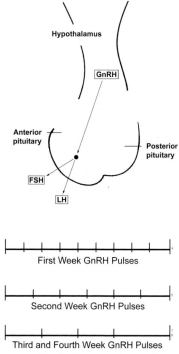

Figure 6-3: The fertility pacemaker. A schematic presentation of the hypothalamus, the anterior and posterior pituitary gland. GnRH pulses at various intervals during the course of the menstrual cycle are shown.

1. *Follicle-stimulating hormone (FSH)* is produced in the anterior lobe of the pituitary gland. FSH production begins to increase at the end of the previous cycle and increases even more at the beginning of the cycle because of the decrease in estrogen and progesterone production at the end of the previous cycle (see Figure 6-1 for reference).

2. The *luteinizing hormone (LH)* also is produced for the same reasons and begins to increase slightly just prior to the onset of menstruation as the estrogen and progesterone levels fall. Both pituitary hormones are suppressed by progesterone and estrogen on the release of these hormones from the pituitary. Once the corpus luteum begins to degenerate and progesterone and estrogen decrease, the inhibitory activity of these hormones is discontinued and FSH and LH begin the cycle all over again.

3. The FSH causes the growth and development of *one ovum* (usually) and a cyst on the ovary called the *follicle.* This is referred to as *the recruitment phase.* Several follicles are "recruited" in response to the early increase in FSH, which occurs between approximately days 3 to 5 of a normal 28-day cycle (or approximately nine to 10 days prior to actual ovulation). It should be noted that 28-day cycles only occur 5 to 10 percent of the time.[2]

4. The *second stage*, following the recruitment of the follicles, is called the *selection phase*. In this phase, *one follicle* (usually) that previously had been recruited is now *selected* to eventually ovulate. Out of the hundreds of thousands of ova present, it is not understood why a particular one would be selected over others.

5. Following that phase, the *final stage* of the development of the follicle, called the *dominance phase*, begins to appear. Here the selected dominant follicle continues to grow and produces rising levels of estrogen, which, in turn, suppress the maturation of the other ovarian follicles.

6. The *LH hormone* stimulates certain cells that line the follicle to produce the *estrogen* hormone.

7. The *estrogen hormone* slowly increases in the blood of the woman until they reach a very high level (the estrogen peak) about one day prior to the release of the ovum (ovulation).

8. The hormone estrogen also causes the endometrium to regenerate during this part of the cycle (*the preovulatory phase*) in what is referred to as proliferative endometrium.

9. It also is the *estrogen hormone* that works on the cells of the *cervix* to produce *cervical mucus* (Type E) and the increased production of progesterone produces various physical changes in this mucus, which stop the flow of the mucus.

10. Up until this point (the estrogen peak), this part of the cycle is variously referred to as the *follicular phase* (pointing to the development of the follicle), the *proliferative phase* (pointing to the development of the endometrium) or the *preovulatory phase* (pointing to the occurrence or timing of ovulation) of the menstrual cycle.

11. The *preovulatory phase* of the menstrual cycle is *highly variable* in length.

12. What often is referred to as mid-cycle (although it is often not mid-cycle at all),[3] the pituitary gland suddenly produces a large amount of the LH hormone. This is called the LH "*surge.*"

13. It is this "surge" in the LH hormone that is thought to *cause rupture of the follicle* and release of the ovum (*ovulation*). The exact mechanism of ovulation is not entirely understood, but it is thought that prostaglandins may play a role in the stimulation of the capsule of the follicle that may be helpful in causing contractions of the follicular wall and its subsequent rupture and release of the egg (ovulation). In fact, with such contractions, the woman will sometimes feel an *abdominal pain* associated with ovulation.

14. Ovulation generally takes place *12 to 24 hours following the LH "surge."*

15. What causes the LH "surge" is not entirely understood. Many people feel that the sudden fall in the production of estrogen, which occurs after the estrogen peak, causes the release of LH. Thus, the close correlation of the estrogen peak with ovulation. This is not the only reason for the LH "surge" and other factors are undoubtedly involved. Suffice it to say that this mechanism is not fully understood at the present time.

16. With rupture of the follicle at the time of ovulation, the follicle collapses and through the influence of the LH hormone, certain cells in the follicle now begin to produce progesterone. This *collapsed follicle* now is known as the *corpus luteum*.

17. The production of *progesterone* increases until about seven days after ovulation when it reaches its peak, stabilizes and then begins to decrease. The *corpus luteum* also produces *estrogen* with a second peak occurring after ovulation, but this peak is not as high as the one that occurs during the preovulatory phase of the cycle.

18. Progesterone acts on the endometrium to stimulate the glands in the endometrium to produce *certain biologic fluids* that are designed to nutritionally support the growth and development of a new human being. This endometrium is now called a *secretory endometrium*.

19. The onset of menstruation occurs when there is a decrease in the production of the hormones, progesterone and estrogen by the corpus luteum. Without the hormonal support of these two hormones, the endometrium essentially degenerates and sloughing or shedding occurs and thus, *menstruation*.

20. The time *from ovulation until menstruation* (the length of the luteal phase) averages about *13 days* but ranges from *nine to 17 days* (*13 ± four days*).[4]

21. This time corresponds to the natural life of the corpus luteum, which begins to degenerate at about eight days following ovulation and completes this process about 13 days following ovulation (on average).

22. The *second half* of the menstrual cycle is variously referred to as the *luteal phase* (pointing to the corpus luteum), the *secretory phase* (pointing to the endometrium) or the *post-ovulatory phase* (pointing to the time of ovulation in the menstrual cycle). The *second phase* of the menstrual cycle is *much more stable in length* than is the preovulatory phase.

23. With the rapid fall of progesterone and estrogen, menstruation occurs. FSH is stimulated and the cyclic process is started all over again.

24. If pregnancy occurs, a hormone is produced at least by eight days after conception and is called *human chorionic gonadotropin* (*hCG*). This hormone

is produced by the early developing placental tissue (this is the hormone that is tested in the over-the-counter urine pregnancy tests and blood tests).

25. *Human chorionic gonadotropin* (hCG) will stimulate the corpus luteum to continue to function, thus preventing its degeneration. As a result, *progesterone continues to be produced* by the corpus luteum early in pregnancy. *Studies have shown that this corpus luteum will continue to produce progesterone all the way through to the end of pregnancy.*

The fine coordination of each of these hormonal events is truly *one of the most amazing events in all of biology.* Our lack of respect for its complexity and the delicacy of its balance has led to a considerable amount of chemical and mechanical interference with it – an affront to human ecology.

Receptors

For hormones to work effectively, they must bind with chemicals within the cell called *receptors*. These receptors are located usually within *the nucleus* of the cell. Thus, they often are referred to as *nuclear receptors*.

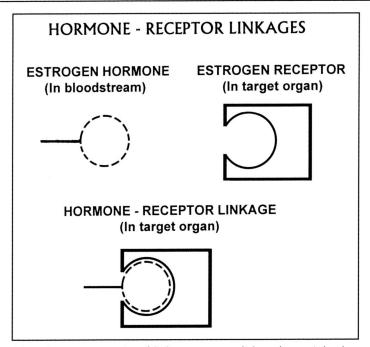

Figure 6-4: A schematic representation of the hormone-receptor linkages that are vital to the important function of any hormone.

These receptors are chemicals located within the target organ that must bind with the hormone in order to make the hormone effective. To have an effective hormone response, one must have *both normal hormone levels, as well as normal receptor levels.* Properly pulsating FSH is generally responsible for the production of the reproductive receptors; however, estrogen prior to the timing of ovulation also is helpful in the stimulation of progesterone receptors.[5] The *steroid receptors* are predominantly located within the *nucleus of the cell* (intranuclear) as opposed to *cytoplasmic* (within the cytoplasm of the cell). The concept of hormone-receptor linkages is depicted in a schematic form in Figure 6-4.

It is good to keep in mind that *hormonal dysfunction* can occur either because the *hormone levels are too low*, the *receptor levels are too low* or *both are too low*. Unfortunately, it is difficult to measure the receptors in the menstrual cycle in clinical medicine at the present time; thus, only indirect assessments of receptors can be made.

Clinical Estimates of the Luteal Phase

The length of the luteal phase can be clinically estimated with either the use of the post-Peak phase with the **CREIGHTON MODEL System** or various basal body temperature systems. Over the years of clinical reproductive medicine the basal body temperature system has been the one that has been utilized the most. Data now shows that the length of the post-Peak phase is the best clinical indicator for estimating the length of the luteal phase. This is important to know because as we begin to talk about **NaProTECHNOLOGY** and the **CREIGHTON MODEL System**, the *post-Peak phase* will be identified as one of the biomarkers.[6] It is an excellent and accurate measure of the length of the luteal phase. It is reproducible and measurable and easy to obtain (and it's free).

Myths, Ignorance and Insults

OFTEN HAVE STATED publicly that when it comes to an opinion about a natural means to regulate fertility, I have never met a physician who does not have an opinion on it. Furthermore, that opinion is usually negative. At the same time, the physicians who hold this view often know virtually nothing about these systems and their scientific foundations. If you think about it, this is really disturbing, because we presume that a physician is going to provide us with a reasoned and studied opinion. In many ways, nothing could be further from the truth. In this chapter, I would like to address some of the *myths, ignorance and insults* that have been placed before this work over the many years of its development. Many of these continue to be applicable at the very time this book is being written.

When I speak to a group of doctors, I will often present to them some of the scientific work that validates and substantiates the very foundation of the **CREIGHTON MODEL Fertility***Care*™ **System** and **NaProTECHNOLOGY** (see Internet Appendix). After painstakingly going through the data and the results of the various scientific investigations, I often get a physician who raises his hand and says, "Your system is not really natural because it removes spontaneity from the act of having intercourse, and, furthermore, it asks people to 'abstain' from intercourse at the time in the cycle when the woman has her highest level of libido." With regard to the issue of "spontaneity," there are any number of things that we otherwise take for granted that interfere with this "spontaneity" on a day-in and day-out basis. For example, when one of the physicians is listening to my lecture, he or she has willingly foregone the issue of "spontaneity" even if they were not using a natural method but were using one of the artificial methods of contraception. To somehow isolate a natural means of fertility regulation as the only thing that interferes with "spontaneity" is an emotional response that denies reality.

The physicians who hold onto the notion that the highest point of a woman's libido is at the time of fertility ignore those studies that show the opposite. In work published by Kingsley Davis,[1] on the rhythms of sexual desire, he found that the highest sexual desire was found immediately prior to menstruation, during menstruation and shortly after menstruation. Furthermore, he also found that the sexual desire of women was actually lowest at the time of anticipated fertility. Such studies were duplicated by Dr. R. D. Hart in 1960.[2]

These studies are of interest because they objectively indicate that the highest interest in a physical sexual encounter is at times other than the time around maximum fertility. There continues to be women, of course, where the maximum sexual desire is described as being around the time of fertility. Thus, it is more important to understand and place into context the meaning of this as opposed to simply denying that such would occur.

When one discusses an increased level of libido, it does indicate an increased interest in a sexual encounter. However, it is not like a set of dominoes that when set in motion lead to one final conclusion. In other words, it does not mean that the increased sexual interest is to be resolved **only** with an act of physical intercourse. This increased sexual interest also is a reflection of a desire to be close – physically and emotionally close to one's spouse. This could be satisfied by being physically close in a non-genital form of physical touching. When done out of love, this is a special form of expression in the human marriage relationship that goes to the deeper meaning of the discovery of the *"inner soul"* of one's human sexuality.[3]

Pope John Paul II, in his exhortation to families titled *Familiaris Consortio,*[3] introduced the concept of the *"inner soul"* of human sexuality. He wrote that:

> "The choice of the natural rhythms involves accepting the cycle of the person, that is, the woman, and thereby accepting dialogue, reciprocal respect, shared responsibility and self-control. To accept the cycle and to enter into dialogue means to recognize both the spiritual and the corporal character of conjugal

communion, and to live personal love with its requirement of fidelity. In this context, the couple comes to experience how conjugal communion is enriched with those values of *tenderness and affection* which constitutes the *inner soul of human sexuality*, in its physical dimensions also. In this way, sexuality is respected and promoted in its truly and fully human dimension and is never 'used' as an 'object' that, by breaking the personal unity of soul and body, strikes at God's creation itself at the level of the deepest interaction of nature and person"[4] (emphasis applied).

This contribution by Pope John Paul II in language and concept is extraordinary. As one reflects upon the discussions of human sexuality that have occurred over the last 40 or 50 years, the one thing that ultimately is missing is a better understanding of its meaning in human relationships, its meaning to the very nature of love and as an expression of that meaning, a discovery of its "inner soul." The **CREIGHTON MODEL Fertility*Care*™ System** has woven within its very fabric these concepts of human sexuality and the teachers of the system become experts in the very fundamental meaning and significance of human sexuality with particular reference to the discovery of its "inner soul."

One of the terms that is often used to describe a natural means to regulate fertility is the term "periodic abstinence." The idea of *"periodic abstinence"* is not at all specific to the use of a natural method. Those who use contraceptives also practice periodic abstinence since they do abstain from genital intercourse between one sexual contact and the next. In fact, they have spent the overwhelming majority of their lives in an abstinent mode. So the idea of periodic abstinence is not a concept that applies exclusively to a natural means to regulate fertility and it should not be used as a description of a natural method.

The decision to either have or not have intercourse is dependent upon *actual choices* one makes to either achieve or avoid pregnancy in the use of the **CREIGHTON MODEL System**. The system uses the term *"selective intercourse,"* which specifically implies the decision-making choices that couples implement while activating the fullness of the system. In their decision making, *they are selecting* in a responsible way *the very best time to have intercourse.* Perhaps even more importantly, *they are mutually selecting* that time. Thus, spontaneous intercourse involves a submission to emotional impulses while selective intercourse subjects itself to choices evaluated and implemented through the incorporation of *the intellect, the will* and *the values* that the couple share. The sharing that is involved in the implementation of the

CREIGHTON MODEL System also is different from contraceptive approaches. These systems do not work unless the couple cooperates with each other. Technological systems are built upon the notion that such cooperation often does not or may not exist. In this latter approach, the basic premise precludes the development of cooperation in this important aspect of the married couple's life. That preclusion can lead to distress, tension, resentment and eventually destruction of the relationship.

This *cooperation of the intellect and the will* is sometimes referred to as *cerebrocentric sexuality.* The focus is primarily *personal* and *internal.* It *maintains the connections between love and life* and it leads to *personalization, humanization* and *physiologic* and *spiritual affirmation.* In the CrMS, we use the acronym *SPICE* to refer to the multidimensional nature of human sexuality, which is *Spiritual, Physical, Intellectual, Creative/communicative* and *Emotional/psychological.* Cerebrocentric sexuality is at the foundation of the commitment to support the natural means to regulate fertility and to *marital bonding. It respects the dignity of both men and women and the integrity of marriage.* It is *genitally affirming* but not extreme in genital functioning (that is to say, it is *ecologically balanced*), and it should be expected to lead to a *decrease* in family violence.

Current contraceptive approaches to family planning involve a *genitocentric* focus in sexuality. As a natural extension of this genitocentric focus, *there is a separation of love from life* and of *life from love.* This we see on a day-in and day-out basis in American (Western) culture. This *depersonalization* leads to *dehumanization* and *psychological* and *spiritual deprivation.* Contraception, sterilization, abortion, the artificial reproductive technologies and pornographic expression are *natural results of a genitocentric view.* As a result of *genitocentrism,* as previously pointed out in Chapter 2, it is absolutely clear that *family violence* has increased to epidemic proportions.

In 1976, a noteworthy book titled "The Curse: A Cultural History of Menstruation" was published. This perpetuated the concept that menstruation was a factor in a woman's life that was to be *dreaded* and had only *negative aspects* associated with it. This appeared to be a carryover of a longstanding, ignorant view of the menstrual and fertility cycle, which truly continues until the present day. In addition, it appeared to be a hangover from what a Harvard physician, in the mid-1960s, referred to as *the toxicity of the menstrual fluid.* Toxic influences in the menstrual blood (referred to as *menotoxins*), which could be harmful to both men and women, were thought to be present.[5]

Also in 1976, unwanted pregnancy was labeled "*the second most common*" *sexually-transmitted disease*.[6] A paper was presented with this title at a scientific meeting of the Association of Planned Parenthood Physicians. Pregnancy, for the very first time, was labeled a disease, and, after all, it had failed the 'cure' – the oral contraceptive.

Over the intervening years, one would have expected some enlightenment to occur. But in September 2003 when the nationally-syndicated television show "Berman & Berman"[7] undertook a discussion of the menstrual cycle, they referred frequently to topics within the discussion as "unmentionables." Then, as late as May 19, 2006, the idea of the menstrual period being a curse once again was resurrected in a story that was written by the Associated Press.[8]

It actually gets worse than that. In the April 2010 issue of Clinical Advisor, a forum for nurse practitioners, it was noted quite seriously that "monthly menstruation is a historic anomaly." What are the historians going to think when they review these last fifty years?

One of the tragedies that we live with in everyday life is a lack of understanding of the menstrual and fertility cycle. There truly are mysteries that exist that women and their physicians have virtually no idea about. It is this ignorance that persists – this large "*blank space*" – that is so prevalent in discussing these issues.

The huge blank space, however, is no longer blank. It has been filled in by scientific investigations that do not see pregnancy as a disease, do not see the menstrual cycle as a "curse" and do not see the mucus cycle as an "unmentionable." For the most part, a woman's cycle and her fertility are conditions of *complete normality* and it is our *lack of knowledge* and our *insecurity* and sometimes our *arrogance* that finds comfort in calling them diseases, curses or unmentionables.

It is true that both the menstrual and fertility cycle can *become* diseased. This should come as no shock. The lungs, the heart, the liver, the kidneys, the brain, the eyes, the ears, the throat, et cetera, also can become diseased, but we would not call them diseased when they are working efficiently and in a healthy fashion. When good investigation is occurring, it begins by an understanding of the normal physiologic processes. This has often not occurred in the field of reproductive medicine.

In **NaProTECHNOLOGY**, we begin by studying the basic concepts of the normal menstrual and fertility cycle. We look at a way of tracking the cycle that is *objective* and *standardized* (see Chapter 8) and, then, we can begin to describe and understand what is normal and what is abnormal or diseased. By taking this approach, we also can find and look for the underlying causes, which then allow us to effectively treat it for long-term health. Indeed, **NaProTECHNOLOGY** uses the **CREIGHTON MODEL System** and its biologic markers that are gained through education to guide its medical and technological resources so they can be used *cooperatively* with the woman's cycle. It is this that allows **NaProTECHNOLOGY** to "unleash the power that exists in a woman's cycle" ... power that is *knowledge and understanding!* Indeed, **NaProTECHNOLOGY** addresses the health problems of reproductive-age women. These are *real problems* and **NaProTECHNOLOGY** provides *real solutions!*

Myths

I have heard well-educated obstetricians and gynecologists say that a natural method will not be effective because women ovulate in response to intercourse or they may ovulate twice or more in a given menstrual cycle. So the question is raised, does intercourse and the complex emotional stimulation that it produces cause a woman to ovulate? Do women ovulate more than once during the menstrual cycle? If the human female ovulated whenever she had intercourse, the natural methods to regulate fertility would, of course, not work. The same could be said of double ovulations if the ovulation events were separated by long periods of time.

Generally there are "*reflex*" and "*spontaneous*" ovulators. Such animals as the mole, cat and rabbit are "reflex" ovulators. That is to say, they ovulate in response to sexual stimulation. Rats, on the other hand, are thought to be "spontaneous" ovulators. That is, they ovulate regularly without influence from the outside environment. Unfortunately, the studies in rabbits have been taken to indicate that human females also are "reflex" ovulators. There is, of course, a significant problem that exists in making the transition from studies done in these types of animals to studies done in human beings. Generally speaking, however, there is no good evidence that shows that ovulation occurs as the result of sexual stimulation.[9-12]

In terms of *double ovulation*, there is no question that this does occur as the presence of fraternal (non-identical) twins would document. Fraternal twins come from the fertilization of two eggs. The evidence, however, would suggest that when double ovulations occur, they occur within the same 24-hour time period. Said in another way, it would be impossible to ovulate today and then a second time next week. When the first ovulation occurs, both the progesterone and estrogen levels begin to rise rather quickly. These hormones, acting together, effectively inhibit a subsequent ovulation. We have studied at the Pope Paul VI Institute nearly 3,000 spontaneous menstrual cycles with daily ultrasounds around the time of ovulation and the only time we have seen either a double or triple ovulation is when the rupture of these two or three follicles also occurs within the same 24-hour time period.

There are any number of ovulation test kits that are currently on the market to determine when a woman is "ovulating." These test kits measure the presence or absence of the LH hormone in a woman's urine. The urine is sampled on a daily basis around the anticipated time of ovulation and the test strip turns a different color when the LH hormone is present. With the presence of the LH hormone documented, it is then thought that this documents the occurrence of ovulation. While these biochemistry tests are actually very reliable in the detection of the LH hormone, they are everything but reliable when it comes to determining if a woman has actually ovulated. In 60 percent of women with regular cycles and infertility, a significant ovulation-related abnormality will occur, which is one of the causes of the infertility problem. In these cases, the LH test kits will show positive, but in fact, either ovulation has not occurred, or the ovulatory process is highly deficient and abnormal. The ovulation test kits are not able to distinguish this. This becomes very problematic when too much emphasis is placed on this particular test.

In addition, there are other factors that contribute to the infertility problem that cannot be detected by the LH test kit. For example, the amount of mucus may be sharply reduced or completely absent in different types of infertility problems. In women who have regular cycles and a diagnosis of endometriosis, 77.6 percent of them will have either dry cycles or what we refer to as limited mucus cycles. These are abnormalities of mucus production, which are associated with abnormal hormone function and abnormal ovulation patterns. All of the hormones, such as estrogen and progesterone, are abnormal in these cycles, but the one hormone that is not is the LH hormone. Thus, if one relies on the ovulation test kits to get information regarding the presence or absence of fertility, they will be gravely misled.[13]

Ignorance

One of the truly great deceptions has been the re-definition of the term *conception*. In referring to conception, for generations, it meant the union of the sperm and the egg, a process also often referred to as *fertilization*. This usually is thought to be the beginning of pregnancy. Through a series of events, however, many textbooks in reproductive medicine and even official medical dictionaries have now redefined conception to mean the time of implantation, which is actually about eight days after fertilization (and after conception).

At the 2nd International Conference on the Intrauterine Device,[14] the mechanism of action of the IUD was candidly discussed. Delegates to the conference expressed concern over the label "abortifacient" being given to the IUD since it would be detrimental in promotion of the device in developing countries where abortion is strongly opposed.[15] Discussion aimed at redefining pregnancy to begin at implantation began as a result of this concern. In other words, the truth for the beginning of life was officially disguised and the public has been deceived ever since with this type of political re-definition. This is sort of like saying that the first 16 to 32 cell divisions of an ovarian cancer are really not ovarian cancer at all. In this case, the first 16 to 32 cell divisions of the beginning of life have been defined out of existence even though they are definitely still there, and, in fact, we have all been through those stages in our own life. In this day and age of "evidence-based medicine" this does not pass muster.

Another one of the incredibly deceptive practices is for physicians to constantly suggest to women that a natural method of avoiding pregnancy simply does not work. A number of the statistical studies that are published in mainstream reproductive textbooks suggest that the "failure rate" of a natural method is in the 28 to 30 percent range. This, if it were true, would of course make this one of the lower-ranking systems currently available.

In coming by those statistics, they include as "failures" all of those women who have become pregnant because with their spouse they chose to use the days that were defined to be fertile. In other words, these were women who were *successful users* of the system and not "failures." Yet, this is a notion that is very difficult for the contraceptive world to understand. They cannot understand the use of a means of avoiding pregnancy to also be used as a means of achieving pregnancy. One would not use a condom, purchase a package of oral contraceptives and start them, place an intrauterine device or get a tubal sterilization with the idea in mind that they would like to achieve a pregnancy. The very idea of that is ludicrous, but, it is no more ludicrous than for the contraceptive world to continually say that those who have used the **CREIGHTON MODEL System** successfully as a means of achieving pregnancy are "failures." Actually, this is an extraordinary group to study so that one can better understand the dynamics of this aspect of its use. But, to call them "failures" is truly absurd. In fact, the **CREIGHTON MODEL System** has been studied extensively with regard to its effectiveness to avoid pregnancy. In a meta-analysis (an analysis of five separate studies of the **CREIGHTON MODEL System** published between 1980 and 1994), a group of 1,876 couples over more than 17,000 couple months of use had a method-effectiveness rate (now currently called "perfect use rate") of 99.5 percent. These couples showed a use-effectiveness rate (currently referred to as the "typical use rate") of 96.8 percent. These data are from couples who are truly using it as a means to avoid pregnancy and those success rates are equal to oral contraceptives.[16]

Insults

It also is interesting to note some other comments that have been made with regard to this work. A friend of mine e-mailed an individual of national stature who appears on television regularly to speak with regard to the various reproductive technologies, almost always in favor of them, and he was asked what he thought about this new science. His response was, "I think this is pure propaganda. Charting is the solution to infertility in women – that is simply silly." He also added as an interesting aside to that: "The infertility industry is full of money-hungry creeps!"[17] I don't remember him saying that on national television though.

Another very prominent physician made the comment that, "Women's observations will never successfully be standardized because women are individuals who operate individually."[18] While women do operate individually, there is absolutely no question that these observations not only have been standardized, but it is the standardization that is inherent in the **CREIGHTON MODEL FertilityCare™ System** that is responsible for the development of this new women's health science.

Another physician wrote to me and said, "Good work, but the name **NaProTECHNOLOGY** will never catch on anywhere… I don't know what it would be, but good luck."[19] Since **NaProTECHNOLOGY** is just reaching out into the medical and lay community, only time will tell whether it will catch on. We will wait with interest.

Recently I was speaking with a female OB-GYN who had an interest in this work. She told me that she had a pregnant patient on progesterone and thought the patient might benefit from the use of "Dr. Hilgers' progesterone protocol." When she told her partners this they told her "He is a quack! We would not recommend anything he does." They conveniently forgot to tell her that they also know nothing about what we do.

This reminds me of another OB-GYN who, after taking our course, began using progesterone to treat postpartum depression with great success. His partners told him that this was not approved by the American College of Obstetricians and Gynecologists (ACOG) and he should stop using this approach. After a couple of years, I asked him how this was going and he told me, "They are all using it now."

One of the most difficult insults I have received came from the medical director of a major health insurance company. My patient had sued them because they would not pay for her diagnostic surgery. The medical director in his deposition said that "Dr. Hilgers' medical judgement was biased because of his religious beliefs." The case went to trial and when the jury finished viewing the videotape of her diagnostic surgery they ruled in favor of the patient and against the insurance company. It raises an interesting question as to whose medical judgement was biased.

I have not identified any of these individuals because I think their anonymity is important to be kept. It does no great service to tell the world who they are, but I do think it is helpful to see some of the comments that have been made over the years relative to this work. I would ask the reader not to be discouraged by them. Almost without question, they come from a framework of ignorance and, to a fairly strong degree, prejudice and bias. In an era of *evidence-based medicine*, these comments also would not "hold up." I am happy to present the medical evidence that supports **NaProTECHNOLOGY** along with its clinical applications and everyday practice, not only for others to scrutinize, but also for its ongoing verification.

A New Understanding

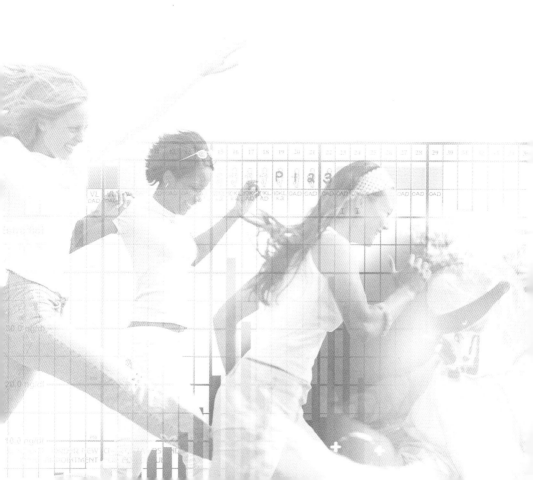

Creighton Model and Its Charting System

The **CREIGHTON MODEL Fertility*Care*™ System** (CrMS) is a standardized modification and legitimate offspring of the original Billings Ovulation Method.[1] It is built on *research*, *education* and *service*, ("The Triangle of Support" for the **CREIGHTON MODEL** user) and is an integrated educational system designed to assure the highest quality-service delivery possible for the new user.

In the **CrMS**, fertility is observed as a part of health, not disease. It is a system that is specifically **not** a natural contraceptive. *It is a true method of family planning...* a method that can be used in two ways: *to achieve*, as well as *to avoid* pregnancy. These principles make this system distinctly different (180 degrees different) from contraception (artificial or natural).

The **CrMS** is a system focused on knowing and understanding the naturally-occurring phases of fertility and infertility. Through this understanding, the couple is able to make decisions (choices) regarding pregnancy. It provides women the added benefit of being able to monitor and maintain their procreative and gynecologic health over a lifetime. **CrMS** teachers (**Fertility*Care*™ Practitioners**) are trained allied health professionals and physicians (**Fertility*Care*™** Medical Consultants) are trained to incorporate the **CREIGHTON MODEL** into their medical practice. It is a system that is completely integrated in its education, research and service orientation. It meets the demands of the allied health and medical professions in the field of the natural means to regulate fertility. It is a system built to accomplish accountability and competency through a *strong, professional infrastructure* and it works within the context of a high ethical and moral service delivery framework.

The **CrMS** allows married couples to consciously cooperate in the achievement of a pregnancy as a component of its use. While an emphasis has been placed on assisting couples with infertility (and the **CrMS** has a very special capability of helping couples with these difficulties), this system is *unique* in its ability to assist couples of *completely normal fertility* to use it throughout the course of their reproductive life for both the achievement, as well as the avoidance of pregnancy. It also is unique in its ability to assist a woman in the long-term monitoring and maintenance of her reproductive and gynecologic health. Therefore, it is, by definition and application, a *lifelong system* (a permanent system) not to be reduced to a fraction of one's procreative life.

The Teaching System

The **CREIGHTON MODEL System** is based upon *individual follow-up* after the couple has attended a group *introductory* session. The individual follow-up assures individual attention, allows for all questions to be asked, and allows the system to be "tailor-made" to the individual couple.[2]

It also is built upon a "case management" concept.[3,4] This is a comprehensive approach to client care and it allows for complex problems to be solved. The case management approach allows for a comprehensive and prioritized approach to the management of difficult cases. It is truly a benefit of standardization and it is completely holistic in its approach.

NaProEducation Technology

NaProEducation TECHNOLOGY (Natural Procreative Education) is a technology that has developed as a result of the commitment to educational research in the **CREIGHTON MODEL System**. It is an *advanced educational technology*, the principles of which have not been previously used in either medical or patient education. The allied health education model and standardized educational content previously mentioned are a part of this NaProEducation Technology. It also involves:

1. Objective and measurable standards that are incorporated into the system.

2. The use of a *Picture Dictionary*[5] that objectively teaches the mucus observations.

3. A *Follow-Up Form*[3] that allows for the standardization of teaching from one teacher to the next and an orderly transfer of knowledge in a way that allows for "equal access" to the vital information to utilize the system properly.

4. A *vaginal discharge recording system (VDRS)* that has been developed out of standardization and allows for a **standardized terminology** to be utilized. There have been developed **standardized observations** and, of course, **standardized charting**.[3]

5. A *Pregnancy Evaluation Form*[4] for the evaluation of any pregnancies that occur during the use of the Creighton Model System.

6. A number of ongoing assessment and evaluation tools that also have been developed and used to improve quality control.[3]

There is no system like it in the world! It is truly unique and individual. It works, has allowed for growth and development of the system and, more and more, has allowed for an increased insight in the advanced personalism of our human sexuality.

The Creighton Model System

The **CrMS** provides the couple with the means to be able to freely express their reproductive potential. It relies upon a sign – *the discharge of cervical mucus* – that is *essential* to human fertility. Because of this, the **CrMS** is the most precise of all natural methods.

The **CrMS** is based upon the fact that whenever a woman is fertile she will experience a characteristic discharge of cervical mucus, which is obvious to her at the opening of the vagina. As ovulation approaches, this discharge undergoes a progressive change that can be easily observed and interpreted. The **CrMS** is unlike other natural methods that monitor only the events occurring after ovulation has passed or relies simply upon past cycle history.

It is a system that can be used at any stage of a couple's reproductive life. It can be used if a woman has *regular* or *irregular* cycles, is *breastfeeding*, is *premenopausal*, or is *discontinuing the use of contraceptive medications*. The system also can be used successfully if the woman is experiencing a *continuous mucus discharge* or is *anovulatory*. In addition, the system offers new hope to the evaluation and treatment of *infertility* and a host of *other reproductive and gynecologic problems*.

The advantages of the **CrMS** are numerous. First of all, it is *safe!* There are no known medical side effects associated with its use. It is *inexpensive!* The cost of **FertilityCare**™ services is considerably less than that of contraceptives. Finally, it is *highly reliable* and it is *natural.* The **CrMS** *cooperates* with the couple's own natural fertility process.

Another important advantage to the system is that it is a *shared method* of fertility regulation. The responsibility for its use is placed equally upon both spouses. To use the method successfully, it is necessary to *make accurate observations* and to *chart them correctly.* In addition, one must follow the instructions of the system, which depend upon the couple's decision to either achieve or avoid pregnancy.

As the couple learns more about their natural phases of fertility and infertility, they will begin to realize how important and vital these gifts really are. Unlike contraceptives, the **CrMS** treats fertility as a normal and healthy process. The challenge to live in harmony with one's fertility is often one of the most exciting and meaningful aspects in the use of this system. Most couples find that the love and respect each holds for the other grows as their understanding and appreciation of their fertility increases. It is a system that is firmly based in a *respect for human life, human dignity and the integrity of marriage.* Indeed, it is the couples who use this method and their families who benefit from this experience.

The **CREIGHTON MODEL** reveals the essential events that occur during the course of the menstrual and fertility cycles. The menstrual period is usually three to seven days in duration. Following the cessation of menstrual flow, a woman will generally observe the absence of any type of vaginal discharge or the sensation of dryness. After the dry days, she will begin to notice the beginning of a very characteristic discharge. This discharge usually begins with sticky, cloudy or tacky, cloudy characteristics and progresses to become clear, stretchy or lubricative in one or two days. The clear, stretchy or lubricative mucus discharge lasts usually three to four days. This, however, will be variable from woman to woman and from cycle to cycle. The *last day* in which the mucus is *clear, stretchy or lubricative* is called the *Peak Day.* After the *Peak Day,* the remainder of the cycle is generally dry.

Charting correctly the signs of fertility is important to the successful use of the **CrMS**. In addition, it is of great assistance to the user in developing confidence. The chart also is an outstanding health record.

Definitions

The following definitions are important during this discussion:

1. **Peak-type mucus** = any mucus discharge that is *clear, stretchy or lubricative*. Any one of these three characteristics, alone or in any combination, results in the mucus discharge being defined as *Peak-type mucus*.

2. **Non-Peak-type mucus** = any mucus discharge that is *not* clear, stretchy or lubricative. All three of these characteristics must be absent in order to establish the identity of *non-Peak-type mucus*.

3. **Peak Day** = the *last day* of any mucus discharge that is *clear, stretchy* or *lubricative*.

The Inside of the Chart

On the inside of the chart (Figure 8-1), there are numbers across the top from one through 35. This tells the day of the menstrual cycle. For each day, there is a box provided for the placement of the proper stamp and another box provided for writing the proper description. In addition, there is a place provided to write the date. The user should chart each new menstrual cycle beginning at the left margin of the chart and continuing horizontally, regardless of how long that cycle might be. On occasion, it will run more than the length of the chart and go to a second or a third line. There is room for six months of charting on each chart.

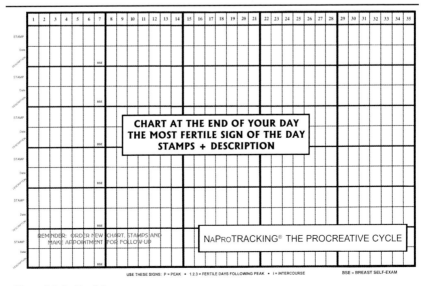

Figure 8-1: Inside of chart.

Stamps

Stamps have been developed for use with the CrMS (Figure 8-2). These stamps are used throughout the world:

Plain red stamps	=	For days of bleeding
Plain green stamps	=	For infertile dry days
White, baby stamps	=	For mucus days
Green, baby stamps	=	For dry days that are fertile (within the count of 3)

In addition to the above stamps, yellow stamps also are sometimes used with the **CrMS**. In this teaching system, yellow stamps are only to be used upon specific indication and then only with the advice of the teacher. A new client coming into a teaching program will not be given yellow stamps in the introductory packet of stamps that they receive. They will be taught directly at the time of follow-up with the **CREIGHTON MODEL Practitioner** (the teacher).

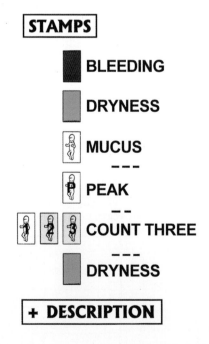

Figure 8-2: Basic stamps used in charting the **CREIGHTON MODEL System**. The "P" and "1,2,3" are written on the chart by the client couple.

Descriptions

For each day of charting, a description is written in the description box. A standardized means for recording these has been developed and is discussed later in this chapter (see Vaginal Discharge Recording System). In addition, the following signs are placed on the chart at the appropriate times:

P = Placed on a white, baby stamp on the Peak Day
1, 2, 3 = Placed on the 3 stamps following the Peak Day
I = An act of intercourse

The descriptions are extremely important. The message of the system is completely within the charting of the descriptions and the stamps allow for an easy way to keep track of those days that are fertile and those days that are not. The user should record the most fertile sign of the day in the box provided. *The CrMS story is told in the day-by-day descriptions of the mucus patterns.*

A Charting Example

The next several figures will show an example of how a cycle is charted. The first chart in this sequence is Figure 8-3. In this case, five red stamps have been placed for the designation of the five days of menstruation. The symbol "H" means heavy menstrual flow, "M" means moderate menstrual flow, and "L" means light menstrual flow. On the day of light menstrual flow, the woman also has recorded *dry*. With experience, most women, if not all, can identify the presence or absence of mucus on the light and very light days at the end of the menstrual flow.

In Figure 8-4, the couple has now recorded the next four days, which are dry. The written description *dry* is placed in each box, and, for these infertile dry days occurring pre-Peak, a plain green stamp is placed in position. The woman has not recorded all of these days at one time, she has recorded each of these days at the end of each particular day.

In Figure 8-5, the woman begins to chart the observation of the mucus discharge. It usually begins as a sticky, cloudy discharge and progresses to become clear, stretchy and/or lubricative. For each day, a written description is placed in the description box. In addition, each

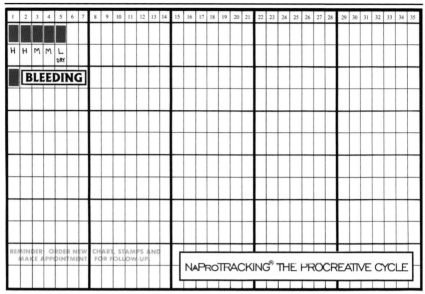

Figure 8-3: First five days of charting showing the use of red stamps for charting the menstrual flow.

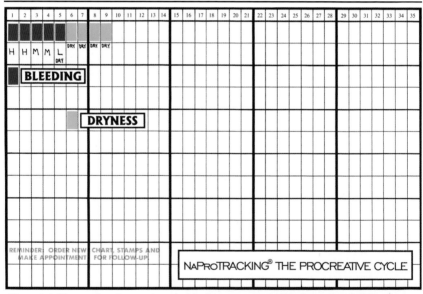

Figure 8-4: The next four days are charted with plain green stamps. The days are pre-Peak dry days.

of these days takes on a white stamp with a baby imprint on it. The *last day* of the mucus discharge that is *clear, stretchy, or lubricative* is called the **Peak Day** and a "**P**" is placed on that stamp. This cannot be placed until at least one day after the Peak Day. When the change in the mucus occurs following the Peak Day, then a "P" can be placed on

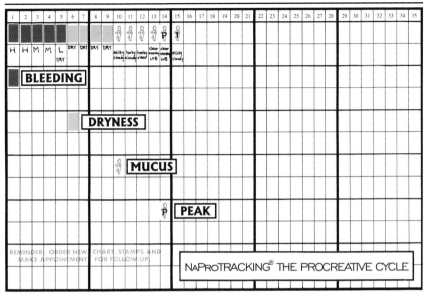

Figure 8-5: With the beginning of the mucus, white baby stamps are used. The Peak is marked with a "P". The day following the Peak is a dramatic change and is a day "1" in the three-day count.

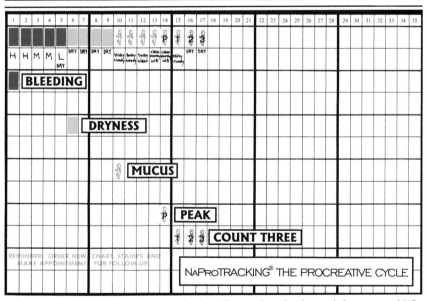

Figure 8-6: Day 2 and 3 after the Peak are dry days. They are charted with green baby stamps and "2" and "3" are written on them to complete the three-day count.

the chart for the Peak Day. In this case, on the day after the Peak, the mucus has changed to a sticky, cloudy-type of discharge. Non-Peak-type mucus days that follow the Peak Day in the count of three take a white, baby stamp.

In Figure 8-6, two additional days have been placed to the previous chart. These next two days are dry days and take on a green, baby stamp. In addition, the numbers 1, 2, and 3 have been placed on the stamps for these three days indicating the three additional days of fertility following the Peak Day.

In the final chart of this sequence, Figure 8-7, the completed 28-day cycle is shown. The remainder of the cycle is dry and this is recorded in the description box. In addition, the woman has placed a plain green stamp in the stamp box for each of the days. The charting is done *daily*, and it should be done at the *end of each day*. The chart should be kept in a convenient and readily-accessible location so that it can be used practically.

This charting example is a 28-day cycle, but it definitely is not a chart that you might expect to have yourself. Keep in mind that the **CrMS** is "tailor-made" to each individual woman. The basic principles of the observations and the charting of those observations are maintained, and even though the chart itself may look somewhat different, do not make the error of presuming that your cycles are going to be identical to the one in Figure 8-7. They might be, but it is quite likely that they will not be. This is actually not a problem. It is one of the nice features of this system because it can be adapted to any type of cycle pattern.

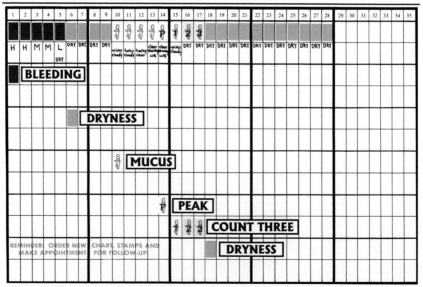

Figure 8-7: The cycle is now complete. The remaining days of this cycle are dry and charted with plain green stamps.

Vaginal Discharge Recording System^{SM}

The descriptions are the most important part of charting. They must accurately reflect the observations the woman makes so that a true picture of the mucus patterns can evolve. The *Vaginal Discharge Recording System*^{SM} (VDRS) has been developed so that charting can be done more easily and its accuracy improved. Every client is encouraged to use the VDRS from the very first follow-up appointment. Experience has shown that it is very easy to learn and use, and with its ready accessibility on the back of the chart, the client always has it for quick reference.

The recording system is outlined in Figure 8-8. While this recording system uses numbers, it should *not* be called a scoring system. In effect, any form of symbolism could be used in the same fashion, but a system of numbers and letters was chosen for this particular system. While there is a general tendency for the higher numbers to be associated with a higher degree of fertility, this should *not* be used in that way. The series of numbers and letters are simply a means of recording accurately the observations that the woman is making. When one becomes familiar with the recording system, it also makes chart reading much easier.

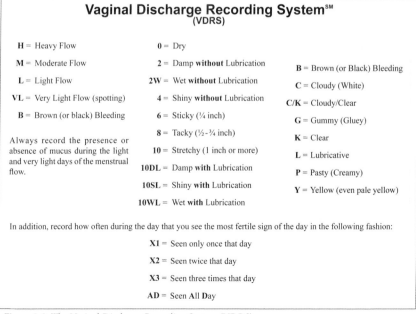

Figure 8-8: The Vaginal Discharge Recording System (VDRS).

During the menstrual flow, the symbols H means heavy, M means moderate, L mean light, VL means very light (or spotting) and B means brown (or black). During the light and very light days of the menstrual flow, an observation of the mucus should *always* be recorded.

The numbers 0, 2, 2W and 4 all relate to observations that have the same significance as dry observations. In these cases, when the client wonders which would be the most fertile sign of the day, she should record the higher number. This is merely a convention for recording purposes and for accuracy in recording. All four of these recordings are generally thought of as dry observations relative to stamp placement and the use of the method instructions.

When the numbers 6, 8 and 10 (sticky, tacky and stretchy) are used, a letter from the right hand column must *always be used*. Either a color or a consistency or both must be present when the mucus is stretchable.

The special categories of Peak-type mucus are recorded as 10DL (damp *with* lubrication), 10SL (shiny *with* lubrication) and 10WL (wet *with* lubrication). Since lubrication is present in all of these observations, the mucus is therefore of the Peak-type and would be of a high degree of fertility. The number 10 in this case does *not* mean stretchy. It is simply a means of recording these special categories of Peak-type mucus.

In addition to the above recordings, it also is important to record how often the *most fertile sign of the day* is observed. This is done by using X1 = seen only once that day; X2 = seen twice that day; X3 = seen three times that day; and AD = seen all day. The latter designation means that the mucus has been observed *four or more* times during the day. Once it has been observed four times, the woman no longer needs to keep a count of the number of times she has observed that most fertile sign. It automatically becomes an all-day (AD) observation.

Examples of the Recording System in Use

1. Dry – seen all day   = 0 AD
2. Damp without lubrication – seen all day   = 2 AD
3. Stretchy, clear, lubricative – seen all day = 10 KL AD
4. Sticky, cloudy – seen once   = 6 C x 1
5. Tacky, gummy, yellow – seen twice   = 8 GY x 2
6. Sticky, pasty, white – seen twice   = 6 PC x 2

In teaching the language of these observations, the **Fertility***Care*™ **Practitioner** (the teacher) will use a teaching tool called *The Picture Dictionary of the* **CREIGHTON MODEL System**.[5] This dictionary shows examples of the mucus observations so that the client can learn the actual objective language that is used in the recording of the observations. *The Picture Dictionary of the* **CREIGHTON MODEL System** was developed in the very earliest days of the development of the System and was one of the major tools responsible for the standardization of the system. The teacher also will use a *General Intake Form*, a *Follow-up Form* and other teaching tools during the course of the individual follow-ups that will be helpful for both the teacher and the new user to learn the system effectively.

Actual Charting Examples

In Figure 8-9, the actual charting of the menstrual and fertility cycle, accomplished through the use of the **CREIGHTON MODEL System**, is correlated to the blood levels of estrogen and progesterone during the course of the cycle. When the mucus cycle is present (days 14–19 of Figure 8-9), the estrogen levels are rising and falling (the black vertical bars). The mucus cycle stops when progesterone (the red vertical bars) begins to rise. When the estrogen levels are low or

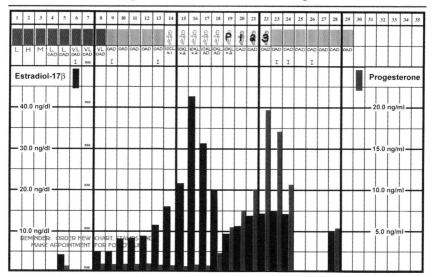

Figure 8-9: The relationship of the levels of estrogen (black bars) and progesterone (red bars) during the course of the menstrual cycle and the occurrence of the mucus sign and the Peak Day (P) in one cycle of a woman with normal fertility. The mucus cycle correlates with the pre-ovulatory rise in estrogen. Refer to page 83 for the Vaginal Discharge Recording System (VDRS).

the progesterone levels are dominant, there is no mucus discharge (dry days). This occurs early in the cycle and then again later in the cycle.

Our fertility depends, then, on the presence of *good sperm, good eggs* and *good cervical mucus.* There are, of course, many other factors involved in the fertility process, however, the presence of good quality cervical mucus is nearly as important to the fertility process as the presence of good sperm and good eggs. We are only beginning to appreciate the clinical role of cervical mucus as it relates to the overall reproductive process. When any one of these three factors is absent, the couple will generally not become pregnant.

In this cycle, the pre-Peak dry days are infertile (days 9-13). In addition, the post-Peak dry days are infertile after the count of three (days 23-29). The days of fertility are the days of the mucus cycle through three full days past the peak day (days 14-22). Also the days of menstruation are initially considered to be fertile (days 1-8 initially) but after two cycles the light and very light days of menstruation can be determined to be fertile or infertile based on the presence or absence of the mucus discharge (in this example, days 1-3 are still fertile while days 4-8 are infertile based on this principle). WARNING: These days of fertility and infertility do **NOT** apply to you. As you begin charting, your **CREIGHTON MODEL Practitioner** (teacher) will "tailor-make" the instructions for your cycles.

This one cycle (Figure 8-9) also begins to show some of the different biomarkers that can be seen when charting. The ones that are present in this particular cycle include:

1. The length of the cycle (29 days)
2. The length of the pre-peak phase of the cycle (19 days)
3. The length of the Post-Peak phase (10 days)
4. The length of menstruation (8 days)
5. The length of the mucus cycle (6 days)

Background of the System

The fundamental principles of the **CrMS** have been known to physicians for many years and are well documented although, as Dr. M.R. Cohen observed, "They have been almost disregarded by gynecologists." In 1952, this group published a schemata of the events that occur relative to the changes in the cervical mucus as ovulation

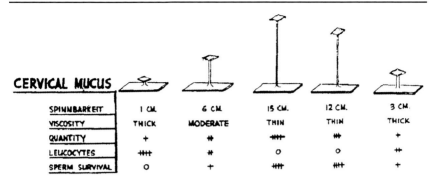

Figure 8-10: Dr. MR Cohen's original schemata for the events that occur in the cervical mucus around the time of ovulation. Of special note is the depiction of the sperm survival and the, de facto, recognition of the role of the cervical mucus as a biological valve (From: Cohen MR, Stein IF and Kaye BM: Spinnbarkeit: A Characteristic of Cervical Mucus. Fertil Steril, 3: 201, 1952).

approaches. This schemata also defined the basic principles of the not yet described **CrMS** (Figure 8-10).

It was noted that as ovulation approached, the stretchability and clarity of the mucus increased along with its quantity of production. At the same time, the viscosity (thinness or thickness) and its content of leukocytes (white blood cells) decreased. The most pertinent observation, however, was the indication that the *survival of the spermatozoa* was directly related to the presence or the absence of an ovulatory or periovulatory type of mucus produced from the cervix.

In the **CrMS**, external vulvar (at the opening of the vagina) observations of the discharge of the cervical mucus, the presence of bleeding and the days when no discharge is present (dry days) all are used to obtain pertinent information on the phases of fertility and infertility and the state of the woman's procreative and gynecologic health. The specially designed *vaginal discharge recording system* (VDRS) is used to accurately record the observations. The use of the VDRS significantly improves the accuracy of the recorded observations.

In the woman with *regular cycles*, the cycle begins with the onset of menstruation (see the first cycle of Figure 8-11). As menstruation tapers there is generally no discharge and the woman observes this as dry. As ovulation approaches, there becomes apparent a cervical mucus discharge that often begins as a sticky, cloudy or tacky, cloudy discharge and eventually becomes clear, stretchy or lubricative. The *last day* of the mucus discharge that is clear, stretchy or lubricative is identified as the Peak Day (and is recorded as a 'P' on the chart).

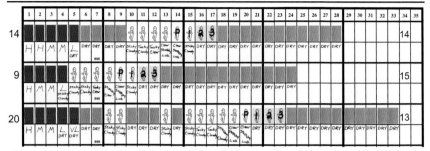

Figure 8-11: Three cycles charted for the CrMS showing the occurrence of menstruation, the pre-Peak dry days, the mucus cycle, the Peak Day (P), and the post-Peak dry days. The pre-Peak phases are variable in length (14, 9, and 20 days) but the post-Peak phases are consistent (14, 15, 13 days). Refer to page 83 for the VDRS.

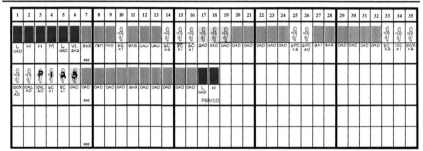

Figure 8-12: The application of the CrMS in long cycles. In this 51-day cycle, the Peak Day (P) occurred on day 38. The post-Peak phase was 13 days in duration. During the pre-Peak phase, "patches" of mucus are apparent. Refer to page 83 for the VDRS.

Because the production of the periovulatory cervical mucus is an estrogen dependent effect and is produced at the time of follicular development, when estrogen is increasing and ovulation approaching, the cervical mucus is produced and will be discharged before and during the time of ovulation.

In long cycles (Figure 8-12) there may be occasional "patches" of mucus prior to the onset of the mucus associated with ovulation. What is prolonged in these cycles is the pre-Peak (or preovulatory) phase of the cycle and what remains relatively consistent is the post-Peak (postovulatory) phase of the cycle.

The same principles apply in anovulatory conditions, such as *breast-feeding* (Figure 8-13). Infant suckling may suppress ovulation and fertility for a number of months. The presence or absence of the characteristic cervical mucus discharge associated with ovulation is then delayed until fertility returns and predicts the onset of the first menstrual period.

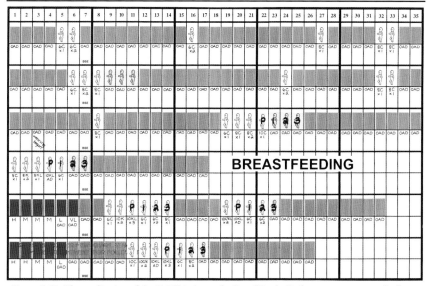

Figure 8-13: The application of the CrMS in breast feeding. "Patches" of mucus occur sporadically, dry days usually predominate, and as fertility returns, the mucus pattern and fertility return. Refer to page 83 for the VDRS.

The *versatility* of the system, clearly one of its strongest features, is found in its fundamental biology. Because it relies on events leading up to ovulation, it defines the times of fertility and infertility in a definitive, day-by-day, *prospective* fashion. Previously difficult cases, such as long and irregular cycles, breast-feeding, coming off of contraceptive pills, anovulatory states and the premenopause, all now can be dealt with in a positive fashion without delay.

Even a woman with a *continuous mucus discharge* (Figures 8-14 and 8-15) can properly identify the days of fertility by using a base infertile pattern (BIP), which is identified with the presence of an unchanging discharge. When fertility begins, *there will be a change in the pattern*, which is easily identified by the woman who has been properly instructed. Thus, fertility is identified.

The **CrMS** is *not* a contraceptive system. It is a system of *true family planning* (see Figure 8-16). The information obtained from monitoring the phases of fertility and infertility can be used to either *achieve* or *avoid pregnancy*. Users of the **CrMS** know their fertility status on any particular day and are given the *freedom* to utilize that information as they so choose. Those who use a day of fertility to achieve a pregnancy are successful users and not failures. A pregnancy can legitimately be observed as the result of the system's successful use.

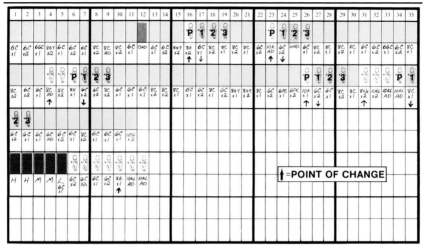

Figure 8-14: The example shows the use of the CrMS in a breast-feeding woman with a continuous mucus discharge. The plain yellow stamps indicate a discharge pattern that is the same from one day to the next. The arrows indicate the points of change and the baby stamps indicate days of fertility.

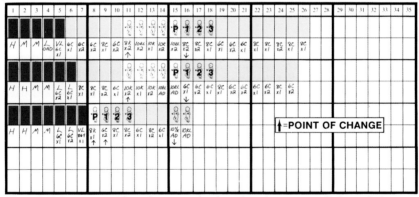

Figure 8-15: In a woman with regular menstrual cycles and continuous mucus discharge, the base infertile pattern is shown up to the point of the change. Peak Day is identified and the pre- and post-ovulatory days of infertility are shown with plain yellow stamps. Refer to page 83 for the VDRS.

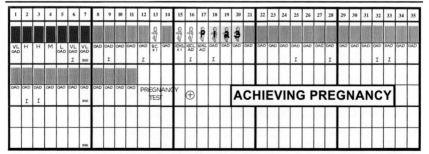

Figure 8-16: In this case, a woman of normal fertility, the system is used to achieve pregnancy. The acts of intercourse in the midst of the mucus cycle (days 16 and 18) should be expected to result in pregnancy as they did in this example. Refer to page 83 for the VDRS.

At the same time, it also can be used by couples, with *a high degree of reliability, as a means of avoiding pregnancy.* The data not only support this, but our own experience with this system shows that even those couples who have very strong medical reasons to avoid pregnancy can use it effectively so long as they are connected to a quality education system for proper training and support (see Internet Appendix).

Because the **CrMS** is based upon *biological markers* that include not only the cervical mucus, but also the absence and the presence of various types of bleeding, it can be used as *a means of monitoring and maintaining reproductive and gynecologic health.* Investigation of this has given birth to **NaProTECHNOLOGY**. Most of the work that has been done in this area has been completed at the Pope Paul VI Institute for the Study of Human Reproduction in Omaha, Nebraska. This reflects the Institute's background and experience in obstetrics and gynecology and in reproductive medicine and surgery. As this system has been used over the years, it has become *an ideal tool for the woman and her physician* (if the physician has been trained properly).

After many years of extensive evaluation, these biomarkers have been shown to reveal the presence or absence of certain types of pathologic or physiologic abnormalities. They give the physician and the patient a "handle" on the menstrual and fertility cycle and allow for its proper evaluation. *It allows one to treat abnormalities in a cooperative (rather than destructive or suppressive) manner.*

The CrMS and the Use of Criteria

In studying the *biomarkers* of the menstrual and fertility cycle as observed through the eyes of the standardized **CrMS**, one recognizes that the **CrMS** is a *criteria-driven system*. In other words, the physician, the **Fertility*Care*™ Practitioner** (FCP) and the woman who is charting her cycles can identify certain biologic events that are occurring by the objective presence of a *biomarker*. Such biomarkers have been associated, with a high degree of clinical correlation, with either one or more abnormal physiologic parameters of either reproductive function or a woman's health. The woman will recognize these biomarkers as patterns that may have been already observed but for which she never had an adequate explanation. The **CrMS** provides those explanations.

The health care provider must recognize the importance of *criteria*. These criteria are *objective signs* that have been studied in such a fashion so that when they are observed in the **CREIGHTON MODEL** charting

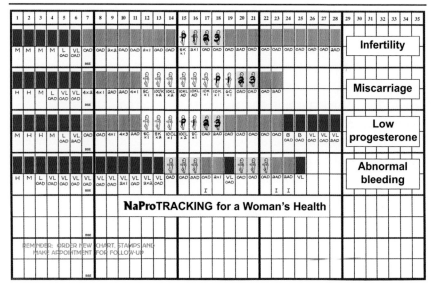

Figure 8-17: The monitoring (NaProTRACKING) of the biomarkers of the CrMS for a woman's health. In the *first cycle*, a limited mucus cycle is observed. This is common in infertility. In the *second cycle*, a short post-Peak phase of 5 days is present. In this cycle, miscarriage would be a very high risk if pregnancy occurred. In the *third cycle*, low luteal phase progesterone is expected from the premenstrual spotting that is present. And in the *fourth cycle*, the unusual bleeding would demand more evaluation. Refer to page 83 for the VDRS.

system they *can be evaluated in an objective fashion.* The discovery of these various objective markers (the presence of certain criteria) will indicate where evaluation should begin and what type of evaluation should be conducted. Furthermore, with a high degree of probability it will give an insight into the potential underlying causes of the clinical abnormality. Some of these variations and their explanations are illustrated in Figure 8-17.

Although the biomarkers of the **CrMS** are not 100 percent correct, they are *strongly suggestive* of a specific problem or set of underlying problems. When these objective parameters – these biomarkers – are identified, the health care provider and the woman who is making the observations will be able to understand more fully *the nature of the underlying problem,* the *type of evaluation that needs to be done* and *eventually the treatment that would be best implemented.* Furthermore, it needs to be stressed that these biomarkers can only be identified with the use of the **CrMS.** It is the objective presence of these biomarkers (referred to as criteria) that has been investigated through research that, at the present time, distinguishes the **CrMS** in the field of **NaProTECHNOLOGY.** Using other forms of natural fertility regulation for these purposes will result in a less effective means of obtaining results and they will not match what is presented in this book.

The **CrMS** is not only a *standardized* system, but an enormous amount of *research* has gone into the basic understanding and correlation of these various biomarkers to underlying physiologic and pathophysiologic events. Thus, nobody should be confused that any other system can provide the same information.

Comprehensive Research and Education Programs

Throughout the history of the **CrMS**, there has been a significant and comprehensive commitment to research and education program development.

In the basic sciences, this has involved hormone-correlation studies of ovulation, endocervical-mucus correlations, use effectiveness studies, ultrasound evaluations of ovulation, and so forth. Many years of research in education led to the development of the core curriculum[6] of the **CREIGHTON MODEL** program and the American Academy of **Fertility***Care*™ Professionals for the *certification* of teachers and *accreditation* of education programs.

American Academy of FertilityCare Professionals

After the establishment of the American Academy of Natural Family Planning, the various presidents and members of the board of directors of the academy over the past 28 years have made an incredible level of commitment to see to it that this organization has functioned and maintained its vitality. It is because of this dedicated and committed leadership that the academy has been able to exist over these past 28 years and carry out its mission of *accreditation, certification, service programs of excellence*, and establishment of its *code of ethics*, along with its mission of providing very important *collegial support* and *interaction*. It does the latter through a series of *national meetings*, which are held on a yearly basis.

In 2001, the American Academy of Natural Family Planning officially changed its name to the *American Academy of Fertility*Care *Professionals (AAFCP)* and became an organization that represented the goals and objectives of the **CrMS** program. The **CrMS** is the only natural system that exhibited the degree of interest that the American Academy requires for its professional activities.

A student entering an FCP training program (or any of the other accredited programs) must be assured that that program is fully accredited by the AAFCP. This accreditation is important because in order to qualify for certification through the academy one of the criteria is the satisfactory completion of an academy-accredited education program. Information on the academy can be obtained by writing:

American Academy of Fertility *Care* Professionals
11700 Studt Road, Suite C
St. Louis, MO 63141
Email: aafcp@aol.com   Web Site: www.aafcp.org

In July 1999, two new organizations were developed for the advancement of the CrMS programs. These organizations were **Fertility***Care*™ **Centers of America** and **Fertility***Care*™ **Centers International**.

Fertility*Care*™ **Centers of America** (FCCA) is a non-profit organization that was established for the primary purpose of promoting the CrMS and the new reproductive science of **NaProTECHNOLOGY** in the United States and Canada.

The purpose was to establish national and international organizations to unite the CrMS services nationwide and worldwide under one general and identifiable name of "**Fertility***Care*™." In this way, the CrMS services could be identified by their name and their unique services could be promoted properly.

As of this publication, there are more than 220 **Fertility***Care*™ **Centers** throughout the United States and Canada. For information, contact:

Fertility*Care*™ **Centers** of America
6901 Mercy Road, Suite 200
Omaha, Nebraska 68106
(402) 390-9167 (tel)
(402) 390-9851 (fax)
www.fertilitycare.org

With **Fertility*Care*™ Centers International** (FCCI), progress is being made on the development of several worldwide regional affiliates. These include **Fertility*Care*™ Centres of Europe** (which was fully affiliated in 2006), **Fertility*Care*™ Centers of Latin America** and **Fertility*Care*™ Centers of Austrailasia**. Over the next several years, this network of **Fertility*Care*™ Centers** will grow and expand.

Finding A Teacher

To learn the CrMS, one *must* attend a one-hour *introductory presentation,* which is usually conducted in a group setting. The learning of the system is, however, "tailor-made" to each couple through a series of *individual follow-up sessions* with the **Fertility*Care*™ Practitioner**. To locate a teacher nearest you (and the system also can be learned through long-distance instruction), log onto **www.fertilitycare.org**.

Action Items

The emphasis in this book is on the many medical applications of the **CREIGHTON MODEL System**. While its use as a family planning system is not the main focus, the reader should be aware that it also can be used very effectively as a means of avoiding pregnancy. In a summary of 5 different studies of the CrMS (a metanalysis), its use by 1,876 couples over 17,130 couple months of use showed a method effectiveness (perfect use) to avoid pregnancy of 99.5 percent and its use-effectiveness (typical use) was 96.8.[7] It was noted that "the system is safe, easy to use, and ethically acceptable to all people." An expanded discussion of the **CREIGHTON MODEL**'s use in family planning can be seen through the Internet Appendix.

Dating the Beginning of Pregnancy

CCURATELY DATING the beginning of pregnancy is recognized to be one of the most important things that can be accomplished in the early days of prenatal care. The more accurate the dates, the less obstetrical interference one can anticipate during the course of the pregnancy. For example, a decreased use of amniocentesis to determine fetal lung maturity prior to repeat cesarean section can be anticipated if the dates are more accurate. This is because a repeat cesarean section can be scheduled because of true confidence that the dates are accurate. In my own practice, amniocentesis for fetal lung maturity has been performed twice in the last 20 years because of my ability to date the true beginning of pregnancy, and neonatal outcomes have been excellent.

The standard textbook in obstetrics, "Williams Obstetrics," states vigorously that "**precise knowledge of the age of the fetus is imperative for ideal obstetrical management!**"[1] (emphasis in the original). And yet, even with all of the available technology, one of the puzzles of modern obstetrics is that the obstetrician has *not yet learned how to accurately* date the beginning of a pregnancy.

Pregnancy can be dated in two different ways. The most common and most often used in clinical obstetrics is the measurement of the *gestational age* of the pregnancy. The gestational age of the pregnancy is measured from the *first day of the last menstrual period.* In this way of dating, the pregnancy is 40 weeks in duration (on average) instead of the *actual 38 weeks*. In other words, it dates the pregnancy, on average, two weeks longer than it actually is.

The other way of measuring the date for the beginning of pregnancy is to measure the *fetal age*. The fetal age of the pregnancy is measured from the *time of conception* or the *estimated time of conception* (ETC). When measuring the pregnancy in this fashion, it will be 38 weeks long or two weeks shorter than the gestational age dates. The fetal age, of course, is the *actual age* of the pregnancy.

Historically, the obstetrician has focused on the first day of the last menstrual period for two reasons. First of all, the menstrual flow is a fairly dramatic symptom that the woman can be expected to remember. In addition, it is easy to teach her to record the first day of the last menstrual period so that when that information is elicited by the physician, at a later time, it is available.

But in the midst of all of this, the obstetrician and many women have missed the point that the *cervical mucus discharge* is very much a *flow* in the same fashion as the menstrual flow. In some countries, they refer to menstruation as the *red flow* and the mucus discharge as the *white flow*. Modern obstetrics has, of course, paid *little attention to the white flow*.

When one is charting the **CREIGHTON MODEL Fertility***Care*™ **System** (CrMS), one can date the pregnancy accurately from the actual or estimated time of conception. Therefore, one can date the pregnancy according to its *true date* (or *true beginning*) or in fetal-age terms. This is measured by evaluating the acts of intercourse that occur during the time of fertility and establishing an estimated time of conception through this approach. Your **Fertility***Care*™ **Practitioner** can help you do this accurately.

When one identifies the ETC, one then can calculate the duration of the pregnancy and the estimated time of arrival (ETA) (the due date). In calculating the ETA with the use of the **CrMS**, the following formula is used:

$$\text{ETA} = \text{ETC} - 3 \text{ months} - 7 \text{ days}.$$

This dating is done in detail at the time of a pregnancy evaluation conducted by a **Fertility***Care*™ **Practitioner** (one of the services provided in the array of services through a **Fertility***Care*™ **Center**).[2] It also can be calculated easily in the physician's office with the availability of the **CrMS** chart. Examples of pregnancies occurring with the **CrMS** are present in Figures 9-1 through 9-3.

We carefully have studied 173 consecutive patients who have been charting the **CrMS** at the time of conception. The ETC and the ETA were calculated in this fashion. In this group of patients, early ultrasound dating of the pregnancy also was obtained. Most of the examinations were performed during the first trimester of pregnancy when the dating of the pregnancy by ultrasound is thought to be accurate within plus or minus three days.

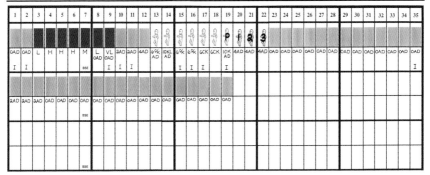

Figure 9-1: A pregnancy occurring in a fairly regular length cycle where the Peak Day occurred on day 17 of the cycle (From: Pope Paul VI Institute research, 2004). Refer to page 83 for VDRS.

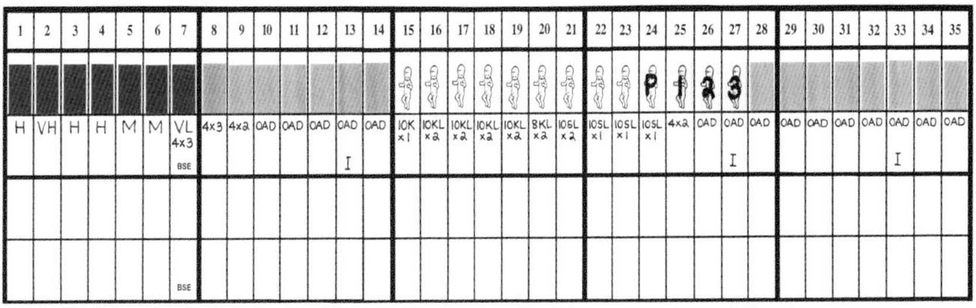

Figure 9-2: A pregnancy occurring in a longer cycle where the Peak Day occurred on day 24 of the cycle (From: Pope Paul VI Institute research, 2004). Refer to page 83 for VDRS.

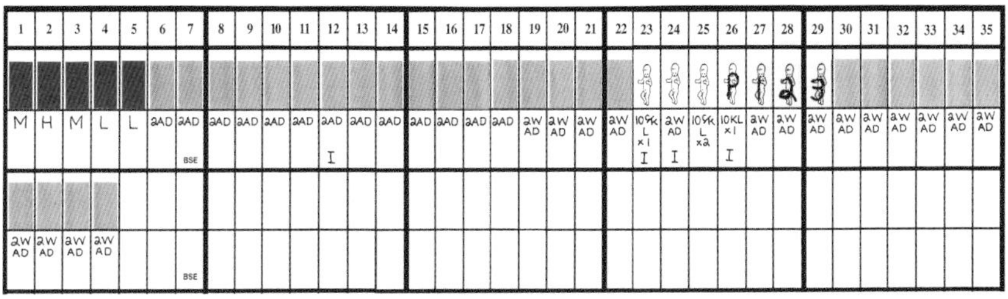

Figure 9-3: A pregnancy occurring in a longer cycle where the Peak Day occurred on day 26 of the cycle (From: Pope Paul VI Institute research, 2004). Refer to page 83 for VDRS.

An accurate date for the beginning of pregnancy can be established with the use of the **CrMS**. This correlates well with the ultrasound (U/S) dates and the estimated due date or ETA. In fact, the **CrMS** dating is correlated, on average, in the following way: **CrMS ETA = U/S ETA + 1.97 days**. The **CrMS** dates were highly accurate with the two being **within 10 days of each other in 100 percent of cases.**

There are other ways to establish an accurate date for the beginning of pregnancy. One way is to have women take their basal body temperature and with the point of the shift in the basal body temperature, one can estimate the possible time of conception. But this has been shown to be not as accurate as the **CrMS** because the shift in the temperature is not as accurate a predictor of ovulation as the occurrence of the Peak Day.[3,4] Ovulation occurs plus or minus two days from the observation of the Peak Day in over 95 percent of cycles.[3]

It is generally recognized that ultrasound is the method of choice for dating pregnancy.[5] The data in this chapter on Peak Day correlation to ETC verify that. And yet, the Peak Day data is easily available and more cost effective. Clearly the use of the LMP for dating pregnancy (which is still a current standard in "modern" obstetrics) carries with it a high degree of error.[6] While ultrasound and the Peak Day were within 10 days of each other in 100 percent of cases studied, it has been shown that the LMP is greater than 10 days different in over 16 percent of cases.[7] This is most problematic in women with long cycles.

Accurately dating the beginning of pregnancy is recognized to be one of the most important things that can be accomplished in the early days of prenatal care. By having accurate dates, one also can better assess the normal progression of the pregnancy and also determine both pre- as well as post-maturity conditions. If induction of labor is a consideration, that decision can be made without added obstetrical manipulation. It is well recognized that increased adverse pregnancy outcomes can be expected if the dates are not accurate.[8,9]

When labor ensues, an accurate judgment can be made with regard to whether that labor is beginning prematurely. If premature labor has started, then aggressive management can be instituted to halt that labor and delay its onset until full term. Again, accurate dates allow for improved judgment in the management of pregnancy, labor and delivery along with the management of a whole variety of medical and obstetrical complications of pregnancy.

It is true that a *cervical mucus discharge* is not a "high tech" idea. But it is an ***incredibly good bioassay*** and it is virtually free! Everyone concerned with prenatal care needs to recognize the accuracy of this bioassay system and the *ease* with which such information is obtained so that its benefits can be better incorporated into obstetrical practice.

Targeted Hormone Evaluation and Treatment

A S EVERY WOMAN KNOWS, the hormones of the menstrual cycle vary from day to day during the course of the cycle and, yet, one of the *most significant defects* in modern reproductive medicine is the inability of physicians to consistently evaluate these hormones. This difficulty arises from the absence of a clinically-relevant marker for the timing of ovulation during the course of everyday clinical practice. This problem has been solved with the advent of the **CREIGHTON MODEL Fertility*Care*™ System** (CrMS) and the research associated with it. *The importance of an ability to target the hormone evaluation of the menstrual cycle cannot be understated.*

The most relevant clinical hormones—estrogen and progesterone—are produced in a cyclic fashion (Figure 10-1). The preovulatory production of estrogen increases as ovulation approaches and decreases after ovulation occurs. Following ovulation and with the development of the corpus luteum, progesterone becomes the dominant hormone. During the postovulatory phase, the progesterone and estrogen levels increase reaching their highest point about one week following ovulation and then decreasing again in the week prior to menstruation. The natural irregularity of the menstrual cycle and the inability of modern medicine to work cooperatively with this has limited the ability to evaluate these very important hormones.

As an *extremely inferior* substitute to a proper assessment of these hormones, a day-21 or day-22 progesterone level is usually drawn (Figure 10-2). Such a practice presumes that all menstrual cycles are

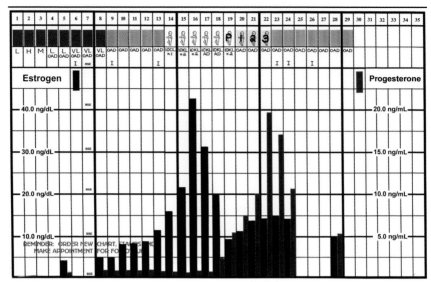

Figure 10-1: A normal CrMS chart with daily levels of estrogen (in black) and progesterone (in red). The hormone curve is within normal limits and it demonstrates the relationships to the mucus cycle (days 14-19), the Peak Day (day 19) and the variations in estrogen and progesterone production during the course of the menstrual cycle. Refer to page 83 for VDRS.

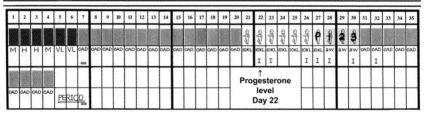

Figure 10-2: In this woman, a progesterone level was drawn on day 22 of the cycle. The level was not helpful in assessing ovulatory function because it was drawn at the wrong time of the cycle. The physician thought that she was "anovulatory" because the progesterone level was still in the preovulatory phase of her cycle. However, because she was charting her cycles with the CrMS, it was easy to determine that the level was simply drawn at the wrong time in her cycle. Refer to page 83 for VDRS.

28 days in duration. The menstrual cycle is 28 days long in only five to 10 percent of menstrual cycles[1] and the natural irregularity of the cycle makes the routine timing of a progesterone level on a particular day of the cycle, for the most part, *worthless*. Furthermore, as the progesterone and estrogen levels increase, reach their peak and then decrease, there are normal levels for each point along the way. At this point in time, the important information that needs to be obtained from an evaluation of these profiles can be obtained only through a **NaProTECHNOLOGY** approach.

A variety of *new therapeutic approaches* also can be identified with the targeted identification of abnormal ovarian function. This can be helpful in treating a variety of women's health conditions. Some of these are *dysfunctional uterine bleeding, recurrent ovarian cysts, premenstrual syndrome and premenstrual dysphoric disorder, recurrent miscarriage, infertility,* and even the *prevention of pre-term birth.* With a proper understanding of an accurately-targeted (or timed) hormone profile, one can institute rational therapeutic programs, which can have a significant impact on a woman's health.

When a woman is charting the **CrMS**, she will identify the various biomarkers of her menstrual and fertility cycles. These include the *menstrual flow,* the *pre-Peak dry days,* the *beginning of the mucus flow through the Peak Day* (the mucus cycle) and the *post-Peak phase of the cycle.* The entire length of the cycle is well documented and a variety of other biological markers of either health or illness can be defined. By identifying a woman's Peak Day, which is very closely associated with the timing of ovulation (ovulation occurs on Peak +/-2 days in 95.4 percent of cycles),[2] the cycle is effectively broken up into pre- and post-ovulatory phases, thus enabling the physician to properly target the cycle for hormone evaluation.

Targeting the Cycle

To target the *preovulatory* estrogen profile, one looks at the previous cycles charted with the **CrMS** and identifies the earliest occurrence of the Peak Day. The woman then comes to the laboratory or the physician's office to have an estrogen level drawn starting on the fifth or sixth day prior to the anticipated Peak Day (P-5 or P-6). These levels are continued *every other day through P+2.* This, along with the targeted postovulatory profile, is illustrated in Figure 10-3.

To target the *postovulatory* progesterone and estrogen levels around the time of ovulation, the woman identifies her Peak Day (P) charting the **CrMS**. Starting on P+3 (see Figure 10-3), the levels are drawn *every other day* for a total of five values (*P+3, P+5, P+7, P+9 and P+11*).

In a series of 193 cycles in which the estrogen levels were targeted as described in this chapter, this approach to targeting the estrogen profile was accurate or gave a reasonable assessment in 96.9 percent of the cycles evaluated.

In a similar study of *post-ovulatory* progesterone and estrogen profiles involving 620 cycles, the cycle was accurately targeted in 609 cycles (98.2 percent).

This targeting of the cycle can be accomplished in most menstrual cycles. In women who have very long and irregular cycles (for example,

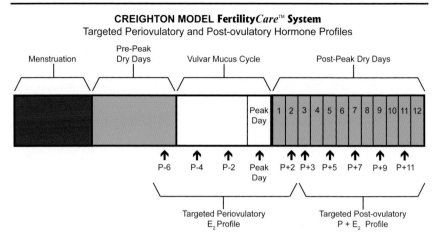

Figure 10-3: This schematic drawing of the CrMS demonstrates how it is used to target the periovulatory and postovulatory hormone profiles.

someone with polycystic ovarian disease), targeting is not very helpful or effective. The hormone profile that one might obtain in a woman with polycystic ovarian disease and long and irregular cycles is different than in one obtained from women with more regular cycles.

In infertility patients who are on treatment to stimulate ovulation with hormones, a progesterone and estrogen level drawn on P+7 (the seventh day after the Peak Day) will adequately *screen* the luteal phase for the purposes of managing medications.

This approach to targeting the cycle is within the scope of practice of the general obstetrician-gynecologist and the specifically-trained family physician, internist, or pediatrician, as well as, the reproductive specialist.

An example of how this can be used is illustrated in Figure 10-4. In this example, the progesterone levels during the post-Peak phase of the menstrual cycle are compared for women of normal fertility with women who have infertility related to endometriosis.

Cooperative Progesterone and Estrogen Replacement

Throughout the course of contemporary reproductive medicine and modern gynecology, the use of either progesterone or estrogen during the menstrual cycle as a therapeutic agent for managing women's health problems has been a foreign concept. The *single most common hormone abnormality in women of childbearing age* is most likely the dysfunctional luteal (postovulatory) phase. This dysfunction

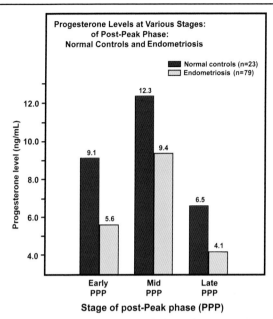

Figure 10-4: These are the targeted progesterone levels during the early, middle and late post-Peak phase comparing patients with endometriosis and infertility with patients of normal fertility. At each point, the progesterone levels in the endometriosis patients were significantly decreased.

will be associated with suboptimal progesterone or with suboptimal estrogen (E_2). In some cases, both of them will be suboptimal.

It is thought that if progesterone or E_2 is supplemented during the course of the menstrual cycle, it will interfere with normal hormone function. This supposition is correct if the physician is unable to *target the cycle* properly with these two hormones. If progesterone or E_2 are provided to a woman during the *preovulatory* phase of her cycle, they will both have a tendency to feed back to the pituitary gland and suppress the hormones. This would subsequently affect follicle-stimulating hormone (FSH) and luteinizing hormone (LH) and have a domino effect on the production of the ovarian hormones and ovulation. Contemporary medicine has missed the fact that both progesterone and E_2 can be supplemented as therapeutic agents during the course of the menstrual cycle in ways that will cause *virtually no harm*, will *improve the woman's health*, and *will enhance fertility* without causing damage to a developing embryo upon achievement of a pregnancy.

In order to accomplish this, however, progesterone and/or E_2 must be used in a *cooperative* fashion. This ultimately will lead to a new concept in medicine that **NaProTECHNOLOGY** calls **cooperative progesterone replacement therapy** (CPRT) and **cooperative estrogen replacement therapy** (CERT). The simple concepts for this therapeutic program can be outlined in the following points:

1. Progesterone and E_2 are produced in a cyclic fashion: E_2 is the dominant preovulatory hormone, while both progesterone and E_2 are produced during the postovulatory phase of the cycle.

2. True replacement therapy can be provided only during the postovulatory phase of the cycle.

3. The preovulatory phase of the cycle is variable in length.

4. Therefore, one must have a simple, but reliable means of determining when the patient is in the postovulatory phase of the cycle.

5. With the use of the **CREIGHTON MODEL System** (CrMS), the Peak Day can be a reliable, reproducible sign for the timing of ovulation and is the hallmark for the woman to know she is entering the postovulatory phase of the cycle.

If one were to start either progesterone or E_2 therapy on a given day of the cycle, it would have adverse effects. The preovulatory phase of the cycle is highly variable. Additionally, o*vulation occurs on day 14 of the cycle in only 13.5 percent of cycles.*[3] The Peak Day, however, is a reliable sign for estimating the day of ovulation (with ovulation occurring on Peak Day +/- two days in 95.4 percent of cycles).[2] Thus, using the post-Peak phase of the cycle as an indicator for the use of progesterone or E_2 supplementation provides an *ovulation-dependent* means of identifying the beginning of the true luteal (postovulatory) phase of the menstrual cycle. Providing either progesterone or E_2 in this way is *cooperative* with the cyclic hormones of the menstrual cycle and ultimately defines CPRT and CERT.

Types of Progesterone Support

Progesterone support can be provided in a variety of different ways. The most critical issue for the use of progesterone is the *timing* during the course of the menstrual cycle. *Progesterone support will not work if it is not given at the right time of the menstrual cycle.* Thus, the cycle must be properly targeted for progesterone support to be of any therapeutic value.

In order to effectively practice medical **NaProTECHNOLOGY**, the physician must be *completely familiar with the use of progesterone in a way that is cooperative with the cycle.* The following are ways in which progesterone support can be provided:

1. Oral micronized progesterone capsules (standard or sustained release)

2. Micronized progesterone vaginal capsules

3. Progesterone by intramuscular injection

4. Human chorionic gonadotropin (HCG)

Oral Micronized Progesterone Capsules

Progesterone, as a hormone, generally is not absorbed from the gastrointestinal tract. Thus, oral preparations of progesterone have not been widely available, although, a pharmacologic mixture of micronized progesterone in peanut oil has recently become available. When a compound is *micronized* it means that the agent is pulverized to very small particles before it is ingested. This micronization increases the ability of the stomach to absorb the hormone. Compounding pharmacies are able to provide a micronized form of progesterone. These can be made up into a standard preparation or a sustained-release form.

Micronized Progesterone Vaginal Capsules

In the original work with the **CrMS**, the only form of progesterone available was progesterone in vaginal suppositories made with cocoa butter or propylene glycol. These suppositories were messy and were confusing to the women who were observing vaginal discharges in the **CrMS**. A standard oral micronized progesterone capsule was substituted for the vaginal suppositories and this became an effective therapeutic strategy.

Progesterone Injections

Progesterone also is available in an intramuscular (IM) depot (long acting) injection form. The progesterone is contained in sesame-seed-oil. This allows it to have a more long-acting effect. The commercial products are available in a dosage of 50 mg/cc of sesame seed oil. A compounding pharmacy with the appropriate equipment also can compound progesterone in oil at a higher concentration of 100 mg/cc. The sesame seed oil form of progesterone is generally less irritating than the peanut oil form.

Human Chorionic Gonadotropin (HCG)

Human chorionic gonadotropin (HCG) also can be used in a cooperative way during the course of the menstrual cycle. HCG is an "LH substitute"; it has LH-like activity (being biochemically very similar to LH) and can be used physiologically as a substitute for the LH hormone, which is not readily available at this time.

When HCG is given during the postovulatory phase of the cycle (the post-Peak phase of the cycle), it will *stimulate the corpus luteum* to produce both progesterone and estrogen. This can be monitored by drawing a Peak +7 progesterone and E_2 level prior to treatment and then following treatment. One can document the increased production of progesterone and E_2 in this fashion. The blood draw on Peak +7 should be performed prior to that day's injection of HCG.

Cooperative Estrogen Replacement Therapy (CERT)

Since E_2 also is produced during the post-Peak phase of the cycle, the physician may want to administer E_2 to the patient in a cooperative fashion. Any estrogen given prior to ovulation will have the effect of *inhibiting ovulation*. This is contrary to the basic principles of good therapeutics, but it can be given post-peak and it will have therapeutic effects because it is being given cooperatively.

CPRT and Regulation of the Menstrual Cycle

A benefit to the use of CPRT is its effect on the menstrual cycle: it has a strong tendency to regulate the cycle. This is demonstrated in Figure 10-5.

In this example, progesterone is started during the post-Peak phase of the third cycle. Before progesterone was started, the mucus cycle ranged from 12 to 15 days in duration. The Peak Days occurred on days 19, 20, and 22 respectively. Following progesterone administration, the mucus cycles shortened to seven and nine days in duration and the Peak Day occurred on days 14 and 17 of the cycle.

The use of progesterone support during the post-Peak phase of the cycle also had an effect on the subsequent menstrual cycle. It shortened

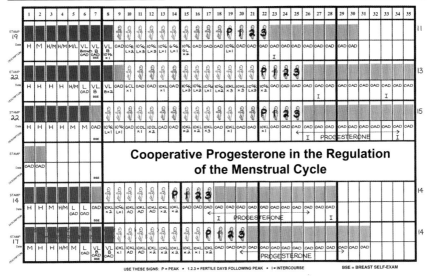

Figure 10-5: In this case, progesterone was given in the third cycle. It is vaginal progesterone given Peak +3 through P+12. The next two cycles are shorter with a shorter pre-Peak phase and a shorter mucus cycle (From: Pope Paul VI Institute research, 2004). Refer to page 83 for VDRS.

the pre-Peak phase and, thus, shortened the entire menstrual cycle. This phenomenon has been observed in a large number of patients to date. Therefore, a form of CPRT (with progesterone vaginal capsules, progesterone oral capsules, HCG injections or even progesterone injections) may assist in the regulation of the menstrual cycle and the normalization of the time of fertility in those patients who have prolonged mucus cycles, delayed Peak Days and longer menstrual cycles. This also will benefit women who have a tendency toward double peaks.

For the Doctor

1. The standard oral micronized progesterone capsules will contain between 200 and 300 mg of micronized progesterone depending on what the physician orders. The sustained-release form contains a 200-mg maximum amount of progesterone in the capsule. Between these two forms of progesterone, the sustained-release form is tolerated better than the standard oral form. Because of its quick absorption, its first pass through the liver and its development of various metabolic by-products, the side effects frequently associated with standard micronized oral progesterone are light-headedness, dizziness and fatigue. The oral sustained-release form is virtually devoid of those side effects, although

the absolute blood levels are lower. The commercial form of oral micronized progesterone in peanut oil also has a high side-effect ratio with the same side effects being observed. Thus, I have preferred the use of oral micronized sustained-release progesterone capsules to be given at a starting dose of 200 mg by mouth every day at bed time from Peak +3 through Peak +12.

This *targeting of the cycle* is designed specifically to cooperate with the luteal phase. The ovulation sequence is over in virtually 100 percent of patients by Peak +3 and the average length of the post-Peak phase of the cycle is 12 days. While physicians often make up their own routine, beginning progesterone earlier (for example on Peak +1) or continuing progesterone through to the time of menstruation should be cautiously avoided. Progesterone must be given in a targeted fashion to be therapeutic. If it is given prior to ovulation, it will be less effective. If it is continued beyond the normal length of the post-Peak phase, it will create its own hormonal abnormality because progesterone is no longer being produced and only exogenous progesterone is available. Thus, for the greatest effectiveness, this protocol for progesterone administration should be used.

It also should be pointed out that oral progesterone is not a strong agent for lengthening the post-Peak phase. Thus, cooperative use of oral progesterone is best suited for those women whose post-Peak phases are reasonably normal in length. If one is treating a woman with a short post-Peak phase (a short luteal phase), oral progesterone is not satisfactory because it does not consistently lengthen the post-Peak phase.

2. When using a vaginal application of progesterone, it is recommended that an oral micronized progesterone capsule (not sustained release) at a dosage of 300 mg be placed within the vagina at night, every day from Peak +3 through Peak +12. This will have a moderate stimulus on the endometrium and the myometrium, so it can be useful in women who have short post-Peak phases or it is useful in pregnancy. Generally, these capsules are easy to use, produce only a minimal discharge the following day, and are not messy. They can be used in cooperation with the family planning uses of the **CrMS**.

Progesterone vaginal capsules occasionally will cause *vaginal dryness* or *vulvar irritation* or sometimes a "cakey" discharge. This can be managed by inserting one or two 400 IU (international units) vitamin E capsules in the vagina along with the progesterone. The vitamin E is packaged in a glycerin capsule, which easily dissolves at body temperature releasing the vitamin E oil to the mucus membranes. Vitamin E has a superb soothing effect on mucus membranes and will resolve either the dryness or irritation. These capsules should be inserted at night so that they will melt at body temperature while the woman sleeps and will create the least amount of disturbance for her.

3. The usual dosage of progesterone when used by injection in CPRT is 100 mg IM on Peak +3, 5, 7, 9 and 11. Alternate dosages also can be used. For example, providing a 50 mg dosage on Peak +3 and 11 along with 100 mg on Peak +5, 7, and 9 will give a boost of progesterone that mimics a physiologic dosage form of progesterone.

When progesterone injections are used, it is extremely important to draw up the progesterone into the syringe with a *different needle* than the needle that is used to inject it. In addition, it is *extremely important* to inject the progesterone over a slow period of time, usually *120 to 180 seconds*. If progesterone is given quickly, it can be very irritating. If it is given slowly and with proper administration, it can be very well tolerated. The hips should be alternated as injection sites and, after the progesterone is injected, it should be massaged into the muscle. If local irritation and itching occurs from the progesterone injection, applying vitamin E oil over the surface of the injection site and the surrounding skin will provide relief. On occasion, injectable progesterone can cause a significant amount of irritation, especially if given too quickly. This is not common if the progesterone is given properly. If this does occur, it may have to be discontinued and an alternate route of administration may have to be selected.

The use of intramuscular progesterone during the *post-Peak phase* of the cycle should be limited to those situations where there is no good alternative. It does have a strong endometrial effect and will usually induce a menstrual period in those women who have long and irregular cycles. Thus, it is useful for women who have long and irregular cycles secondary to polycystic ovarian disease; in this situation, it can be used 100 mg IM on day 18, 21 and 24. While this is not CPRT, this protocol is a legitimate use of progesterone because it is being used to counteract the otherwise unopposed estrogen effect that is common in this situation. Three injections of progesterone in a given cycle, if properly administered, are very well tolerated.

4. HCG is given by intramuscular or subcutaneous injection and it is well tolerated. It is easily administered and a *very predictable medication*. Few side effects are associated with its use. The usual dose is 2000 units on Peak +3, 5, 7, and 9. A goal in the administration of HCG is to bring the progesterone and E_2 levels well within the normal range and to keep the length of the post-Peak phase normal. If the progesterone and E_2 levels are too high or the post-Peak phase is too long, the dosage can be reduced to 1000 units on Peak +3, 5, 7, and 9, or to 2000 units on Peak +3, 5, and 7. Our practice has been to teach spouses to give the injections of either progesterone or HCG. With proper training by our nursing staff, the spouses do well. This makes receiving the medications very tolerable and very cost effective.

5. If the luteal phase E_2 level is suboptimal, cooperative estrogen replacement

therapy (CERT) can be used. In doing this, an oral micronized E_2 form is available and is active (Estrace). The usual dosage is 0.5 or 1 mg by mouth every day at bedtime from Peak +3 through Peak +12. On occasion, the dosage may be increased to 2 mg from Peak +3 through Peak +12.

An alternative formulation for CERT is the use of triestrogen. Triestrogen is a compounded form of natural human identical estrogen that contains 80 percent estriol, 10 percent estradiol and 10 percent estrone. If using this for the purposes of CERT, the dosage is 2.5 mg by mouth every day at bedtime, Peak +3 through Peak +12 or 5 mg in the same timing. These dosages are well tolerated with no apparent side effects. One can measure the increased level of E_2 by monitoring the E_2 level on Peak +7. This allows for the appropriate adjustment of the dosage for that particular patient. When monitoring the E_2 level in this case, the estrogen preparation is not discontinued prior to the measurement of the E_2 level.

THE ACCURATE EVALUATION of ovarian function continues to be a significant puzzle to those involved in the provision of reproductive health care. In fact, there are literally millions of women who go about their daily lives with abnormal ovarian function and don't even know about it. If they would go to their doctor and ask if this could be evaluated, and this is especially true for those women with regular menstrual cycles, very little would be offered them.

If you happen to be a woman who has experienced infertility, miscarriage, premenstrual syndrome, recurrent ovarian cysts and other abnormalities of ovarian function, it becomes even more important that this be evaluated. If you are currently experiencing any of these conditions, it is almost universal that the function of your ovaries has not been assessed. I have even had patients plead with their reproductive specialists to have a hormonal analysis performed that would test their ovarian function while the specialist gazes out in space saying basically that such an evaluation is not necessary, when they really don't know how to go about doing a meaningful assessment. In fact, just the other day a patient once again informed me of a reproductive specialist who wanted to draw her progesterone level on day 21 of the cycle.

It should be noted that in most infertility evaluations, one of the main questions asked is: "Is she ovulating?" But in over 56 percent of women with both infertility *and* regular cycles *the ovulation is either absent or defective.* The traditional means through which a woman is tested to see if she is ovulating include the following: (1) a shift in the basal body temperature, (2) an endometrial biopsy that shows secretory endometrium, (3) an elevated "mid-luteal phase" progesterone level, and/or (4) a positive urine test by one of the "ovulation test kits." *Each of these four tests will not determine if the ovulation is normal, defective or whether ovulation has occurred at all.*

Ovarian function can be evaluated in any number of ways, but it must take into account the variations of the hormones of the menstrual cycle that occur from one day to the next during the course of the cycle. This, ultimately, is where the current problem lies. The modern physician does not really know how to go about evaluating the various hormones of the menstrual cycle, given the fact that these hormones are at different levels from day to day throughout the cycle. The key to such an evaluation is *the ability to target the cycle properly* for the evaluation of these hormones (see Chapter 10). Thus, the **CREIGHTON MODEL System** introduces a means by which this can be done and the patient participates in her own care by tracking the biomarkers of the system.

Over the last 30 years, I have been involved in the study of ovarian function from several points of view. Of course, the **CREIGHTON MODEL System** itself gives us some insight into the variations that can occur with regard to the function of the ovaries. Two additional approaches also can be used. One of these approaches could be considered the evaluation of the *function* of the ovaries and it is based on a survey of the woman's hormone levels during the course of her cycle.[1] The second could be considered an evaluation of the *anatomy* of ovulation and the various abnormalities or defects that might exist that also could cause problems.[2]

Over this time frame, I also have been involved in the evaluation of literally thousands of cycles of spontaneous ovarian function in women who have various pre-existing abnormalities. The Pope Paul VI Institute has evaluated more than 3,000 menstrual cycles with the use of daily ultrasound examination around the time of ovulation to assess the presence or absence of an ovulatory defect. I am quite sure that there is no center in the world that has this extensive degree of experience. In addition, these women have been evaluated closely with the measurement of the hormones that are produced in the ovaries. In order to complete both of these approaches to evaluation, one must understand the basic principles outlined in Chapter 10 of this book where the ability to *target* the various phases of the cycle are made so easy.

The Function of the Ovaries

The ovaries produce two major hormones—*estrogen and progesterone*—during the course of the menstrual and fertility cycle. This has been detailed in Chapters 5 and 6 of this book.

The production of estrogen is evaluated as it approaches the time of ovulation and then again during the postovulatory phase of the cycle. These are the two main times in the cycle where estrogen production by the ovary is important. The production of progesterone is evaluated during the postovulatory phase only because that is the major time that the progesterone hormone is produced. So much can be learned from this type of an evaluation.

We will start with the postovulatory phase of the cycle first. There are several different types of abnormalities that have been observed. These often are referred to as *luteal phase defects* because they involve a deficiency in the function of the *corpus luteum*. Furthermore, these different types of luteal phase deficiency have been labeled Type I, II, III, IV and V. Of these deficiencies, four of them are abnormalities in progesterone production and one is an abnormality in estrogen production.

The *Type I* luteal phase deficiency specifically involves the abnormal production of progesterone by the corpus luteum. In this case, the progesterone level begins to increase following ovulation, but within a very short period of time, it decreases suddenly and a menstrual period begins. The time from ovulation until menstruation is very short (usually eight days or less). This also will result in a short post-Peak phase. Such an abnormality often is associated with women who have repetitive miscarriages, but also can be seen in women with infertility (Figure 11-1 in the "For the Doctor" section).

The *Type II* luteal phase deficiency involves a specific decrease in progesterone during the entire postovulatory phase of the cycle, but the length of the postovulatory or post-Peak phase is normal. In other words, the corpus luteum produces abnormally low amounts of progesterone. This is one of the more common types of abnormal ovarian function seen in women with regular cycles and infertility (Figure 11-2 in the "For the Doctor" section).

The *Type III* luteal phase deficiency involves the progesterone hormone as well. In this case, the hormone begins to increase following ovulation and usually is even higher than normal. But beginning about

Peak+7 or one week prior to the onset of menstruation, there is an abrupt drop in the production of progesterone and that decrease in progesterone continues until the beginning of the next menstrual period, which is about a week later. This type of deficiency often is referred to as a *late luteal defect*. This condition is seen in women who have infertility, miscarriages and premenstrual syndrome (Figure 11-6 in the "For the Doctor" section).

The *Type IV* luteal phase deficiency is quite rare. It involves a decrease in the amount of progesterone being produced on P+3 and P+5 and by P+7 it returns to normal status. Its significance is not yet fully understood and requires more study.

The *Type V* luteal phase deficiency is a specific decrease in estrogen production during the postovulatory phase of the cycle when both the estrogen levels before ovulation and the progesterone levels after ovulation are either normal or near normal. This is a very interesting form of luteal phase deficiency, which has not been studied very well. In my textbook on **NaProTECHNOLOGY**, I describe this for the very first time. The singular decrease of estrogen during the postovulatory phase of the cycle does have a certain clinical impact. It appears to have something to do with the fertility process, although the exact nature of that is not yet fully understood. It also appears to be present in women who have a *decreased bone mineral density*, which is a precursor to *osteoporosis*.

When studying the postovulatory phase of the cycle, it is important also to study the estrogen levels around the time of ovulation. The reason for this is fairly simple. As the follicle grows and develops and produces estrogen in the time leading up to ovulation, it is the same tissue that becomes the corpus luteum in the postovulatory phase of the cycle. Thus, if there is an abnormality in the production of progesterone during the postovulatory phase of the cycle, there is often an abnormality in the function of the developing follicle. A basic principle in reproductive biology shows that the function of the developing follicle and the function of the corpus luteum tend to go hand in hand. While there are exceptions to this, it generally is a true statement.

In looking at the estrogen levels around the time of ovulation, one can see that in the Type I and II luteal phase deficiencies, there also is a pre-existing *follicular phase deficiency*. In these cases, the function of the follicle as measured by the production of estrogen is clearly abnormal. This is illustrated in Figures 11-1, 11-3 and 11-5 in the "For the Doctor" section.

The *Type III* luteal phase deficiency is one of the exceptions to the basic principle of the function of the follicle being related to the function of the corpus luteum. In this case, the function of the follicle is nearly normal as exhibited in Figure 11-5 in the "For the Doctor" section. This suggests that the cause of this late decrease in progesterone is not specific to the developing follicle itself. The exact mechanism is not understood, but it may involve a deficiency of important enzymes in the function of the corpus luteum during the postovulatory phase of the cycle.

We know the least about Type IV and V luteal phase deficiencies, but they do exist and they are definitely worth additional study.

Anatomic Defects of Ovulation

When studying the function of the ovaries from the point of view of the function of the developing follicle and the corpus luteum, it brings one to an obvious interest in whether or not the status of the ovulation is normal or abnormal. In certain types of situations, such as women who experience infertility problems, *the anatomic abnormalities* of ovulation (as determined by daily ultrasound examination) are really significant with a normal ovulatory pattern being present in only 43 percent of cycles. Thus, in order to have a good understanding of the underlying causes of the infertility problem (or miscarriage problem), a good understanding of the process of ovulation also is important.

By evaluating the growth and development of the follicle with the use of ultrasound technology, we can see the developing follicle grow and develop up until the time that it ruptures. We also can see that the follicle has ruptured when these examinations are performed on a daily basis around the time of ovulation. This may require four to seven daily ultrasounds to determine if a woman has an ovulation-related defect. As a result, we have developed a classification system for the various types of abnormal ovulation events. This classification system is outlined in Table 11-1.

This classification system has been very helpful in evaluating the various abnormal ovulation-related events. For example, when an unruptured follicle is identified, this makes the cycle anovulatory. In

---

Table 11-1: Working Classification System for the Disorders of Human Ovulation as Determined by Serial Ultrasound Assessment

---

I.   Mature follicle ($\geq$ 1.90 cm) (– or Re C.O.)
        MF: –, Re

II. Luteinized unruptured follicle (+ or – C.O.)
        LUF: +, –

III. Immature follicle (< 1.90) (+, – or Re C.O.)
        IFS: +, –, Re

IV. Partial rupture ($\leq$ 0.75 cm rupture) (+, –, Re C.O.)
        PRS: +, –, Re

V.   Delayed rupture (+, –, or Re C.O.)
        DRS: +, –, Re

VI. Afollicularism
        AF

---

other words, the egg, which is inside the follicle, is trapped because the follicle never releases it. In our years of study, we have never seen a pregnancy in a woman who had an unruptured follicle in the cycle being evaluated. All of these conditions are associated with infertility in various ways. In addition, the small follicle, the immature follicle, is associated with miscarriage.

These various abnormalities of ovulation also are associated with underlying hormonal deficiencies. In Figure 11-7, the estrogen levels around the time of ovulation are seen for the six different ovulation abnormalities. All of the estrogen profiles are abnormal (significantly decreased from the normal control group), except for the delayed rupture group (which also is the least common of all of the ovulation-related abnormalities). This suggests the presence of a *follicular phase deficiency* in most of these defects.

Interestingly, the postovulatory progesterone profile for these same six abnormalities is significantly low for all of them (and it is statistically significant) (Figure 11-8 in the "For the Doctor" section).

It makes sense that if the ovulation sequence is anatomically abnormal, it also would be functionally abnormal. In fact, that is what our studies have shown. In considering treatment of any of the ovulatory defects, one must consider some degree of stimulation of the ovary that will correct the underlying hormonal deficiencies and the defects in ovulation. This is often, but not always, effective. While we have a number of medications that will stimulate the follicle, a perfect medication has not yet been developed.

Final Comment

The study of ovarian function from both the functional and anatomic point of view is a cornerstone of medical **NaProTECHNOLOGY**. Our ability to perform these tests, especially the hormone tests, is made possible because the women are charting their cycles using the **CREIGHTON MODEL System**. This allows the physician to measure different hormone levels at different phases of the cycle knowing full well that the various changes in the production of these hormones can be definitively identified. The gap that exists in modern reproductive medicine is simply that the physicians have given up on the ability to properly target the cycle. This capability, however, is fully within the range of all physicians interested in reproductive medicine and it is not adequate for a physician to simply say, "That can't be done."

One of the really interesting features of all of this is the question of how many women of reproductive age actually have abnormal ovarian function that they do not know about. What I often tell patients is that measuring the ovarian hormones is not like measuring the thyroid hormone. When one wants to test the thyroid gland, one can get a blood level at almost anytime and it will be helpful. Because of the various changes in the reproductive hormones during the course of a woman's menstrual and fertility cycle, the physician must have a simple and yet easy way to be able to target the cycle properly to measure the hormones so that the results take on meaning. The **CREIGHTON MODEL System** allows us to do that and then, with the interpretation of the results, **NaProTECHNOLOGY** takes over and provides treatment for these types of difficulties.

For the Doctor

1. To assess the periovulatory estrogen profiles in the cycle, one is instructed to have their blood drawn every other day from six days prior to the anticipated Peak Day through Peak+2 (for the estrogen levels around ovulation time). Then she needs to get her blood drawn for both post-Peak estrogen and progesterone on Peak +3, 5, 7, 9 and 11. This will accurately assess their luteal phase production.

2. To have an ovulation series by ultrasound, the woman should have a pelvic ultrasound examination using both an abdominal and a vaginal ultrasound probe. This examination should be done on day 5 of the cycle as a baseline and then every day beginning five days prior to the anticipated ovulation day (the anticipated Peak Day) through the day of follicular rupture (ovulation). A Peak+7 ultrasound also should be done to assess the status of the endometrium during the middle of the luteal phase.

3. The shape of the hormone curves (preovulatory estrogen and postovulatory progesterone) are shown in graphs A through F. The periovulatory estrogen profiles and postovulatory progesterone profiles for the six ovulation defects are shown in graphs G and H.

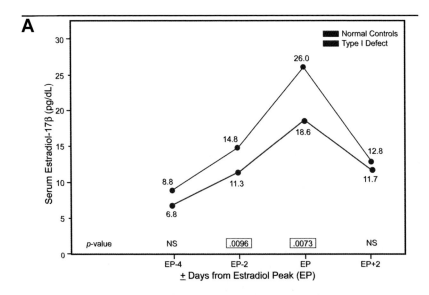

Figure 11-1: Periovulatory estradiol-17β levels, normal controls vs. Type I luteal phase deficiency (N=20).

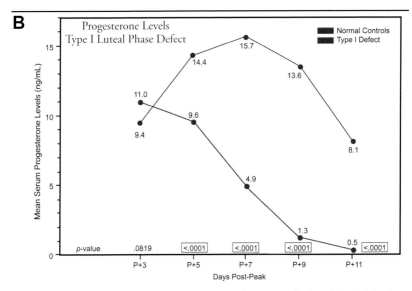

Figure 11-2: Deficiencies in luteal phase progesterone, short post-Peak phase (Type I) (N=20).

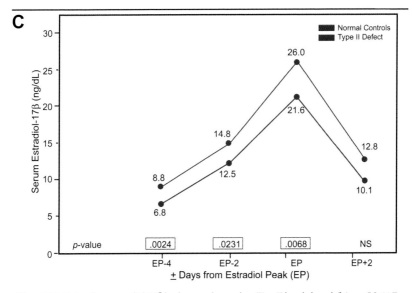

Figure 11-3: Periovulatory estradiol-17β levels, normal controls vs. Type II luteal phase deficiency (N=115).

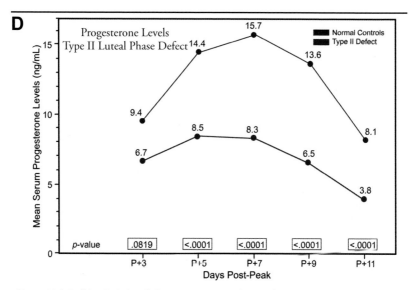

Figure 11-4: Deficiencies in luteal phase progesterone, suboptimal progesterone (Type II) (N=115).

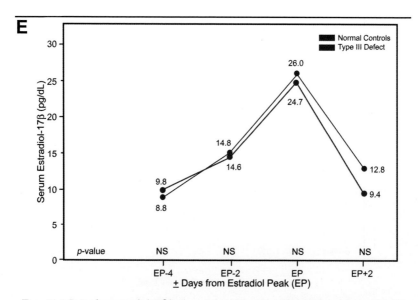

Figure 11-5: Periovulatory estradiol-17β levels normal controls vs. Type III luteal phase deficiency (N=41).

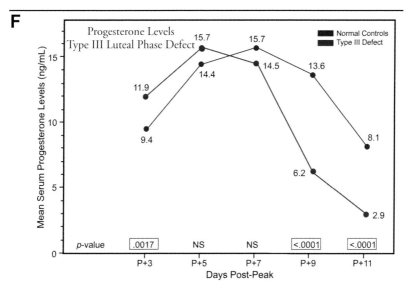

Figure 11-6: Deficiencies in luteal phase progesterone, late luteal defect (Type III) (N=41).

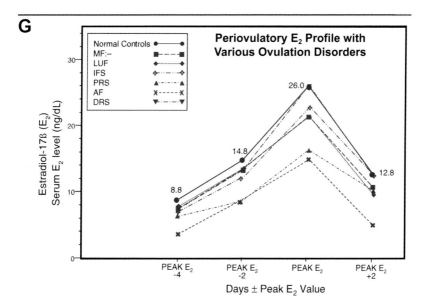

Figure 11-7: A summary of the periovulatory E₂ profile as seen with the various ovulation disorders.

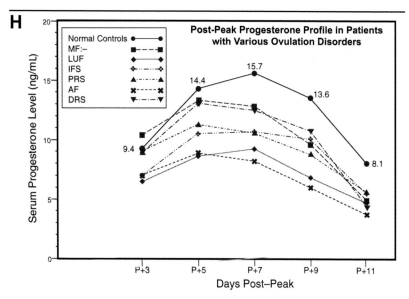

Figure 11-8: A summary of the post-Peak progesterone profile in patients with various ovulation disorders.

Hormones vs. Artimones

THE CLASSIC DEFINITION of a hormone is a substance that is released into the bloodstream at one special tissue site and travels to a distant set of cells where the substance exerts its characteristic effects.[1]

Over the last century, an extraordinary amount of work has been done in relation to the ovarian hormones estrogen and progesterone and their various artificial substitutes. In the first half of the century, most of the work focused on the identification and production of the hormones *that are naturally produced in the body.* In the second half of the century, an overwhelming majority of the research has gone into the production of *artificial substitutes* for progesterone and estrogen.

This work in the latter half of the 20th century has been stimulated by two major factors. The first is that the pharmaceutical industry has focused on developing compounds that can be protected by patent and thus can be profitable. Secondly, the introduction of the oral contraceptive in 1960 led to a strong funding base for the pharmaceutical industry to pursue a variety of different formulations.

Unfortunately, this has led to *one of the single-most inexact biochemical, physiological and pharmaceutical applications in all of medicine.* The medical literature is replete with the use of the terms "progesterone" and "estrogen" even when they do not apply to the hormones normally manufactured in the body. In fact, professional medical meetings that deal with the hormones of the menstrual cycle or reproduction attest to the extensive misuse of terminology in this area.

In the last half of the 20th century, the focus in reproductive biochemistry and pharmacology has been on the use of *artificial hormone substitutes* rather than the use of the naturally-occurring hormones as they chemically exist. This has been stimulated by the absence of fundamental research in developing systems that would allow for the targeted use of hormones in the menstrual cycle. Since both estrogen and progesterone are produced in a cyclic fashion during the course of the menstrual cycle, they cannot be taken on a daily basis like other hormones. Rather, their use must be specifically targeted in the menstrual cycle. The absence of research in targeted reproductive hormone use has generated a focus on substitutes that *suppress or destroy normal hormone function* and make it appear simplistically that such targeting is unnecessary.

The **CREIGHTON MODEL Fertility***Care*™ **System** (CrMS) and **NaProTECHNOLOGY** provide a simple and reproducible means by which the menstrual cycle can be targeted, thus re-emphasizing the use of *hormones* that are *naturally produced in the body.* To use such hormone preparations, the physician and patient need to have a sound understanding of the importance of such use along with the differences between the various applications.

Effects of Progesterone and Estrogen

The name progesterone refers to *a single compound* that is identifiable by its molecular structure. The term estrogen, on the other hand, refers to *a family of compounds* that have a general group of predictable physiological effects. Progesterone is a naturally-occurring C_{21} steroid; testosterone is a naturally-occurring C_{19} steroid; and the estrogens are naturally-occurring C_{18} steroids.[2]

Progesterone inhibits the effects of estrogen on the mucus-producing crypts of the cervix and stimulates the production of Type G mucus mostly during the postovulatory phase of the cycle and during pregnancy. This type of mucus acts as a barrier to sperm penetration in what often is referred to as a closure of the biological valve. In pregnancy, it also inhibits access of various bacteria into the cavity of the uterus.

Progesterone does not interfere with the beneficial effects of estrogen on either high-density lipoprotein cholesterol (HDL-C) or low-density lipoprotein cholesterol (LDL-C) profiles. It is metabolized in the liver and these metabolites then are eliminated in the urine.

Progesterone has a fairly short half-life. It also has anxiolytic (anti-anxiety) and antidepressant effects on the central nervous system.[2] Progesterone also may protect against fibrocystic breast disease, endometrial (uterine) and breast cancer, and osteoporosis. It promotes fat burning for energy and can act as a diuretic.[3]

The estrogens are important in the development of secondary sexual characteristics in females. This includes the growth and development of the vagina, uterus and fallopian tubes. Along with other hormones, estrogen also will cause enlargement of the breasts through promotion of ductal growth, stromal development and the accretion of fat. It contributes to the molding of the body contour, shaping of the skeleton, and pubertal growth spurt of the long bones; it also has positive effects on bone mass. The growth of axillary and pubic hair and the pigmentation of the genital region (as well as the nipples and areola during pregnancy) also are estrogen-related effects. In pregnancy, it also induces the breast ducts to mature. Estrogen increases HDL-C while decreasing LDL-C and lipoprotein-A.[2]

In the preovulatory phase of the cycle, estrogen stimulates the growth of a new uterine lining following the shedding of the lining during menses. It will stimulate the cervical crypts to produce Type E mucus, which is essential for sperm migration and penetration through the cervix and for fertility (referred to as opening the biologic valve). Estrogen also will increase rhythmic uterine contractions, which can be identified during the preovulatory phase of the cycle with the use of real-time ultrasound. These contractions may assist sperm transport.[2] Estrogen also will increase the contractive ability of the tubal muscle.

Following ovulation, high estrogen levels cause a feedback to the hypothalamic-pituitary axis to decrease follicle-stimulating hormone (FSH) and luteinizing hormone (LH) production. This is one of the major postovulatory effects of estrogen production. Estrogen also enables the induction of progesterone receptors and induces the maturation of cells in the lining of the vagina. Estrogen undoubtedly has an effect on the secretory cells in the endometrium during the postovulatory phase of the cycle, but its exact role has not been clearly elucidated. Further research in this area may be very important in the future development of strategies for the treatment of various reproductive abnormalities.

Hormones vs. Artimones

With the development of the oral contraceptive and its widespread marketing and distribution in 1960, a considerable amount of effort has gone into the research and investigation of a series of biochemicals that have both *estrogen-like* and *progesterone-like* properties, but are *neither* estrogen *nor* progesterone. The first orally-active estrogen substitute was the non-steroidal compound diethylstilbestrol (DES), which was synthesized by E.C. Dodds in 1938.[4] Subsequently, it was found that an alteration of the testosterone molecule yielded an orally-active compound that had some progestational-type activity.[5] In 1952, norethynodrel was synthesized and later, norethynodrel was selected as a potential oral contraceptive agent for testing in a small group of women. It later was shown that norethynodrel had the ability to suppress ovulation, but irregular spotting and bleeding were common, so the estrogen mestranol was added to the norethynodrel pill to yield a combined medication marketed under the name Enovid. This pill, *Enovid,* was the *first marketed birth control pill.* Thereafter, the number of available preparations proliferated.[5]

In 1964, ethinyl estradiol was introduced as an alternative to mestranol as the estrogenic component of many birth control pills. Several other progestational agents also became available. Growing evidence of an association between the estrogen component's potentially catastrophic side effects accelerated the trend toward "low-dose" combination pills containing less than 50 μg of ethinyl estradiol. Since then, a variety of different combination preparations have been marketed. These contain varying ratios of the estrogen and progesterone *substitutes* across a 21-day period of administration in order to minimize the clinical side effects.[5]

From a clinical point of view, *this has created a blurring in the minds of physicians* as to what estrogen and progesterone really are. Are they the same as that manufactured in the human body? The blurring of the distinctions between these two has become so significant that, in reading the medical literature, the distinction between what is the naturally-occurring hormone and an artificial substitute, which is *not* the naturally-occurring hormone, has been obscured. On December 15, 2006, NBC's Today Show's in-house medical expert Dr. Nancy Snyderman made the comment that "hormones are hormones" and that "bioidentical hormones are like choosing a different flavor of ice cream – but they are still ice cream."[6] Nothing can be further from the truth!

To deal with this in **NaProTECHNOLOGY**, new terminology needs to be introduced to allow one to speak factually about the various preparations. The new terminology includes the terms *isomolecular hormone* (IMH) and *heteromolecular artimone* (HMA). These are defined as follows:

Isomolecular Hormone (IMH):

This is a chemical that is chemically (by nature of its molecular structure), biologically, physiologically and pharmacologically *identical* to the hormone that is manufactured naturally in the human body. While these often are referred to as "natural hormones," the actual origin of the chemical is not as important as the isomolecular nature of it. These chemicals can be synthesized from various precursors and made to be identical to the human hormone. In fact, there are virtually no isomolecular hormones in use at the present time that are natural in the sense that they have been derived from a natural source. These hormones also are properly referred to as *bio-identical.*

Heteromolecular Artimones (HMA):

These are chemicals that are distinct and different from the isomolecular hormone to which they often are confused. In the case of reproductive hormones, they may have estrogen-like or progesterone-like activity, but invariably that activity is not the same as the isomolecular hormone. Furthermore, they also have chemical activities in the body that are distinctly different from the isomolecular hormones. These HMAs are substitutes for the "real thing." Chemical compounds with biological activities that are progesterone-like have been variously referred to in the literature as progestins, progestational agents, progestagens, progestogens, gestagens or gestogens. Often, however, the term progesterone is used to refer to these hormones and that is inaccurate. Thus, it is appropriate to refer to these substitutes as *artimones* (artificial hormones) or more specifically *HMA progestins* and *HMA estrins.*

The distinctions between these different chemicals can be demonstrated. In Table 12-1, the relative potencies of the IMH progesterone and various HMA progestins are shown. The HMA progestins are significantly more potent than the IMH progesterone and this demonstrates at least at one level, how wrong Dr. Nancy Snyderman was in her characterization of the two types of chemicals (IMH and HMA). *Birth control pills contain only HMA progestins,* the most

**Table 12-1: Relative Potencies of IMH Progesterone
and Various HMA Progestins[1,2]**

Progesterone (IMH)	1
Dydrogesterone (HMA)	10x
Medroxyprogesterone acetate (Provera) (HMA)	50x
Norethindrone (HMA)	500x
L Norgestrel (HMA)	4,000x

1. The relative doses required to elicit responses similar to those seen in premenopausal, secretory endometrium.
2. Kina RJB, Whitehead MI: Assessment of the Potency of Oral Administered Progestins in Women. Fertil Steril 46: 1062, 1986.

common of which is *norethindrone*. Most of the 19-nortestosterone progestational agents (HMA progestins) have significant *androgenic* (male-hormone-like) activity.

The HMA progestins and HMA estrins (estrogen-like compounds) are widely used in reproductive and postmenopausal medicine at this time. They are all approved by the Food and Drug Administration (FDA) and yet the distinctions between the isomolecular *hormones* and heteromolecular *artimones* continue to be blurred even at the FDA level.

A number of clinical effects are associated with the HMAs used in contraceptive medications. They include HMA estrin-related effects such as adverse mood changes, the enhancement of thrombosis, increased blood pressure, venous thromboembolism and hepatocellular liver adenomas. HMA progestin-related effects also include adverse mood changes in addition to weight gain, acne and nervousness. The combination of the two HMAs has resulted in increased myocardial infarction in smokers over the age of 35, a delayed time to conception after the discontinuation of the HMA, and a lower return of the fertility rate. Breast cancer diagnosis and invasive cervical cancer also are increased.

Isomolecular Hormones

A variety of isomolecular *hormones* for both progesterone and estrogen are available commercially and available through compounding pharmacists. These are listed in Table 12-8. These sometimes are referred to as *bioidentical hormone preparations*, which means they are biologically and physiologically identical to the hormones naturally produced in the body. The term "bioidentical hormone" is a good and accurate term for referring to these preparations. All of the ingredients in these preparations are approved by the FDA, although some combinations of them have not yet received official FDA approval. Much of this relates to the availability of good research in these areas. While a considerable amount of research has been done, only a minimal lobby exists specifically to promote the isomolecular hormones at the FDA level. Thus, the adequate review of these products has been slow.

Clinical Effects of Isomolecular Hormones

In 1960, the same year that the oral contraceptive became available, the *Merck Index of Chemicals and Drugs* listed the following medical uses for progesterone: functional uterine bleeding, amenorrhea, premenstrual tension, dysmenorrhea, habitual abortion, menopausal syndrome, and infertility.[7] Since that time, with the introduction of the HMAs, the usage of progesterone and IMH estrogen has changed.

At this time, these hormones mostly are used during the postmenopausal years, where most of the data exists. Progesterone also has been used to a limited extent in the support of pregnancy, the treatment of habitual spontaneous abortion and in infertility. With the introduction of **NaProTECHNOLOGY**, IMH progesterone and estrogen now have multiple new applications for postmenopausal *and* premenopausal women.

Progesterone is a unique progestational agent being the only available bio-identical and physiologically active progestational agent. Medroxyprogesterone acetate (MPA) is the most commonly prescribed HMA progestin. While the change in the chemical structure between the two appears to be small, the difference in chemical structure produces significantly different effects.

For a complete and detailed review of the variation in effects on the cardiovascular system, lipid metabolism, vasomotor symptoms, the effects on the breast, brain and bone, and various other effects, the reader is referred to "The Medical & Surgical Practice of **NaProTECHNOLOGY**."

Delivery Forms, Dosing Amounts and Dosing Schedules

Various forms of IMH estrogen and progesterone are available from compounding pharmacists. This allows the physician to tailor therapies to fit patients' needs. Some oral and intramuscular versions of IMH estrogen and progesterone, however, are available commercially. Intramuscular forms of progesterone also can be compounded in higher concentrations.

A micronized form is used for capsules of IMH estrogen or progesterone. This has an ultra-fine consistency. By decreasing the particle size with micronization, aqueous dissolution in the gastrointestinal (GI) tract is increased and absorption is enhanced. This increases bio-availability. The micronized powder also can be compounded with a slow-releasing agent, such as methylcellulose. This provides a prolonged, even delivery of the hormone and, especially with progesterone, can reduce side effects significantly.

Lozenges (troches) also can be compounded, but patients have less satisfaction with these forms. Vaginal suppositories also have been produced. Standard suppositories generally have been fairly messy and have been unusable with patients who also are charting their cycles using the **CrMS**. The micronized form compounded into an oral gelatin capsule also can be inserted into the vagina and used as a vaginal suppository. This method is less messy and does not interfere with the woman's mucus observations.

A number of skin creams are available with progesterone, but the amount of progesterone in most of the over-the-counter creams is extremely small. In order to obtain a reasonable level of progesterone, a compounded version produced by a compounding pharmacist is preferable.

Absorption Patterns of Progesterone

Over the years, there has been a considerable amount of work done on evaluating the various absorption patterns for the use of IMH progesterone by different modes of delivery.

Figure 12-1 illustrates the peak levels of serum progesterone following the administration of progesterone by a variety of different forms and routes. This work, done at the Pope Paul VI Institute, is fairly consistent with published reports. Serum levels with the over-the-counter skin creams are very low; vaginal progesterone and troches did not reach very high peak levels; oral progesterone in various formats reached mid-levels; progesterone in peanut oil (Prometrium) reached the highest levels for oral progesterone administration. The highest levels of all were obtained with 200 mg of progesterone given by intramuscular injection.

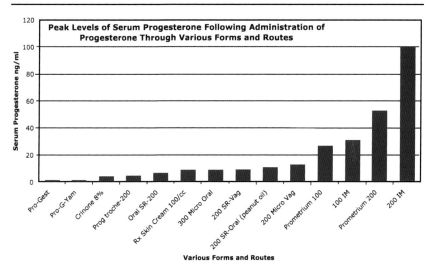

Figure 12-1: The peak levels of serum progesterone following administration of progesterone through various forms and routes. SR = sustained release, IM = intramuscular (From: Pope Paul VI Institute research, 2004).

Progesterone Support During Pregnancy

ROGESTERONE HAS BEEN used to support pregnancy for more than 60 years, having received its start with medical research dating back to the 1940s.[1,2] Its initial use was in patients who had recurrent miscarriages caused by luteal phase deficiency. Luteal phase deficiency is due to a failure in the proper function of the corpus luteum. The production of progesterone from the corpus luteum is thus decreased. There is evidence to support the idea that progesterone given in *early pregnancy* may be useful in some women with recurrent miscarriage[3-5] and that the measurement of progesterone in early pregnancy can be a marker for the further assessment of abnormal pregnancies.[6,7]

The administration of progesterone *later in pregnancy* has been considered to be justified because of an association of premature labor with decreased progesterone concentrations and the observation that progesterone reduces the intensity and frequency of uterine contractions.[8-12] It is thought that the administration of progesterone might therefore reduce uterine contractions and help prevent preterm labor.

This idea has received a considerable boost from recent widespread publicity given to two research papers that both showed *a significant reduction in pre-term delivery rates* with the administration of either progesterone[13] or 17 α-hydroxyprogesterone caproate.[14] While this was portrayed as a "major breakthrough" by the national media, in reality, data on the use of progesterone (or 17 α-hydroxyprogesterone caproate)

137

for the prevention of preterm labor has appeared in the medical literature for over the last 30 years.[15-21]

In conjunction with estrogen, progesterone has the following important functions:

- It stimulates the growth of the uterus.

- It causes "maturation" (i.e. differentiation) of the endometrium (the lining of the uterus), converting it to a secretory type.

- It stimulates the decidualization of the lining required for implantation.

- And it *inhibits contractions* of the uterine muscle.[22]

The corpus luteum is the major source of progesterone during the first nine to 10 weeks of pregnancy. Over the last several decades physicians have been taught that there is a shift in the production of progesterone production from the corpus luteum to the placenta between the sixth and the 12th week of pregnancy. During the second and third trimester of pregnancy, it has been universally thought that the placenta is the major source of progesterone production, thus it also has been taught that because the placenta takes over the production of progesterone at this time, supplementation of the pregnancy with progesterone is completely unnecessary after the 10th to 12th week. It also has been shown in a virtually ignored research study[23] that the corpus luteum of pregnancy *continues to produce progesterone* all the way to the end of pregnancy. Progesterone concentrations in the peripheral vein of women at full term were shown to be the same as the progesterone concentration in the ovarian vein coming from the ovary where there was *no corpus luteum.* The progesterone concentrations from the ovary in which a corpus luteum was present, however, were *more than twice that* of the progesterone levels in the peripheral vein.

Progesterone is produced in very large amounts during pregnancy. In the near-term pregnant woman, progesterone is produced in the amount of 250 mg/day and up to 600 mg/day in women with multiple pregnancies. This extraordinarily-large production of progesterone needs to be taken into consideration when determining the dosage of progesterone support.

In women who have preterm labor, both serum levels of progesterone and 17 α-hydroxyprogesterone are decreased significantly during the second and the third trimester of pregnancy.[16] Since progesterone has an inhibitory effect on the ability of the uterine muscle to contract,[24-29] this would be expected. In fact, it has recently been found that progesterone inhibits contractions of human uterine muscle while 17 α-hydroxyprogesterone caproate dos not.[29] Progesterone also is found in very large concentrations within the muscle of the pregnant uterus[30] and that concentration can be increased further with the oral administration of micronized IMH progesterone.

Indications for the Use of Progesterone in Pregnancy

One only can speculate as to how common progesterone support in pregnancy is used at the present time. There are no studies to show the frequency of its use. It has been suggested that the exposure to progestational agents of all kinds has decreased significantly over the last 20 to 30 years.[31,32] It recently has been pointed out that this may be the result of the significant late-appearing side effects that were documented following the *in utero* exposure of the fetus to the potent steroid artimone diethylstilbestrol (DES) and that this bad experience cast "a long shadow."[33] In spite of this, the use of progesterone, at least in early pregnancy, does appear to be widespread in artificial reproduction programs.[34-38]

Keeping perspective, the use of progesterone during early pregnancy (the first 10 to 12 weeks) has been in use for nearly 60 years. Indications for its use have included a documented luteal phase deficiency, history of recurrent pregnancy loss, or vaginal bleeding during the first six to eight weeks of pregnancy.

While the use of progesterone during the second and third trimesters of pregnancy has increased in the last few years because of the recent publication of articles suggesting its benefit in the prevention of pre-term labor,[13,14] it generally has not been used during the second and third trimester of pregnancy. This perhaps is best expressed in this commentary published in 1991:

> "The use of progesterone in ongoing pregnancy… is a thornier problem. While it is clear that some viable pregnancies are characterized by lower serum progesterone levels than others, it is unclear whether or not therapy is beneficial or even necessary for their continued well being."[39]

This comment and the attitude toward the use of progesterone in the second and third trimester in pregnancy is troubling. **For some reason, the intensive investigation of the role of progesterone in pregnancy during the second and third trimester has gone virtually**

unapproached or ignored over the last 25 to 30 years. And yet, a considerable amount of data suggests that progesterone production is clearly decreased in a variety of pregnancies where obstetrical complications exist. What is troubling is that further research has not been forthcoming and investigation of this important area has been left unattended. The recent publication of the effectiveness of progesterone in the decrease in prematurity[13,14] has led to such comments as, "I think it's going to awaken people to an old idea that kind of slipped away." While promising studies in this area have existed since the 1970s, it has been difficult to interest pharmaceutical companies or government agencies to fund more comprehensive experimentation. It literally has been "sitting on the pharmacists' shelf for more than 30 years."[35] And yet, *it continues to be an edict of contemporary reproductive medicine* that progesterone should not be administered after the first trimester. In this day of "evidence-based medicine," there is **no evidence** on which to base this edict. In fact, the evidence that does exist actually *supports its use* during these stages of pregnancy in selected cases.

For the last 30 years, I have been supplementing pregnancies with IMH progesterone. This project began with the use of progesterone in early pregnancy in patients with infertility or a previous history of miscarriage. The goal of progesterone therapy was to decrease the incidence of miscarriage in subsequent pregnancies.

As this project began to grow, it was difficult to determine the dosage of progesterone that should be given and an objective means by which the pregnancy could be monitored. This led to the measurement of serum progesterone levels during the course of pregnancy. Eventually, a standard curve for progesterone in normal pregnancy (a normogram) was developed and the ability to objectively assess progesterone became possible. While the progesterone level was found to be decreased in women who had spontaneous abortion (a finding that others had previously observed), an extensive data base was established that documented the decrease in progesterone during the second and third trimester of pregnancy in patients who had various obstetrical complications. As a result of this project, a specific set of indications for the use of progesterone in pregnancy could be identified.

Those patients who have a previous pregnancy *history of spontaneous abortion, stillbirth, preterm delivery, premature rupture of the membranes, pregnancy-induced hypertension or toxemia, or abruption of the placenta* are considered candidates for the use of progesterone in pregnancy through the Pope Paul VI Institute protocol for progesterone support in pregnancy. In addition, those patients who, during the course of their pregnancy, develop signs or symptoms of *threatened premature labor* or objective signs of cervical dilatation and effacement to which a *cervical cerclage* is necessary also are provided progesterone support. *All multiple pregnancies or pregnancies with a major congenital uterine anomaly* are supported throughout the entire course of pregnancy. Patients with a documented history of *infertility* also are supported. In some cases, progesterone is monitored as a matter of routine to assess further the potential use of progesterone in a given pregnancy. For example, women who have a history of *premenstrual syndrome* where there is a documented luteal phase deficiency of progesterone during the postovulatory (post-peak) phase of the menstrual cycle, even though they have not had previous pregnancy difficulties, would be a candidate for assessment of serum progesterone in pregnancy. The result is then plotted on the normogram and a determination is made with regard to the use of the progesterone.

Assessment of Progesterone during Pregnancy

Much of the work that has been accomplished on the assessment of serum progesterone in normal pregnancy was done from the early 1950s through the 1970s.[41-51] Furthermore, most of the assessment of progesterone in pregnancy, as it relates to various complications of pregnancy, was accomplished from the early 1960s through the early 1980s.[50-64] In spite of improvements in the accuracy and precision of progesterone assays since that time and a better ability to date pregnancy and establish more accurate gestational ages, very little subsequent work has been done in this area.

It has been known for a long time that progesterone is decreased during the first trimester of pregnancy in patients who have spontaneous abortions. It long has been thought that the placenta takes over for the production of progesterone during the second and third trimesters of pregnancy,[65] but a decrease in progesterone production, presumably by the placenta and likely by the defective corpus luteum during the second and third trimester of pregnancy in a variety of different pregnancy-related complications and previous pregnancy historical events, also has been observed.[66] This suggests that the role of progesterone as an indication of placental function may be more significant than what had been previously appreciated and especially is important into the second and third trimesters of pregnancy.

It is not new that a variety of pregnancy-related complications are associated with decreased progesterone production. For example, it has been shown previously that serum progesterone levels are decreased in intrauterine fetal death,[52] premature labor, threatened premature labor, premature rupture of the membranes, amnionitis, and abruption of the placenta.[56,57] Increased levels of progesterone also have been observed in twin pregnancies,[42,45,54] Rh isoimmunization[49] and hydatidiform mole.[64]

As early as 1951, the urinary excretion of pregnanediol, the main urinary metabolite of progesterone, was evaluated extensively in normal and abnormal pregnancies.[67] In these studies, decreased levels of pregnanediol were observed in a variety of pregnancy-related complications somewhat similar to the studies on progesterone. Decreased levels of pregnanediol were observed in spontaneous abortion, missed abortion, intrauterine fetal death, premature labor, placenta previa and accidental hemorrhage and intrauterine growth restriction.[67-71] Pregnanediol levels also were observed consistently to be decreased in patients with toxemia of pregnancy and pregnancy-induced hypertension.[67-69,71]

In our study, we also observed a decrease in second and third trimester progesterone levels in patients with certain types of abnormal reproductive histories.[66] These included: a history of *polycystic ovarian disease* (also decreased in the first trimester), *induced abortion, one previous spontaneous abortion, three or more spontaneous abortions and premature birth.* The data would suggest that patients with these histories should be considered at risk for placental insufficiency in subsequent pregnancies.

Also, a number of new, *current* pregnancy problems were observed in our study to have decreased progesterone production.[61] These conditions, not previously reported, include: patients with *adherent placentae, low-lying placentae or placenta previa* (observed by ultrasound), *midtrimester abruptions* (observed by ultrasound), *smokers, postpartum hemorrhage, fetal distress, low Apgar scores, meconium-stained amniotic fluid, decreased biophysical profiles, intrauterine growth restriction and oligohydramnios.*

The data in this very large and systematic study of progesterone in pregnancy suggests that the ***more significant progesterone deficient*** *time period in pregnancy is actually after the first trimester and into the second and third trimesters.* This "flies in the face" of what "modern" reproductive medicine says about progesterone in pregnancy and yet the work conducted at the Pope Paul VI Institute is unique in this field and the surveys are very large (see: The Medical & Surgical Practice of **NaProTECHNOLOGY**).

Observed Effects of Progesterone Support

With the use of progesterone support in pregnancy, a number of positive effects have been observed over the years. The incidence of both gestational hypertension and toxemia of pregnancy are quite low with the use of progesterone with the PPVI protocol as compared to published standards. What perhaps is even more dramatic is the apparent decrease in the incidence of mild forms of gestational hypertension and mild and severe toxemia. Such an impact of progesterone on these conditions has been observed previously and it was noted that this effect was observed only when the progesterone was administered no later than mid-pregnancy.[75] When compared to placebo, progesterone has been observed to cause a significant reduction in blood pressure suggesting that progesterone has an anti-hypertensive action.[76-78]

The incidence of postpartum depression is reduced significantly in progesterone-supported program patients. The general incidence of postpartum depression is considered to be in the 10 to 15 percent range. With the PPVI Protocol, only 2.2 percent of supplemented patients had postpartum depression.

In addition, meconium-stained amniotic fluid was found to be reduced in the PPVI program with an incidence of 6.1 percent compared to about 16 percent in published studies.[79]

Progesterone support is a mainstay of the Pope Paul VI Institute Prematurity Prevention Program. This is discussed in detail later.

Safety of Progesterone Use in Pregnancy

It has been pointed out that the problems identified with the use of diethylstilbestrol (DES) has cast "a long shadow" on the use of hormonal supplementation in pregnancy.[33] In addition, there appears to be an extraordinary amount of confusion related to the use of progesterone support in pregnancy. Furthermore, the Food and Drug Administration (FDA), which is quite capable of relieving this confusion, has continued instead the confusing story, and some of this needs to be addressed.

In the recent labeling of progesterone products for the FDA, one of the contraindications to the use of oral progesterone is listed as "known or suspected pregnancy."[80] And yet, no such contraindication is identified for the use of progesterone gel.[81] In fact, while oral progesterone has been contraindicated specifically in "known or suspected pregnancy," progesterone gel is indicated for progesterone supplementation or replacement as a part of an artificial reproductive technology (ART) program for the treatment for infertile women with progesterone deficiency in the early stages of their pregnancies. In an odd twist, while the oral progesterone is contraindicated in "known or suspected pregnancy," its official labeling also states that this oral progesterone "should be used during pregnancy only if indicated (see contraindications)."[80]

The commercially-available oral progesterone preparation is recognized as a pregnancy Category B substance by the FDA and, "several studies in women exposed to progesterone have not demonstrated any significant increase in fetal malformations."[80]

The confusion worsens when one looks at the labeling for progesterone injection USP in sesame oil. Here the labeling becomes frightening:

> "**WARNINGS**: The use of progestational drugs during the first four months of pregnancy is not recommended. Progestational agents have been used beginning with the first trimester of pregnancy in attempts to prevent abortion, but there is no evidence that such use is effective. Furthermore, the use of progestational agents, with their uterine-relaxant properties, in patients with fertilized defective ova may cause a delay in spontaneous abortion.
>
> Several reports suggest an association between intrauterine exposure to progestational drugs in the first trimester of pregnancy and genital abnormalities in male and female fetuses. The risk of hypospadias (5 to 8 per 1000 male births in the general population) may be approximately doubled with exposure to these drugs. There are insufficient data to quantify the risk to exposed female fetuses, but insofar as some of these drugs induce mild virilization of the external genitalia of the female fetus and because of the increased association of hypospadias in the male fetus, it is prudent to avoid the use of these drugs during the first trimester of pregnancy."[82]

In the "Warning for Women" section of this FDA-approved labeling, it states: "Therefore, since drugs of this type may induce mild masculinization of the external genitalia of the female fetus, as well as hypospadias in the male fetus, it is wise to avoid using the drug during the first trimester of pregnancy."[82]

This role of the FDA in perpetuating this confusion is unnecessary. In the past, the Obstetrics and Gynecology Advisory Committee to the FDA has recommended that the restricted use of progesterone and 17-OHP-C in early pregnancy be lifted.[83] Unfortunately, while this recommendation was made in 1984, it never has been heeded completely.

Much of the confusion surrounds a *user-unfriendly nomenclature* as it specifically relates to *progestational agents.* The term "progesterone" is often used loosely to refer to any progestational agent. But progesterone is progesterone and nothing more.[84] It is produced naturally in the human body along with other naturally-occurring progestational agents, such as 20 α-dihydroprogesterone, 20 β-dihydroprogesterone, and 17 α-hydroxyprogesterone. Progesterone is the only known natural progestational agent with major biologic significance and 17 α-hydroxyprogesterone is so weak that it is virtually inert.

To help clarify the nomenclature, those progestational agents that are *natural to the human body*, i.e., actually are manufactured physiologically within the body, are best referred to as **hormones** and by their specific name. Those progestational agents that are *artificial to the body*, i.e., are not manufactured physiologically in the body, are best referred to as **artimones** (artificial substitutes for naturally occurring hormones - see Chapter 11). In this way, one can begin to distinguish between those compounds that are naturally occurring to the body and those that are foreign to it. This becomes important as one looks at the overall question of safety. Progesterone is a C_{21} *steroid* deriving from the *pregnane nucleus.* There are certain artimones that also are C_{21} compounds. These include 17-hydroxyprogesterone caproate (17-OHP-C) and medroxyprogesterone acetate (MPA) (Figure 13-1).

There also are C_{19} steroids derived from the *androstane* nucleus. *Testosterone* is the prototypical C_{19} steroid. While testosterone is a naturally-occurring C_{19} steroid with obvious androgenic properties, there are a number of artificially-derived C_{19} compounds that are less androgenic, but also have progestational activity. These include compounds such as norethindrone (19-nor ethinyl testosterone), norethynodrel, norgestrel and ethisterone (ethinyl testosterone). These 19-nortestosterone derivatives *unequivocally can masculinize the female*

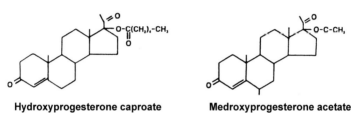

C₂₁-Steroid (Pregnane)

Progesterone

C-21 Progestins

Hydroxyprogesterone caproate

Medroxyprogesterone acetate

Figure 13-1: The C_{21} pregnane nucleus and the chemical structure of progesterone and the C_{21} artimones 17-OH-progesterone caproate and medroxyprogesterone acetate.

fetus if given in high doses at susceptible times in the development of the embryo.[31,83-85]

The confusion or lack of understanding of the pharmacology involved still is producing erroneous conclusions regarding progesterone as a teratogenic agent. **Progesterone is an antiandrogen**, not an androgen. The C_{19} artimones do have androgenic potential. The C_{21} artimones may show long-acting progestational effects because they are not rapidly removed from the circulation and metabolized like progesterone.[85]

The effect of these 19-nor compounds was recognized by Drs. L. Wilkins and H.W. Jones, et al, in 1958 and this study continues to be cited and is a cause for confusion.[86] This study, from Johns Hopkins University, presented 21 cases of females that showed evidence of masculinization of the external genitalia. In 12 of these cases, there was *in utero* exposure primarily to the C_{19} artimone ethisterone (ethinyl testosterone). In three cases, no steroids were used in pregnancy and in the remaining six cases IM progesterone was used. Of those six cases, three also were exposed to ethisterone and one to methyltestosterone, explaining the defect. In the other two cases, the women also received stilbestrol. There is now evidence that this also can exert a masculinizing influence.[87-89]

In an extensive review of the fetal effects of progestational agents (both natural and artificial), it has been concluded that despite many studies, there remains **little reason to suspect that progestogen exposure in utero exerts a deleterious effect on fetal development.** The sole exceptions are the 19-nortestosterone derivatives, which in high doses (10 to 20 mg daily) can cause genital virilization.[31] The evidence is considerable that orally-ingested progestogens do not cause a general increase in birth defects, are not cardiac teratogens, do not cause limb reduction defects, and do not cause neural tube defects or hydrocephalus. The frequency of esophageal atresia has not been increased in any of the studies, and *in utero* exposure is unlikely to result in abnormal development of the male genitalia. Other reviews have come to similar conclusions.[90-92]

With specific reference to medroxyprogesterone acetate (MPA) (Provera), animal studies have suggested an increased risk of facial clefts and masculinization of female fetuses and feminization of male fetuses. These effects were observed, however, *only* at high doses (8 mg/kg/day and 10 to 40 times the human dose). No similar increased risk was found for either progesterone or 17-OHP-C. It should be noted that when early mouse and rabbit concepti were cultured with mega-doses of progesterone (2,000 and 10,000 ng/mL) they failed to undergo further cleavage until cultured in a progesterone-free medium. This finding is nonspecific and does not bear on the likelihood that progesterone will cause birth defects in intact animals.[84] Furthermore, it is noted that these concentrations do not appear in nature. In human teratology studies, both 17-OHP-C and MPA[93] generally have shown no increased risk in anomalies with the possible exception of one case of transient clitoral enlargement with MPA (in 166 cases) and retrospective reports of hypospadias with 17-OHP-C and MPA. *In the human studies on progesterone, no increase in anomalies has been observed, including cardiovascular anomalies.*

As an interesting aside, the fetal umbilical artery blood levels of progesterone have been noted to be higher in male infants than in females. The female umbilical vein levels were the same. Thus, the difference between the two is greater in female fetuses suggesting that they metabolize more progesterone than the male.[94]

It also has been suggested that the administration of progesterone may accelerate early childhood development and enhance academic performance,[95,96] but this has not been confirmed[97] and others have argued against it.[98]

As noted earlier, progesterone is produced in large quantities during the course of pregnancy, increasing as the pregnancy advances. During the last trimester, the placental production of progesterone is approximately 250 to 300 mg/24 hours. While maternal plasma total progesterone levels also increase during this period of time, fetal serum levels are nearly seven-fold higher than maternal serum levels.[99] In addition, progesterone is released into the retroplacental blood pool (the blood behind the placenta) and concentrations are several times higher than maternal serum levels[100] (even with intramuscular progesterone). *Thus, the fetus is exposed naturally to very high levels of progesterone, even higher than what one would anticipate with the administration of progesterone either oral or by intra-muscular injection.*

The question of whether excess progesterone may affect neural development can be raised and has been studied. Essentially no conjugation or metabolism of these steroids occurs in nervous tissue. Furthermore, fetal tissues appear saturated with progesterone and probably do not have the capacity for additional progesterone uptake.[101]

In our own experience with the use of progesterone in pregnancy, the incidence of fetal anomalies in patients on progesterone (2.2 percent) versus those who were not taking progesterone (2.7 percent) was actually lower (although the difference was not statistically significant). We observed one male infant with hypospadias with an incidence of 0.2 percent. But this is significantly lower than the quoted incidence of 5 to 8/1000 (0.5 to 0.8 percent) and even more significantly different than the claim that progesterone may be associated with a doubling of that frequency.[82] We also observed one female infant with mild labial fusion treated effectively with estrogen cream (incidence of 0.2 percent). But this, too, is much lower than the reported incidence of 1.8 percent. This series of patients is one of the largest, if not the largest, ever reported for progesterone supplementation in pregnancy. Furthermore, nearly all of these patients had exposure to progesterone during the first four months of pregnancy and no increase in any of the anomalies was observed.

It has been shown that in animals progesterone at five times the daily level had no apparent effect on fetal weight.[102] In our own experience, we found no significant difference in the birth weight of those babies born after exposure to progesterone support. The average weight for those exposed to progesterone support was 7.82 pounds and for those not on progesterone support 7.81 pounds.

In conclusion, specifically as it relates to the naturally-occurring hormone progesterone, **there is no credible evidence to suggest that its use to support pregnancy, whether that support be in the early days or months of the pregnancy or later in the pregnancy, is in any way teratogenic or responsible for any genital malformations**. In fact, all of the available evidence **strongly** supports its safety when used in pregnancy.

In the discussion on this subject in our textbook, "The Medical & Surgical Practice of **NaProTECHNOLOGY**," over 2,000 pregnancies were reviewed or reported with the use of progesterone support in pregnancy with *no increase in birth defects or genital anomalies*. Progesterone support in pregnancy can be considered completely safe!

For the Doctor

NaProTechnology Progesterone Support Protocol

The **NaProTECHNOLOGY** Progesterone Support Protocol now has over 30 years of experience supporting its use. There are several important features with regard to this protocol:

- First and foremost is its ability to objectively monitor the dosage of progesterone based upon the serial monitoring of serum progesterone levels during pregnancy.

- Its selection of progesterone over the use of 17-hydroxyprogesterone caproate.

- Its use during the course of pregnancy where supplementation of progesterone can be objectively quantified. Thus, it is not limited to use in only the first trimester of pregnancy, but often extends into the second and third trimesters.

- Its proven safety.

Progesterone has been selected as the hormone of choice for the support of pregnancy over and above 17-hydroxyprogesterone caproate (17-OHP-C), 17-hydroxyprogesterone hexonate (17-OHP-H) or medroxyprogesterone acetate (MPA). The selection of progesterone is based on the following factors:

1. Progesterone is the main natural-support hormone of pregnancy.

2. 17-OHP-C, 17-OHP-H and MPA are all synthetic analogues (artimones) of 17-hydroxyprogesterone and progesterone and are chemically different from natural progesterone and this likely decreases their ability to bind to myometrial progesterone receptors.[72]

3. 17-OHP-C, 17-OHP-H generally are not available. 17-OHP-C, the most commonly used and the subject of one of the recent revival papers,[15] was manufactured under the trade name Delalutin (Bristol-Meyers-Squibb Company), but its manufacture was discontinued in 1986 because of a declining market share.[73]

4. 17-OH-progesterone is a much weaker hormone then progesterone.

5. While 17-OHP-C can be considered safe in pregnancy (as is progesterone), MPA still has a few lingering questions remaining with regard to safety.

6. Progesterone is a completely natural hormone. That is, it is a hormone manufactured in abundance by the human body during pregnancy, while the others all are foreign to the body and not manufactured by it.

The key to the objective supplementation of progesterone during pregnancy is the availability of a *meaningful standard curve* (or **normogram**) for the production of progesterone during the course of pregnancy. These curves are not available in most laboratories. The National Hormone Laboratory of the Pope

Paul VI Institute, however, has developed such a curve in the many years of its work in the use of progesterone-supported pregnancy. The standard curve for normal pregnancy is shown in Figure 13-2. While a standard curve such as this is somewhat difficult to compile, they are not at all out of the reach of most laboratories. It does require a consistent effort to monitor serum progesterone levels in patients whose pregnancies are completely normal and to do that with the assay that is being used within the laboratory. There are differences between assays from laboratory to laboratory (even if it is the same assay system) and, of course, differences between different assay systems. In some cases, these differences may be quite significant and they need to be accounted for in the clinical use of such assessments.

The standard curve that we developed is flanked by two dotted lines that represent one standard deviation away from the average. By placing that marker to flank the average progesterone level during pregnancy (by gestational age at two weekly intervals), the hormone level that is drawn on an individual patient can be plotted in a way that is gestational age-specific. The curve can be broken up into *four zones* (Zone 1 through Zone 4). This is illustrated in Figure 13-3.

In using progesterone in pregnancy, only **human-identical progesterone** is utilized, and, over the last 30 years, the intramuscular injection of progesterone has been the main route of administration. The original protocol for this was published in 1991.[74] Progesterone should be administered to the indicated populations *as early as possible* at the beginning of pregnancy. This is best

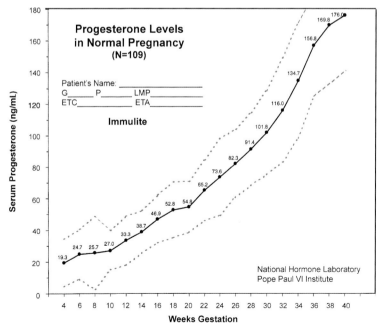

Figure 13-2: Progesterone levels in normal pregnancy with the mean and one standard deviation shown (DPC-Immulite).

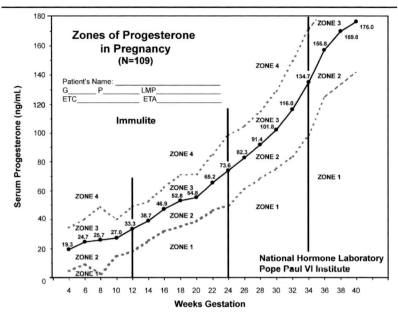

Figure 13-3: The four zones of progesterone shown using the DPC-Immulite assay.

accomplished in those women who are charting the **CREIGHTON MODEL System** (CrMS). As a matter of routine, when the woman reaches 16 days post-Peak (Peak +16), a pregnancy test can be performed and, if necessary, progesterone support initiated.

During the course of pregnancy, progesterone levels are drawn on a two-week basis and progesterone is supplemented based upon the progesterone level. The dosage of progesterone administered is determined on the zone that the progesterone level is in. When the progesterone level is drawn, it *always* should be drawn *immediately prior to the administration of the subsequent progesterone dose.* In this way, the progesterone level is drawn at the bottom of the natural absorption pattern of the administered progesterone. In this way, a best estimate of the baseline production of progesterone during the course of that pregnancy can be obtained and an objective decision can be made relative to the next dosage of progesterone to be administered. *The goal of treatment is to see that the serum progesterone level during pregnancy reaches either the average level or is in Zone 3 or Zone 4.*

If the woman is taking either oral progesterone or vaginal capsules or suppositories of progesterone, she should not use those the night before she gets her progesterone level drawn. Again, with the monitoring of progesterone levels every two weeks, an objective assessment of the dose of progesterone can be obtained.

The supplementation protocol for the use of progeserone in pregnancy for each of the zones of progesterone and the time of the pregnancy is found in the medical textbook "The Medical & Surgical Practice of **NaProTECHNOLOGY**."

When progesterone is administered intramuscularly, it can, on occasion, create local irritation, redness and swelling (along with associated itching). These side effects can be reduced greatly with the proper administration of the progesterone. If the progesterone is drawn up with one needle and administered with a second needle, and the progesterone is given very slowly (over two to three minutes) in the hip and according to instructions, these side effects can be reduced greatly. In the 30 years of our experience, we have never seen an abscess either infected or sterile with the administration of progesterone. We have, on occasion, seen induration and an inflammatory reaction. This almost always has responded to the local administration of heat and time. On occasion, the injections have to be discontinued and then either oral or vaginal or a combination of the two are used. Again, it cannot be stressed enough that the IM administration of progesterone must be given properly. In the majority of cases, we instruct the husbands to give these injections to their wives and they come in for a specific shot instruction given by our registered nurses. If there is localized itching at the site of the injection, vitamin E oil applied to the site can be very helpful in relieving those symptoms.

Examples of Progesterone Support in Pregnancy

In Figures 13-4 through 13-7, a number of examples are given of the assessment of progesterone during the course of complicated pregnancies, and the outcomes of those pregnancies are described.

A number of years ago, Dr. John Rock recommended that a national registry be created to document fetal outcome following progesterone-support therapy.[103] Such a registry was never undertaken to my knowledge, but it clearly makes sense that a national registry of this type, or at least a collaborative registry, should be undertaken for the ongoing assessment of this issue because of its overall importance. It is time to make a concerted commitment to see that this gets done.

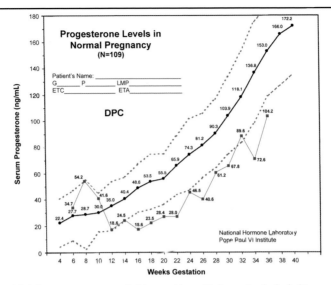

Figure 13-4: A progesterone curve of a 34-year-old, gravida 2, para 1, who had a history of having had an emergency cesarean section at term for severe fetal distress that ended in a neonatal death. She was an infertility patient with endometriosis and polycystic ovarian disease and was a heavy smoker. In the above pregnancy, her progesterone production was clearly suboptimal after looking quite favorable during the first trimester. She was supplemented with progesterone and had a healthy male infant at 38- weeks gestation by repeat cesarean section.

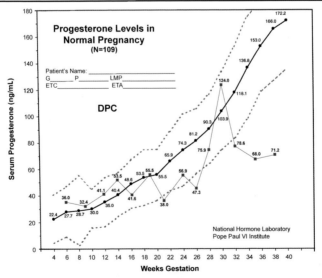

Figure 13-5: This 36-year-old gravida 4, para 2 with one previous miscarriage developed severe IUGR during the above pregnancy. At birth, the baby weighed 4 lbs. 14 oz. She was supplemented with progesterone and her levels in the second and third trimester were mostly Zone 1 and lower Zone 2. The placental weight at delivery was 197.0 grams (<10th percentile). She delivered spontaneously at 38 weeks a small but healthy infant with Apgars of 9 and 9.

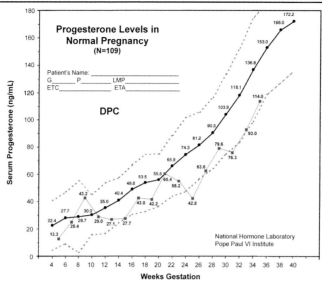

Figure 13-6: This 42-year-old gravida 1, para 1 achieved a pregnancy seven months after evaluation and treatment with NaProTECHNOLOGY. Prior to coming to the Pope Paul VI Institute, she had two failed attempts at IVF. In those attempts, her endometriosis and hormone dysfunction was left undiagnosed. In her pregnancy, she had a suboptimal progesterone profile usually in Zone 1 or lower Zone 2. With progesterone supplementation, she delivered a healthy female infant at 39 weeks.

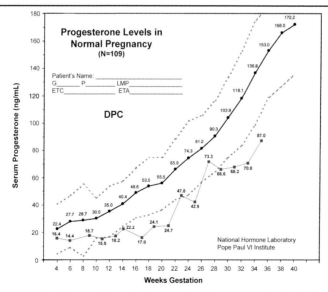

Figure 13-7: This is a 39-year-old, gravida 4, para 1 who had an intrauterine fetal demise at 26 weeks associated with very severe hypertension. She also had one previous miscarriage. In this pregnancy, which was supported by progesterone, she had a healthy female infant at 38-weeks gestation. She weighed 8 lbs. 15 oz. Apgar scores were 8 and 9. She was normotensive throughout the course of her pregnancy.

Surgical NaProTECHNOLOGY:
Surgery of the Heart

URGICAL **NaProTECHNOLOGY** is a specialized form of gynecologic surgery whose primary aim is to reconstruct the uterus, fallopian tubes and ovaries in such a way that pelvic adhesive disease (scarring) can be eliminated and not caused by the surgical procedure itself. It is, in a sense, a *"near adhesion free"* form of surgery.

The principles of this *"near adhesion-free"* type of surgery can be applied to many different types of conditions that can be associated with infertility, recurrent miscarrage, severe menstrual cramps, pelvic pain, recurrent ovarian cysts, heavy menstrual bleeding, and ectopic pregnancy. This approach is helpful especially in treating endometriosis, pelvic adhesive disease, polycystic ovaries, uterine fibroids, and various occlusions of the fallopian tubes. The details of this approach to surgery are presented in 262 pages and 21 chapters of my textbook, "The Medical & Surgical Practice of **NaProTECHNOLOGY**."

About 30 years ago, the American Board of Obstetrics and Gynecology approved three new subspecialties in the field of obstetrics and gynecology. These subspecialities were gynecologic oncology (care of cancers of the female reproductive system), perinatology (care of high-risk pregnancies), and reproductive endocrinology (care of women with infertility and other hormone-related problems). It was the hope when these subspecialities were developed that they would advance those three areas of women's health.

The development of the reproductive endocrinology training programs originally started with an emphasis on reconstructive pelvic surgery. But in 1978, when the first baby was born by *in vitro* fertilization (IVF), the specialty changed dramatically. Its focus over the last 30 years has been on the development of the skills needed for IVF. As a result, many younger reproductive endocrinologists (infertility specialists) do not, at this time, have the surgical skills necessary to do some basic and most advanced reconstructive pelvic surgeries.

Over a decade ago, the Society of Reproductive Surgeons, a group within the American Society for Reproductive Medicine (formerly the American Fertility Society), began to recognize this deficiency and fostered the development of postgraduate fellowship programs that would have as one of their major emphases training in pelvic surgery, microsurgery, laser surgical applications, and so forth. These training programs have grown slowly over the past 10 years and have evolved now into training programs with an emphasis on *operative laparoscopy*. These procedures tend to leave behind more scar tissue than what can be obtained with surgical **NaProTECHNOLOGY** approaches.[1] Thus, for women with infertility, that is not desirable.

One of the best examples of a surgical procedure that has been lost in the transition to *in vitro* fertilization is ovarian wedge resection. This is a procedure that many years ago carried with it 66 percent pregnancy rates.[2] It was well known to be associated with a high incidence of the formation of pelvic adhesions (scar tissue). As a result, when clomiphene citrate became available in the middle 1960s, this procedure was all but abandoned because of the stated reason that it created significant scar tissue. And yet, the pregnancy rate following clomiphene therapy was *significantly less* than that associated with ovarian wedge resection.[3] Furthermore, ovarian wedge resection made a major contribution to the long-term treatment of some of the hormone and menstrual cycle abnormalities associated with women who had polycystic ovaries. The use of clomiphene citrate has no such long-lasting effect. More recently, *in vitro* fertilization has been utilized for this purpose, and yet the pregnancy rates are even lower and the health benefits absent.[4]

In the meantime, a good deal of progress has been made in the prevention of pelvic adhesions. Work done at our center and by others now has shown that ovarian wedge resection can be done in such a way that it not only carries with it high pregnancy rates, but also is associated with a very low incidence of the formation of pelvic adhesions. In addition, it can be done through a fairly small surgical incision with a low incidence of surgical complications. A good deal can be gained from its positive hormone and cycle effects. Thus, surgical **NaProTECHNOLOGY** is an important development in the field of reconstructive pelvic surgery *with its major emphasis on adhesion prevention.*

In many ways, this portion of **NaProTECHNOLOGY** has been developed within the standard practice of gynecologic pelvic surgery, but there are very few programs around the United States that actually implement the strategies involved in this surgical subspecialty. It is not that some brand new way of performing a surgical procedure has been invented. Rather, it is a surgical subspecialty that has been refined by incorporating a number of different, but currently available, applications that have as their end result the prevention of pelvic adhesive disease (scarring).

Qualifications of the Physician

A physician who engages in surgical **NaProTECHNOLOGY** should be, at the very least, a board-certified obstetrician-gynecologist with a very special interest in these surgical applications. A board-certified general surgeon with these interests also would be basically qualified. In both cases, additional expertise in the use of laser and in microsurgical applications also is necessary. Continuing medical education instruction is important, and obtaining added experience through a surgical **NaProTECHNOLOGY** fellowship will be very helpful. The Pope Paul VI Institute in affiliation with Creighton University School of Medicine offers a one-year fellowship for training in this area (see *www.popepaulvi. com*). In addition to these basic medical and surgical requirements, a special interest and dedication to these surgical principles is strongly recommended.

Selection of Patients

In reviewing the surgical procedures of the Pope Paul VI Institute, approximately 60 percent of those patients who have endometriosis will be able to have a corrective surgical procedure with laser at the time of their diagnostic laparoscopy. The type of surgical procedure used will depend on the extent to which the pelvis is involved with endometriosis and adhesive disease. In mild endometriosis, 85.6

percent were treated by laser laparoscopy while all of those with severe endometriosis needed a laser laparotomy (an open surgical procedure).

In surgical **NaProTECHNOLOGY**, the main goal is to *make a good diagnosis* that then will lead to a better form of treatment. When it is treated effectively, the goal is to do it in such a way that there is the greatest opportunity for the disease to be removed with a limited exposure to the formation of adhesions. Thus, it is unusual to combine the diagnostic laparoscopy with a major surgical procedure. The one exception to this may be patients who require an ovarian wedge resection in a situation where this is the *only disease process* present or there is just a limited amount of endometriosis that can be laser vaporized at the time of the laparoscopy. Combining those two surgical procedures is often not too complex or difficult and can be scheduled properly.

There are several difficulties in doing the laparoscopy and a major surgical procedure at the same operation. The first of these is the length of time it takes to do the major surgical procedure. These procedures often can take three or four hours (sometimes longer) and when combined with a diagnostic laparoscopy can make the entire surgical procedure too long. One of the other major problems is the planning that goes into most of these surgical procedures, including such things as preparation of the bowel and advanced discussion about the nature of the surgical procedure and the complications with which it might be associated. Thus, it is the practice at our center to do the diagnostic laparoscopy and if laser laparoscopy cannot be performed at the same time, then the procedure is videotaped and the patient is scheduled for a *laparoscopy review (comprehensive management review).*

At this visit, usually lasting 45 to 60 minutes, the entire nature of the patient's case is presented from the point of view of **NaProTECHNOLOGY** and what it can offer the patient in terms of treatment. If further surgery is contemplated, then a complete discussion of those surgical procedures and their possible complications are presented.

At this laparoscopy review, the videotape of the laparoscopy is viewed with the patient (even if major surgery is not contemplated, the laser laparoscopy is shown). The **CREIGHTON MODEL** chart is reviewed for various biomarkers that are important to be resolved relative to their infertility or miscarriage history, and a review of the entire hormone evaluation is undertaken.

The ultrasound evaluation of ovulation then is discussed and presented to them. If there are abnormalities, they are presented in the context of the entire problem. Additional factors, such as the results of any biopsies, the seminal fluid analysis, also are presented. By placing this into its total context at one visit, a comprehensive approach or strategy for treatment can be developed and explained to the patient. From this review, the recommendation of the physician is made, discussion with the patient is undertaken and questions are answered.

In surgical **NaProTECHNOLOGY**, once again, the goal is "near adhesion-free" surgery while at the same time removing the disease that is present. It is a form of surgery that is in some ways similar to plastic surgery because of its goal to reconstruct the pelvic tissues in such a way that they resemble tissues that have never been adversely affected. While we are not entirely capable of doing this in all cases, in nearly all cases we are able to approach it. And in those cases, the overall situation will be greatly improved. The surgical challenges are exciting and what can be accomplished to assist the patient is extremely satisfying.

"Near-Contact" Laparoscopy

Over the last 20 years, the skill in diagnostic laparoscopy has improved significantly because of the work of individuals, such as Drs. Goldstein,[5] Redwine[6] and Martin.[7] Laparoscopies continue to be performed, however where the *potential* for the diagnostic tool is *not being fulfilled.* I have observed on many occasions a diagnostic laparoscopy that was considered normal, but when it was repeated, a high incidence of abnormalities was identified. In a series of 46 such cases, 41 of them (89.1 percent) had endometriosis and in two cases adhesive disease was identified (4.4 percent). In only three cases (6.5 percent) was normal pelvic anatomy identified.

Improved training in diagnostic laparoscopy for individual practitioners is necessary. Experience in laparoscopic sterilizations in a residency program is *inadequate* for subsequently performing diagnostic laparoscopy. The two skills are quite different.

It has been shown that using the magnification of the laparoscope for a close-up view can improve one's ability to detect various conditions.[5] Dr. Redwine introduced the term "near-contact" laparoscopy (NCL).[6] In this approach, the laparoscope is placed close to the tissues being examined ("near contact") as opposed to the more

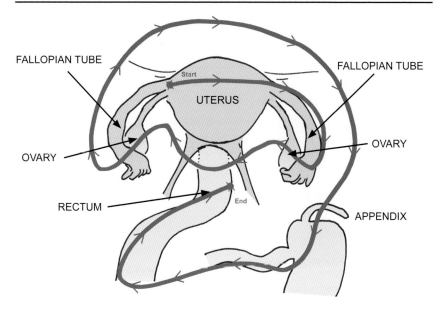

Figures 14-1: In this diagram, an orderly sequence for evaluation of the pelvis tissues, which is essential to doing good diagnostic laparoscopy, is illustrated. The technique begins at the left posterior fundus and proceeds in a clockwise, somewhat spiral fashion around to the right and circulating in the way illustrated. In this way, if this becomes routine, the ability to miss important diagnostic features of the pelvis is reduced significantly. The surgeon should choose some means of proceeding in every diagnostic laparoscopy with a systematic, routine approach that carefully evaluates all of the tissues within the pelvis, including the appendix, cecum, terminal ileum and rectosigmoid colon.

traditional approach where the scope is left at some significant distance from the tissues. This technique allows for a much better diagnostic approach. In addition, the laparoscope is used in an orderly sequence so that no area is left without being evaluated (Figure 14-1).

Selective Hysterosalpingography and Catheterization of the Fallopian Tubes

One of the most difficult aspects of the infertility evaluation is to study the anatomic and functional integrity of the fallopian tubes. It is common to perform hysterosalpingography (HSG), an x-ray test where dye is injected into the uterus and followed out the fallopian tubes. But a better way has been introduced. This technique injects each fallopian tube separately and measures the pressure inside the tubes. It is referred to as **selective hysterosalpingography** (SHSG).

The first effort to evaluate the fallopian tubes selectively using contrast material was published by Drs. Corfman and Taylor in 1966.[8] This procedure has been popularized more recently by others.[9-12] A

number of other investigators also have added to the procedure various aspects of transcervical catheterization of the fallopian tubes (TCFT).[13-16] Dr. N. Gleicher[12] first reported on a standardized tubal perfusion technique. It was suggested that the evaluation of tubal perfusion pressures could provide important diagnostic information, and further investigation of this area was encouraged. In 1999, Drs. Hilgers and Yeung[17] described a group of patients for whom the intratubal pressure (ITP), at the time of the SHSG, was obtained before and after TCFT.

The average intratubal pressure for freely-patent tubes is 0.53 ATM (atmospheres) and for partially-obstructed tubes 1.23 ATM. The completely-obstructed tubes had an average pressure of 2.79 ATM. Some degree of obstruction is quite common in women with infertility problems.

With TCFT the pressure can be lowered to normal in women with partially-obstructed tubes, but in completely-obstructed tubes, the pressure will remain unchanged or reduced only slightly. A surgical procedure to correct that problem has been developed.

The adequate evaluation of the fallopian tubes in patients with infertility has been a problem for many years. Because the fallopian tubes are not readily accessible, direct access to them generally has not been possible. But with the advent of SHSG, it now is possible to assess the fallopian tubes more thoroughly and get more accurate information. In our **NaProTECHNOLOGY** practice, it has completely replaced HSG as a diagnostic approach.

In partially-obstructed fallopian tubes, it has been reported that an amorphous material of unknown cause often is present in the form of a caste within the fallopian tube.[18] Such "plugs" may be the cause of the partial-tubal occlusions that have been observed. This also could explain why the normalization of the ITP after TCFT occurs in such a high percentage of cases. It also may explain why with standard hysterosalpingography the observation often is made that dye will not initially go down the fallopian tube. With additional pressure, injecting the dye, the dye is then seen to go down the tube and spill into the abdominal cavity (all observed with x-ray). Before the use of SHSG and TCFT, tubal spasm usually was given as the explanation for this observation, but these "plugs" are a more likely explanation.

It also has been reported that intrauterine pregnancy rates after SHSG and TCFT range from nine to 37 percent.[19,20] While pregnancy rates were not the focus of the Hilgers and Yeung study, SHSG and

TCFT now are considered to be important components of a basic evaluation for women who have had difficulty achieving pregnancy. It is a significant improvement over hysterosalpingography without losing any of the component aspects of the traditional HSG.

The average exposure to x-ray in this procedure is well within the range of radiation safety.[21] The safety margin is adequate even if a second procedure is necessary. Delivery of medications to the fallopian tube also has been described.[22]

Preventing Pelvic Adhesions

In those patients who were operated on with severe pelvic adhesive disease using the basic **NaProTECHNOLOGY** anti-adhesion techniques from 1985 through 1993, the total adhesion score at the time of the initial surgery was 33.8 (this scoring system was developed and advanced by the American Fertility Society.[23] The higher the score, the worse the adhesions). At second-look laparoscopy, the adhesion score significantly decreased to 18.1.

In the mid-1990s, more extensive use of Gore-Tex (Teflon) anti-adhesion barrier was implemented in our surgical **NaProTECHNOLOGY** program. A follow-up group of patients who had a total adhesion score of 33.3 at the time of initial surgery (not statistically different than the previous group), had follow-up adhesion scores at second-look laparoscopy of 6.0. When comparing the total adhesion score at second-look laparoscopy between the earlier group (1987-1993) and the later group (1994-2005), there was a further significant reduction in adhesion formation. A total adhesion score of 6.0 (with a mean score of 3.0 per side) would be considered minimal adhesions according to the American Fertility Society classification system.[23] More recently we have introduced some additional techniques and the adhesion score was decreased to 2.5. This was accepted for publication, and it was published in the March 2010 issue of the Journal of Gynecologic Surgery.

It is clear that standard approaches to the surgical treatment of endometriosis, polycystic ovarian disease and pelvic adhesive disease generate adhesions in a far greater amount than what is desirable.[24] In fact, laparoscopic surgery has been shown to not reduce adhesions in gynecologic procedures.[1] With the introduction of surgical **NaProTECHNOLOGY** approaches, with their main emphasis on the prevention of surgical adhesions, one can confidently approach major surgical procedures in such a fashion so as to not only eliminate the adhesions that are present, but with a high degree of likelihood reduce or eliminate the reformation or recurrence of adhesions. *In order to accomplish this, it requires the adherence to good anti-adhesion surgical technique.* If these techniques are followed properly, the outcomes should be excellent. This book cannot outline all of these techniques, but for those who might be interested, they are detailed in my textbook.

I often tell my operating room staff that we are performing "heart surgery." This is not surgery "*on* the heart" but, rather, surgery "*of* the heart." We are working in an area that has deep meaning to patients as we are helping them to become prepared to carry a new baby. A baby is so very important to people that we are truly doing "surgery of the heart."

Conditions, Diseases and
NaProTECHNOLOGY

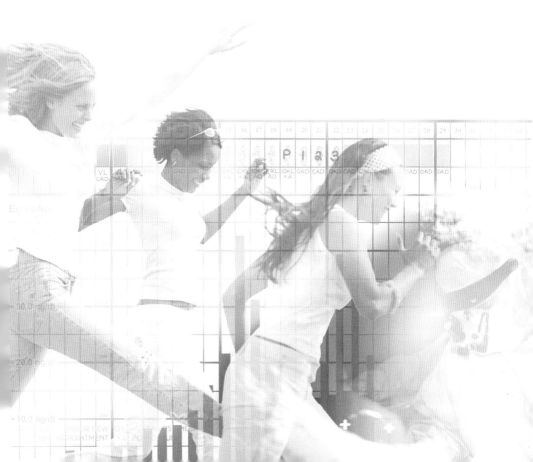

STRESS HAS AN ENORMOUS impact on the ovulation and menstrual cycle. The stress may be *physical* or *emotional*. It may be *acute* or *chronic*. Examples of **physical stress** include such things like *sickness, strenuous activity and travel*. Examples of **emotional stress** could be *change of job, bereavement, major decisions, holidays, relatives visiting, weddings and exams*.

Many other stressors can occur in an individual's life. Those types of stress that are *rapid in their onset and fairly short-lived* are called **acute stressors**. Those stressful events that are *slow in onset and prolonged* are called **chronic stressors**.

Most of the above examples are acute stressors. But a change of job that puts one into a stressful situation can become a chronic stressor. Most chronic stressors are related to *stressful relationships* in the workplace, in a premarriage or marriage environment, or with relatives and friends.

Stress can cause a variety of changes in the charting system. The classic example is the "double" Peak. This is a situation in which stress delays ovulation and the "second" Peak occurs after the stress is relieved. Ovulation occurs with the "second" Peak. It is a situation that can happen to any woman; it may be a protective mechanism at work, delaying fertility until the stress is relieved.

There are a number of other effects of stress. Some women may experience a prolonged Peak-type mucus buildup while others may have a delay in the Peak Day and ovulation. In others, the charting

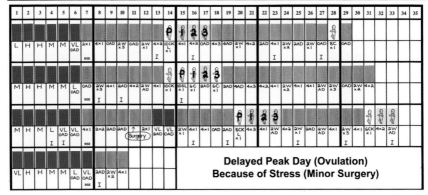

Figure 15-1: A delay in the Peak Day in the third cycle due to stress of minor surgery (see text) (From: Pope Paul VI Institute research, 2004). Refer to page 83 for the Vaginal Discharge Recording System (VDRS).

pattern may become totally dry, or limited mucus cycles may develop. Examples of the various effects of stress are observed in Figures 15-1 through 15-4.

In Figure 15-1, a woman who has undergone a minor surgical procedure on day 11 of her third cycle of charting has a Peak Day occurring on day 20 of the cycle or nine days after the surgery. The cycle itself is the longest (measuring 33 days in duration) she has had in several cycles. It is thought that the surgical procedure and the stress leading up to it were sufficient to delay ovulation, and this delay in ovulation shows up in her charting. Her Peak Day occurred on day 14 and day 15 of the two previous cycles.

In Figure 15-2, the young woman has a normal length mucus cycle with a normally-occurring Peak Day. But during the third cycle of this chart, her grandfather died (on day 15). Because this was Easter week, the funeral was delayed until day 22 of the cycle, as can be seen in the charting example. Her Peak Day did not occur until day 27. This was followed by a normal 15-day post-Peak phase, but the cycle length itself was prolonged at 42 days in duration. The mucus cycle leading up to the Peak Day was 20 days in duration. Both the overall cycle length and the length of the mucus cycle were prolonged significantly. The stressful event occurred at a time when she would normally ovulate, and so it held the actual ovulation event in abeyance while ovarian function continued to produce a Peak-type continuous-mucus discharge. Again, when a cycle like this is observed, the stressful events usually can be pieced together to explain the charting situation. Another interesting feature of Figure 15-2 is that it took about two

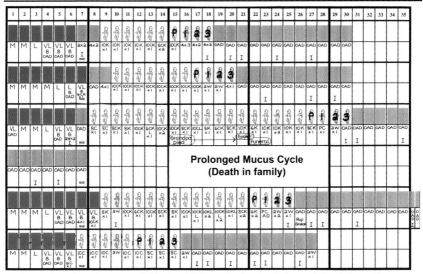

Figure 15-2: Prolonged mucus cycle (third cycle) due to death in family (see text). By the last cycle, stress had been relieved and cycles reverted to normal (From: Pope Paul VI Institute research, 2004).

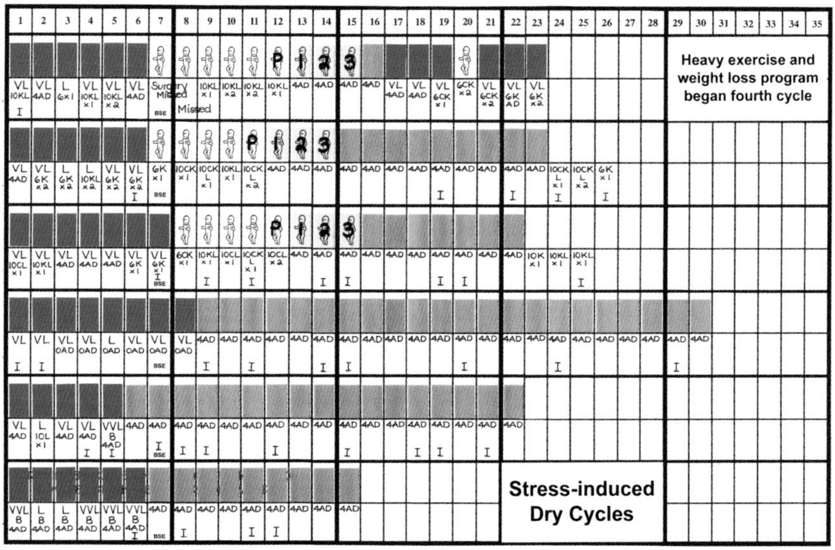

Figure 15-3: Stress-induced dry cycles (starting with fourth cycle) because of new diet and exercise (see text) (From: Pope Paul VI Institute research, 2004). Refer to page 83 for the VDRS.

cycles for her ovulation and fertility cycle to recuperate once the stress was relieved.

In Figure 15-3, a woman's chart is shown with a normal mucus cycle during the first three cycles of charting, but in her fourth, fifth and sixth cycles of charting she has reverted to a completely dry pattern. This woman began a 45-minute jazzercise program with sit-ups and leg lifts at the beginning of her fourth cycle of charting. At the same time, she also went on a weight reduction diet and lost 10 pounds (from 122 lbs. to 112 lbs.). These events are stressors and the cause of her dry cycle pattern.

This same woman was told at the age of 20 that she could not become pregnant because of extensive pelvic inflammatory disease and adhesions (scar tissue). She was told that she needed a hysterectomy. She underwent surgical reconstruction of her pelvis through the Pope Paul VI Institute and the charting that is observed in Figure 15-3 is the charting following her surgery. Because of the weight loss and exercise programs, she converted her cycles to infertile ones. Thus, it was suggested to her that she discontinue the strenuous activity and dieting. When she did this, she reverted back to having normal mucus cycles. A few cycles later, she became pregnant and, from that pregnancy had a healthy baby boy.

The chart of a young woman who was under stress while she was planning her wedding is shown in Figure 15-4. In the first two cycles, stressful activity was taking place in preparing for her wedding. This is one of the classic appearances of a stress-induced "double" Peak situation.

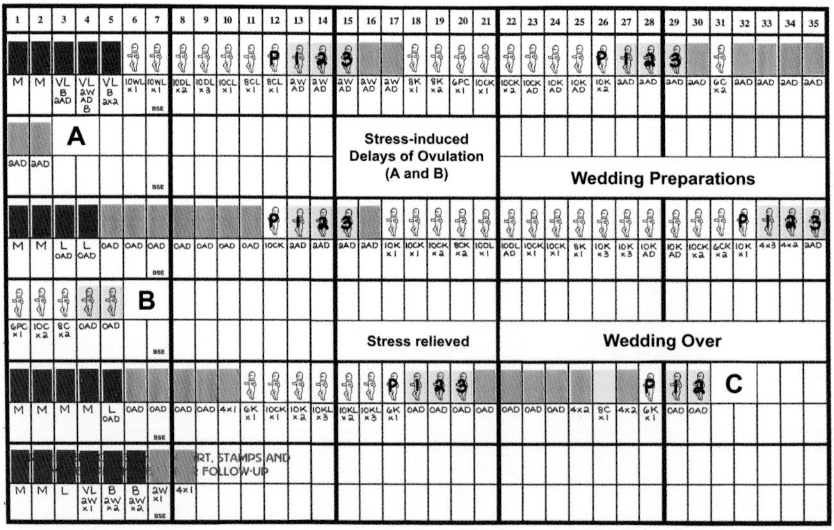

Figure 15-4: Stress-induced delays of ovulation because of stress associated with preparations for a wedding (From: Pope Paul VI Institute research, 2004). Refer to page 83 for the Vaginal Discharge Recording System (VDRS).

In her second cycle of charting (a 40-day cycle), she has a prolonged mucus buildup that concludes on day 32 of her cycle. She has a very short post-Peak phase numbering only eight days in duration. This suggests that the entire cycle was hormonally abnormal.

In her third cycle of charting, when much of the stress was relieved following the wedding, her cycles reverted back to normal. In this cycle, she had a seven-day mucus buildup to the Peak Day, and her Peak Day occurred on day 17 of her cycle. Her post-Peak phase was 13 days in duration and the overall cycle length was 30 days.

With the self-knowledge that comes with charting the **CREIGHTON MODEL System** (CrMS), women may be able to look at their lifestyle and see what changes may or may not be necessary to help reduce stress in their lives.

The reasons why stress causes these effects are not entirely known at the present time. We do know that stress has many hormonal and physiologic effects. The exact relationship to the reproductive system is not well understood. One of the theories is the possibility that β-endorphins play a role in blocking the normal pulsatile production of FSH and LH from the pituitary gland. This blockage, while not complete, is sufficient to cause ovulatory dysfunction. Such ovulatory dysfunction is what may produce delayed ovulation and some long cycles.

Recurrent Ovarian Cysts

IGNIFICANT NUMBERS OF surgical procedures continue to be performed on reproductive-age women for ovarian cysts.[1-4] Oral contraceptives are promoted as a form of treatment, but studies have shown oral contraceptives have little or no effect on the resolution of ovarian cysts.[5] Most of these cysts result from an underlying hormonal dysfunction. By understanding the basic principle involved in the formation of these functional cysts, one can reduce the need for surgical intervention. Almost universally, women with functional cysts will *not require surgery.*

The **CREIGHTON MODEL System** often enables the identification of various types of ovarian cysts. The ovarian cysts that are identified are *persistent follicular cysts* or *persistent luteal cysts* (luteinized unruptured follicles).

While advances have been made in the diagnosis of ovarian cysts with the use of ultrasound,[6] the methodology for studying these cysts generally has been defective. Most studies using ultrasound parameters are studying the ovarian cysts at the time they are causing problems rather than tracking them from their origin. With the experience accumulated in our program with the daily ultrasound evaluation of ovulation, progress has been made in the development of a better understanding of the cause of many ovarian cysts.

Persistent Follicular Cysts

With a persistent follicular cyst of the ovary, the **CrMS** will reveal a prolonged Peak-type mucus discharge and a delayed Peak Day (Figure 16-1). *Persistent follicular cysts* often are associated with chronic pelvic pain, which is usually on one side, but also may be on both sides. The chronic pelvic pain usually is not so significant as to require surgery.

Follicular cysts have, as one of their hallmarks, the dominant and prolonged production of estrogen that is unopposed by progesterone. This is the reason for the prolonged Peak-type mucus discharge and the delayed Peak Day as evidenced in the **CrMS** chart. By disrupting the estrogen dominance with an injection of progesterone, a subsequent menstrual period will occur in three to five days. Once menses occurs, the follicular cyst usually disappears. Use of progesterone also is associated with *a marked reduction in pain* caused by the ovarian cyst.

The case presented in Figure 16-1 was an 18-year-old who had already had two surgical procedures for recurrent ovarian cysts. She had been placed on oral contraceptives for two years and was brought to our program because she no longer wanted to be on oral contraceptives for treatment of this condition. The chart in Figure 16-1 shows her first 39 days of charting. At the time of the first visit, she already was having pelvic pain and, on pelvic examination, she seemed to have an ovarian cyst. She was sent for a pelvic ultrasound examination and a follicular cyst was identified. She was given an injection of progesterone and, on day 5 of her next menstrual period, she had another ultrasound. In this examination, the area where the cystic structure previously was located showed that the cyst had disappeared.

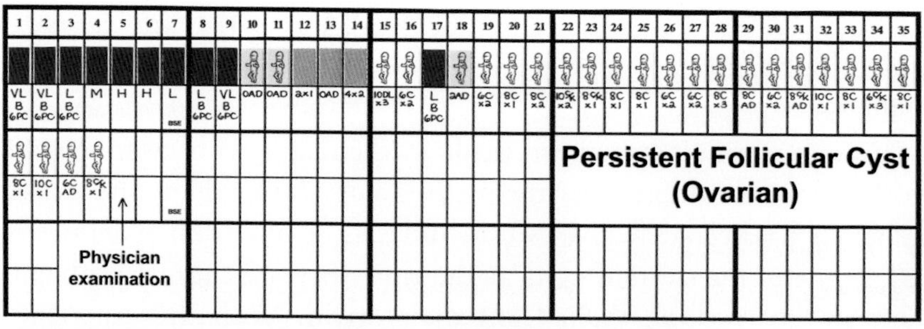

Figure 16-1: This CrMS chart from an 18-year-old shows a prolonged mucus cycle with variable return of Peak-type mucus (VRPM). On the day of the physician examination, she has pain. Ultrasound examination confirmed the presence of a persistent follicular cyst (From: Pope Paul VI Institute research, 2004). Refer to page 83 for the Vaginal Discharge Recording System (VDRS).

Persistent Luteal Cysts

A *persistent luteal cyst* also is referred to as a luteinized unruptured follicle (LUF syndrome). In this situation, the follicle grows and develops to the time of ovulation, but ovulation does not occur. The follicle remains unruptured and a cyst forms and increases in size during the remaining portion of the cycle. Varying degrees of internal debris will form within the follicle suggesting some amount of hemorrhage within that cyst. These also are called hemorrhagic luteal cysts.

Progesterone is produced by the cyst and a Peak Day is observed. The amount of progesterone being produced generally is decreased, and this apparently plays a role in its recurrent nature.

If the patient is charting her cycles using the **CrMS**, the post-Peak phase of the cycle may be prolonged to 16 or more days in duration. This prolonged post-Peak phase is suspicious for the presence of an unruptured follicle (persistent luteal cyst) (Figure 16-2). In the absence of pregnancy and in the absence of the misidentification of the Peak Day (which is quite rare), interpreting this chart as one that reflects a persistent luteal cyst is accurate in the majority of cases. A pelvic ultrasound examination on Peak +16 or 17 or a pelvic examination at that time can verify the presence of the cyst.

In Figure 16-2, the patient underwent ultrasound examinations to study her ovulation sequence. It was documented as an unruptured follicle because of these daily examinations.

The cause of the unruptured follicle is not known entirely, but it is related to a dysfunctional hormone pattern. For example, both the

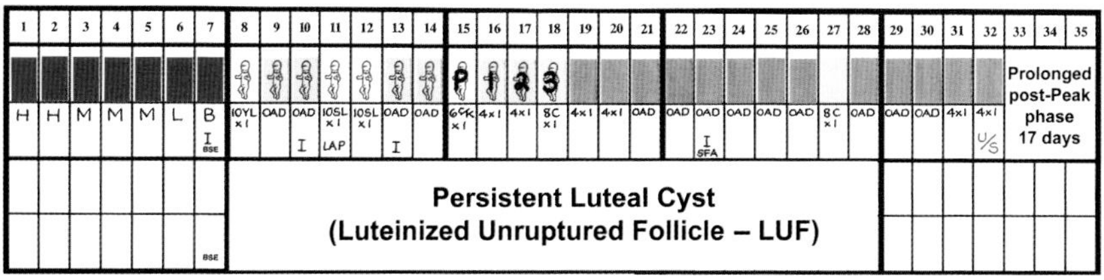

Figure 16-2: In this cycle, a 17-day post-Peak phase was observed and a persistent luteal cyst was documented by serial ultrasound examination (luteinized unruptured follicle, LUF) (From: Pope Paul VI Institute research, 2004). Refer to page 83 for the Vaginal Discharge Recording System (VDRS).

follicular phase estrogen and the postovulatory progesterone levels are decreased in this patient population.

The natural course of events with an unruptured follicle is for that cyst to resolve once menstruation begins. These cysts almost are *universally gone* by the fifth day after the beginning of the next period. A follow-up pelvic examination or ultrasound examination on day 5 of the next cycle is indicated to document its disappearance.

As with follicular cysts, physicians commonly treat unruptured follicles with oral contraceptives. But oral contraceptives suppress the hypothalamic-pituitary axis and may be detrimental to the already dysfunctional hormone pattern. This is unnecessary if one understands these functional cysts and further understands the **CrMS** and **NaProTECHNOLOGY**.

In the cases where a woman experiences pain in association with these cysts, progesterone can be valuable. As with the persistent follicular cysts, pain associated with luteal cysts is diminished significantly once the progesterone is initiated. Pain relief can be expected within an hour.

While a prolonged post-Peak phase is indicative of an unruptured follicle (or a persistent luteal cyst), a *normal-length* post-Peak phase does *not* indicate that the woman has actually ovulated or that an LUF has not occurred. Most LUFs actually occur in cycles where the post-Peak phase is normal in length. Those cystic structures that become medically problematic will most often reveal themselves with a prolonged post-Peak phase.

Ovarian Cyst Assessment

In 45 patients who were evaluated for what appeared to be an ovarian cyst on ultrasound examination, all were treated with IM progesterone. In 38 of these, the cystic structure disappeared by day 5 of the next menstrual period. In seven patients, the cystic structure remained. Follow-up on these seven patients showed that three had serous cystadenomas, two had very large (greater than 5 cm) peritubal cysts, one had a mucinous cystadenoma, and one had a mucinous tumor of borderline malignancy. Thus, the use of progesterone as a treatment for functional ovarian cysts has proved to be helpful in resolving the cystic structure without surgery and in identifying those cases in which further investigation is necessary. Some patients do still need surgical intervention, but **CrMS** charting and the use of IM progesterone clarifies those cases that require further investigation. Experience suggests that this is a better treatment than the use of suppressive oral contraceptive therapy.

Any surgical procedure on the ovary carries the potential for adhesion (scar tissue) formation (especially if done within the context of standard gynecologic surgical techniques). In these women, many of whom are young in age and prior to considering child bearing, *it is crucial that their fertility be preserved and not injured.* Thus, surgical **NaProTECHNOLOGY** techniques always should be used.

If cysts do not disappear by day 5 of the menstrual cycle with the above approaches to treatment, then these cysts need to be carefully monitored. Understanding these principles assists in the early recognition of suspicious ovarian cysts that may have a potential to be cancerous.

Recurrent Ovarian Cysts

The dysfunctional hormone patterns that have been discussed here tend to be repetitive. Functional cysts tend to be recurrent. Because they are recurrent, a form of treatment designed to help suppress ovarian function (oral contraceptives) has been promoted. But if the woman is taught how to chart her cycles using the **CrMS**, has a hormone evaluation during the post-Peak phase of her cycle, and receives subsequent post-Peak progesterone therapy on a long-term basis, these recurrent ovarian cysts can be controlled. Experience suggests that improved ovarian function results.

In treating patients with recurrent ovarian cysts, the use of IM progesterone may be necessary for the initial or acute situation where pain is involved. On a long-term basis, however, the use of oral, sustained-release progesterone usually is satisfactory. The use of vaginal progesterone usually is not necessary, but is an alternative that can be helpful.

Premenstrual Syndrome

THE CONDITION NOW referred to as **premenstrual syndrome** (PMS) has a long and varied history among medical investigators. This history dates back to the time of Hippocrates,[1] and the first reference in a scientific journal was by Frank in 1931.[2] In 1964, Dr. Katherina Dalton brought attention to this condition with her first book on PMS, which promoted the theory that this condition was caused by either a progesterone deficiency or an imbalance in the estrogen-progesterone ratio.[3] Later, she also extensively promoted the use of progesterone therapy for its treatment.[4]

While its medical aspects have been difficult to crystallize, PMS has been locked in with various political and legal views. For example, murder convictions and felony charges have been reduced to manslaughter and misdemeanors respectively because of the argument that the accused woman suffered from PMS. Feminists have voiced concern about this trend indicating that the use of PMS as a defense in criminal or civil matters could result in a negative impact on women's push toward equality with men.[1] Feminists plead that generalizations about women should not be made when assessing the legal or political aspects of this condition.

My own point of view is that this condition has held many women back over the years. This has prompted an interest and concern about finding the underlying causes and treating them effectively, so that the women who suffer from premenstrual syndrome also are given full access to opportunities. Furthermore, PMS is a condition that has destroyed relationships, has led to divorce and child abuse, and has created numerous stereotypes about the behavior of women.

181

Real People, Real Problems, Real Solutions

In 2001, at the age of 44, we decided to have some hormonal blood tests to evaluate what my fertility picture was like in this premenopausal state. I contacted Dr. Hilgers at the Pope Paul VI Institute. The nurse called to let me know that my hormone values were low, very low; so low, in fact, that I had only one-third of the normal estrogen and progesterone for a woman my age.

Then the nurse asked one of the most important questions that I had ever been asked of me in my life. In fact, a question that eventually changed my life for the better! "Debbie, your hormone levels are so very low. Are you ever depressed?" I couldn't believe my ears. "Yes! I am depressed," I answered. "I am very depressed. It started three years ago and has gotten progressively worse." I felt that I was coming out of the dark to even admit that. Who admits to being depressed? Obviously, something was wrong with me. But I thought it was my mind, my psyche; not my body! Never in my wildest dreams, even as a nurse, with a history of low progesterone and repeated miscarriages did I think my depression was biological in origin. "Can it be cured?" I asked. "Yes! We put many women on hCG and they feel better after the second shot," the nurse answered.

I couldn't believe my ears! That month I was placed on hCG on Peak Day +3, +5, +7 and +9. Four injections every month, which my husband or I administer. These shots have helped my ovaries produce appropriate levels of estrogen and progesterone.

My depression disappeared immediately and has not returned. I am now 46 years old. I can laugh again. The children are my joy. My husband said he saw a mask lifted from my face. I love this life!

I went to the staff of the Pope Paul VI Institute three years ago trying to find out about my fertility. Because of the awesome expertise of the nurses, they had the knowledge to ask the million-dollar question that helped me learn about and leave hormonal depression.

Another confirmation of the physiological basis of my depression came to me over a year ago when we were in the process of a move. Due to the hectic time, I missed my medication. The symptoms of depression came flooding back. They disappeared again the next month when I got on my hCG regimen.

God allowed me to go through the dark days of hormonal depression and find hope in treatment. Now I have been able to help others. When women come to me complaining of depression, I tell them to get a baseline medical exam to evaluate their hormone levels before they assume their depression is only in their minds.

The Institute and Dr. Hilgers and staff have helped and will help innumerable women. I, for my part, owe a debt of gratitude to them for the healthy birth of my youngest daughter, and my deliverance from a serious hormonal depression to a life of joy.

Debra M. Brock, RN
Falls Church, Virginia

Some symptoms (both physical and emotional) prior to the onset of the menstrual period are common.[5] These may occur in 50 to 75 percent of women. Moderate to severe premenstrual symptoms that disrupt a woman's lifestyle may occur in 20 to 30 percent of women, and severe, debilitating symptoms are seen in two to 10 percent.

Premenstrual syndrome is related to the diagnosis of *premenstrual dysphoric disorder* (PMDD). The diagnosis of these two conditions is different since one is defined by the 10th Revision of the International Classification of Diseases (ICD-10) and the other is identified by criteria from the 4th Edition of the Diagnostic and Statistical Manual of Mental Disorders (DSM-IV). This latter book is used mainly by psychiatrists. The diagnosis of PMS *requires only one symptom* to be present for its diagnosis, while the diagnosis of PMDD requires *at least five symptoms* to be present *at least one week prior* to the beginning of menses. In both cases, the conditions tend to decrease after menstruation has occurred. They have characteristic appearances during the premenstrual phase of the menstrual cycle. The use of the term PMS is preferred by obstetrician-gynecologists and primary care physicians while psychiatrists and other mental health providers tend to prefer PMDD. Some have argued that PMDD poses a risk for *major depressive disorder* (MDD) and that it may be a causal risk factor for MDD.[6]

Premenstrual symptoms sometimes are more prominent during the preovulatory and periovulatory phases of the menstrual cycle, and this is sometimes referred to as "reverse PMS." While the degree of premenstrual symptom severity varies within the population, it tends to be relatively constant within the individual woman. In addition, it can be influenced by age, race/ethnicity and health status. In a recent monograph,[7] the Association of Professors of Gynecology and Obstetrics (APGO) and the APGO Medical Education Foundation reported the most common symptoms of PMS as listed in Table 17-1. They also indicated that the use of vaginal progesterone suppositories could no longer be advocated. They reported that oral progesterone had been found to be no more effective than placebo in the treatment of PMS (see further discussion later in this chapter).

Table 17-1: Common Symptoms of PMS[1]

- Anger (irritability)*
- Anxiety
- Bloating or weight gain*
- Breast tenderness*
- Depression*
- Decreased concentration
- Decreased self-esteem
- Decreased interest in activities
- Fatigue*

- Food cravings*
- GI complaints
- Headaches*
- Impulsivity
- Mood swings
- Muscle and joint pain
- Insomnia*
- Tension

---

1. APGO Educational Series on Women's Health Issues. Premenstrual Syndrome and Premenstrual Dysphoric Disorder: Scope, Diagnosis and Treatment. APGO, Washington, DC, October 1998.
* Also included in Pope Paul VI Institute criteria.

Exercise and Nutrition:
Non-Pharmacologic Approaches to Treatment

A variety of non-pharmacologic approaches to treatment have been recommended. These include dietary modification such as decreasing caffeine, chocolate, salt, and alcohol intake and increasing complex carbohydrates. Calcium supplementation, vitamin B_6, aerobic exercise, cognitive behavioral modification, relaxation training and group therapy also have been recommended.[7]

It has been reported that conditioning exercise over a six-month period of time may decrease premenstrual symptoms.[8] With the gradual initiation of a running exercise program over a six-month period, a decrease in overall premenstrual symptoms specifically related to breast tenderness and fluid retention was demonstrated.

A specially-designed multivitamin nutritional supplement could have an impact in reducing the symptoms of the various forms of premenstrual syndrome.[9-12] Such supplementation possibly could result in an increased production of progesterone during the postovulatory phase.[10]

It also has been postulated that a magnesium, zinc or calcium deficiency may play a role in the development of premenstrual symptoms.[13-15] Supplementing with magnesium might assist in treating the condition.[14] Calcium imbalance could emanate from inadequate calcium absorption, resulting either from low dietary calcium intake or insufficient vitamin D.

Vitamin B_6 and vitamin E along with the agnus castus fruit extract all have been shown to assist in the treatment of premenstrual syndrome.[16-18] Improvement in PMS symptoms and estrogen metabolism also have been reported using a formulated "medical food" that combines protein, fiber, carbohydrates, fat, and a variety of micronutrients.[19] I have found that exercise and nutrition programs overall are helpful mostly for those women who have mild symptoms.

Pharmacologic Therapy

A variety of drug-treatment approaches have been used in women who have PMS and PMDD. It should be pointed out that oral contraceptives have been considered inadequate for managing women with PMS although they are frequently prescribed for it.[20] Most of the emphasis over the last 10 years has been on the use of alprazolam (Xanax) or one of many antidepressants. A number of studies have shown that alprazolam can be helpful in relieving some of the symptoms of PMS.[21-23] In one famous study published in the *Journal of the American Medical Association*, alprazolam was compared to placebo and oral progesterone in the treatment of severe PMS.[23] In this study, alprazolam was found to be significantly better than placebo or progesterone for total premenstrual symptoms. This particular study had a *methodological flaw,* which is commonly found in studies of therapeutic agents for PMS. All medications were administered from day 18 of the cycle until the first day of menses with a tapering of the medication on the first two menstrual days. Using progesterone in this fashion is *not targeted to the postovulatory phase* and is *not being given cooperatively* with the menstrual cycle.

In 1987, a correlation was found between decreased serotonin levels and depression scores in women who had PMS.[24] This led to the use of a variety of SSRIs (selective serotonin reuptake inhibitors) as the "first line of treatment"[7] for PMS. The initial studies were with fluoxetine (Prozac).[25,26] This led to the marketing of Prozac (fluoxetine hydrochloride) under a new name of Sarafem specifically for reaching those women who had PMS. The product information on Sarafem itself points out that at the standard dose of 20 mg, *only 6 percent of women have marked improvement* and *37 percent have moderate improvement,* for a *total improvement rate of only 43 percent.* While this was indeed greater than the placebo group (15 percent of the placebo group showed marked or moderate improvement), it cannot be considered a highly efficacious treatment.

While alprazolam has been promoted as a routine treatment for PMS, it should be kept in mind that it is one of the most common prescription drugs responsible for admission to drug-dependency units.[27]

Progesterone Treatment

In October 2001, the *British Medical Journal* published a systematic review of the efficacy of progesterone and progestogens (chemicals that have some progesterone-like activity, but are not progesterone) in the management of premenstrual syndrome.[28] This study concluded that the evidence from their meta-analyses (a method of analysis that combines or evaluates the results of a number of studies to investigate a particular issue) did not support the use of progesterone or progestogens for managing PMS. This systematic review did not address, however, the issue of *the timing of progesterone therapy* during the course of the menstrual cycle. *Timed progesterone therapy* is an *extremely important issue* in the evaluation and treatment of this condition. In fact, in the original publications by Dalton,[3,4] she recommended that treatment begin based upon the day of the menstrual cycle and be continued through the beginning of the next menstrual period. This was a *methodological flaw* in her approach to the treatment of this condition as well.

There have been six double-blind placebo-controlled trials of progesterone therapy in women with PMS.[29-34] In five of these studies, no improvement could be identified with the use of progesterone support in the treatment of PMS, while in one of the studies significant improvement was identified.[31] *It is noteworthy that the one study that produced results showing significant improvement with progesterone used properly-timed progesterone administration within the menstrual cycle.*

In these studies, *the methodological flaw in the design of the study*, which has been consistent throughout the history of PMS studies, involves the timing of the administration of progesterone in the cycle. Usually these flawed studies begin the administration of progesterone on day 14 or 16 of the cycle and then continues its use until the beginning of the next menstrual period. In actual fact, the percentage of cycles in which ovulation occurs prior to and including the 14th day of the menstrual cycle is only 34.7 percent. Ovulation occurs following the 14th day in 65.3 percent of cycles. Even at day 20 of the cycle, 7.6 percent of cycles still await ovulation.[35]

The significance of this is diagramed in Figures 17-1 and 17-2. These two figures explain the difference between *non-targeted* progesterone therapy (Figure 17-1) and *targeted* progesterone therapy (or *cooperative progesterone replacement therapy*)(Figure 17-2). In the first instance, progesterone is started on *a given day of the menstrual cycle* (Figure 17-1) — on day 16 in this example (typical of most studies). The progesterone then is continued until the beginning of menses or, in some cases, one or two days after menses. When ovulation occurs on day 14 of the cycle, the beginning of the progesterone

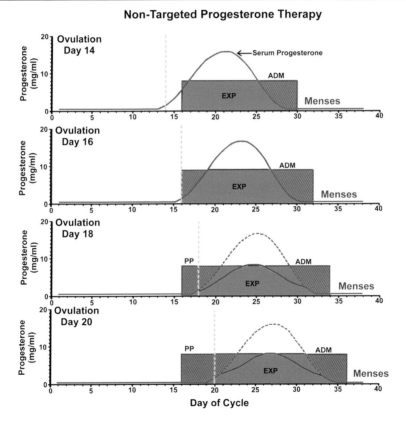

Non-Targeted Progesterone Therapy

PP= Preovulatory Progesterone
EXP= Exogenous Progesterone
ADM= Artificially Delayed Menses

Figure 17-1: A schematic outline of the use of *non-targeted* progesterone with ovulation occurring on days 14, 16, 18 and 20 of the cycle with the progesterone starting automatically on day 16 of the cycle and concluding at the start of menses (From: Pope Paul VI Institute research, 2004). The red area demonstrates the time when the patient is taking her progesterone and (unrelated to when her body actually needs progesterone) how the progesterone administration is out-of-sync.

therapy will be fairly coordinated with the beginning of the naturally-occurring rise in progesterone. *When ovulation occurs later in the cycle, the progesterone will be given in advance of ovulation and thus will have an impact on follicular growth and development. This would be expected to lower artificially the natural production of progesterone by causing the development of a dysfunctional corpus luteum (as the result of an interference in the developing follicle). In addition, the progesterone environment created from the continuation of progesterone until the start of menses artificially delays menses through its impact. In effect, a non-targeted approach to progesterone therapy creates its own hormone*

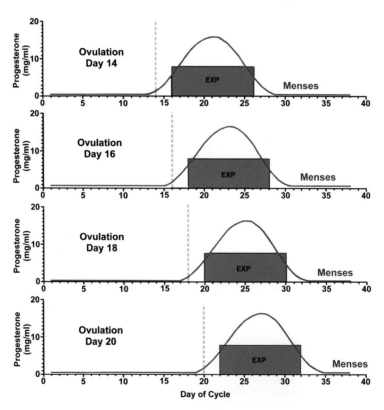

EXP= Exogenous Progesterone

Figure 17-2: A schematic illustration of the use of targeted-progesterone therapy with ovulation occurring on days 14, 16, 18 and 20. Progesterone is given from Peak +3 through Peak +12 or HCG is provided on Peak +3, 5, 7, and 9 and both are finished prior to the onset of menses (From: Pope Paul VI Institute research, 2004).

abnormality as a result of the progesterone being administered in a way that is not in synchrony with the cycle.

This can be corrected, as shown in Figure 17-2, when progesterone is given in a *cooperative* fashion during the course of the menstrual cycle. In this way, progesterone *always is given* following the occurrence of ovulation and discontinued almost always prior to the onset of menses. Supplementation of progesterone or support of the luteal phase in this way will be *cooperative with the women's own production of progesterone* during the course of the postovulatory phase of the cycle. It will maintain the synchrony of the cycle and be therapeutic.

This solves the greatest challenge in the treatment of a variety of women's health conditions. Progesterone-replacement therapy at the wrong time in the cycle represents the single, most important methodological difficulty in the studies done to date on PMS and in a variety of other women's health issues. Targeting of the luteal phase has been, from the beginning of this era of reproductive medicine, grossly in error. This can be corrected when a woman charts her menstrual cycle, identifies her Peak Day with the **CrMS** and begins the progesterone in a cooperative fashion with the post-Peak phase of her cycle.

Other Associated Findings

Drs. Chuong, Coulam, and others studied premenstrual β-endorphin levels in women with PMS and found them to be significantly lower in the postovulatory phase. This finding has been corroborated by others.[37] The PMS patients showed a decrease in β-endorphin the week preceding menses and during the first days of the menstrual flow. The β-endorphin levels regained normal values during the next follicular phase.

These findings of decreased β-endorphin led to a clinical trial of the drug Naltrexone (Trexan, ReVia). A double-blind, placebo-controlled crossover study was used to evaluate the efficacy of this oral opiate receptor antagonist.[38] Using the menstrual distress questionnaire as an objective tool, a significant decrease in symptom expression during the premenstrual phase of the menstrual cycle was found with the use of Naltrexone. It was suggested that this may represent an effective treatment for this syndrome.

NaProTechnology Evaluation and Treatment Protocol

The background provided in the first part of this chapter lays the foundation for the successful **NaProTECHNOLOGY** approach for the treatment of women with PMS. Data in this evaluation is presented on a group of 147 patients who came to us because of PMS and on the first 88 of those patients that we have treated. Data also is presented on hormone profiles for both progesterone, estrogen, and β-endorphin on subgroups of these populations.

The diagnosis of PMS at the Pope Paul VI Institute includes the following list: *irritability, breast tenderness, bloating, weight gain, carbohydrate craving, crying easily, depression, headaches, fatigue and insomnia.* The important aspect to diagnosis is that these symptoms must begin *at least four days prior to the onset of menses.* If they occur within three days of the onset of menses, they are considered to be normal premenstrual symptoms[5] (Table 17-2). In addition to these 10 core symptoms (most of which also are a part of the ICD-10 and the DSM-IV symptom complex), other symptoms also were documented in this group of patients. These included being violent, self-abusive, feeling suicidal, feeling 'wired,' feeling anxious, having panic attacks, feeling confused, feeling paranoid, being anorexic or bulemic, being obsessive-compulsive, having an increased frequency of seizures, and having an increased frequency of sinus infections.

In Table 17-3, the incidence of the 10 core symptoms for these 147 patients is listed. The most common symptoms, occurring in over 75 percent of cases, included irritability, bloating, crying easily, fatigue, depression, carbohydrate craving, breast tenderness and weight gain. Headache and insomnia were frequent but less common than the others.

The average length of time that these symptoms began prior to the onset of menses was 9.4 days. In over 50 percent of patients, the

---

Table 17-2: Diagnosis of Premenstrual Syndrome (PMS)
– NaProTECHNOLOGY

Any of the following symptoms occurring four or more days prior to the onset of menses and fading after menses starts:

• Irritability	• Weight gain	• Depression
• Insomnia	• Bloating	• Crying easily
• CHO craving	• Headaches	• Breast tenderness
• Fatigue	• Other	

Table 17-3: Incidence of Symptoms Associated with Premenstrual Syndrome (PMS) (N=147)

Symptoms	%	Symptoms	%
• Irritability	92.6	• CHO craving	83.7
• Bloating	91.7	• Breast tenderness	82.7
• Crying easily (teariness)	90.2	• Weight gain	75.6
• Fatigue	89.1	• Headache	64.4
• Depression	88.0	• Insomnia	49.2

symptoms started 10 days or more prior to the onset of menses and, in over 90 percent, seven days or greater. This symptom complex and timing is thus very consistent with the more serious condition of premenstrual dysphoric disorder (PMDD).

In evaluating patients, the 10 core symptoms are elicited at the time of entrance into the program. Additional symptoms also are collected if the women have experienced them. The patients then are referred to the **Fertility*Care*™ Center** to begin charting the CrMS so that they can obtain a properly-targeted post-Peak hormone profile. After two cycles have been charted, they return for a complete physical examination and for the ordering of the appropriate blood tests to further evaluate their condition. Once the blood levels are drawn and interpreted, an appropriate treatment regimen is instituted.

This program, from point of entry until the cycle of treatment, requires three cycles with treatment coming in the fourth cycle. Physicians often are frustrated by the length of time from the patient's point of entry to treatment, but when the process of evaluation and eventual treatment is described to patients (who usually have suffered from these symptoms for many years and have seen multiple physicians without adequate assistance) at the point of entry, they are more than willing to participate in their own care so that a diagnosis can be established and proper treatment can be implemented. Part of the approach of **NaProTECHNOLOGY** is to *educate* patients properly so that they understand what is happening within their bodies and can become co-participants in their own evaluation and eventual treatment.

The data that we have obtained on the post-Peak progesterone and estrogen profiles in patients with PMS were compared to a control group of patients who specifically *did not have* PMS and had either exhibited previously normal fertility or had a normal ovulation pattern by ultrasound. The progesterone levels were *significantly decreased* on Peak +7, Peak +9, and Peak +11 and the estrogen levels were *decreased significantly* on Peak +9 and Peak +11.

Beta-endorphins generally increase in the normal patient prior to the onset of menses. That increase in β-endorphin, however, is blunted in patients who have PMS. This is observed by a *significant decrease* in β-endorphins when compared to the control population on Peak +9.

Based on this data, a treatment program for patients who have decreased β-endorphin levels has been developed that uses targeted luteal-phase support (either HCG or preogesterone) as its cornerstone of treatment and Naltrexone, an opiate receptor antagonist, as an additional supportive treatment.

Generally, patients stay on treatment for at least one year and, after that time, consideration can be given to discontinuing the treatment. The treatment commonly needs to be re-instituted long term. I have had patients on post-Peak HCG for as long as 10 years without any difficulties or problems. The husbands often are given instruction on how to administer the injections. Single women are instructed to use subcutaneous injections, which can be self-administered.

For those who received HCG support, 86.5 percent had either *marked* or *moderate improvement* (Table 17-4). In 78 percent of those who received only progesterone support, moderate or marked improvement was observed. The improvement in PMS symptoms with targeted-hormone support then was compared to the published data on fluoxetine hydrochloride (Prozac) 20 mg. Only 43 percent of patients taking fluoxetine had moderate or marked improvement, most

Table 17-4: Premenstrual Syndrome (PMS) Comparison or Response to Treatment — Targeted Hormone Therapy vs. Fluoxetine Hydrochloride

Improvement Response	Fluoxetine 20 mg %	Progesterone Support %	HCG Support %	Placebo %
Marked	6	26.8	51.4	4
Moderate	37	51.2	35.1	11
Total	43[1]	78.0[2]	86.5[3]	15[4]

1. Data based on 95 patients reported in product literature of Sarafem (fluoxetine hydrochloride).
2. Based on 41 patients treated with targeted-progesterone support (with and without lower dose naltrexone), Pope Paul VI Institute.
3. Based on 37 patients treated with targeted-HCG support (with and without lower dose Naltrexone).
4. Data based on 94 patients treated with placebo and cited in product literature of Sarafem (fluoxetine hydrochloride).

of which was just moderate. This is significantly lower than the improvement observed in targeted-hormone support for PMS in the **NaProTECHNOLOGY** protocol. _With the addition of the Naltrexone, 90.4 percent had marked improvement and 95.2 percent had marked or moderate improvement._

Chart analysis (**CrMS**) on patients with and without PMS show that the mucus cycle scores are lower for the PMS group (8.3 vs. 10), but it is not statistically significant (see For the Doctor). On the other hand, the variation in the length of the post-Peak phase is significantly greater for the PMS group (62.5 percent four days or greater variation vs. 10 percent for the group without PMS). This biomarker is consistent with the decrease in progesterone levels previously cited.

One other significant observation is the relationship of premenstrual symptoms in patients who have _infertility_ or a history of _spontaneous abortion (miscarriage)_. While the symptoms in infertility are not as prominent as in women who suffer from PMS specifically, the profile is very similar. In women who have had previous spontaneous abortions, the profile of symptoms is lower than those women who have PMS and infertility, but the profile also is very similar. Overall, about 75 percent of patients with infertility problems will experience significant premenstrual symptoms. This is similar to a previously-reported incidence of 74.6 percent change of mood in patients who have infertility.[39] This raises the possibility that the underlying hormone abnormalities and other changes that occur in women who have infertility problems, spontaneous abortions, and PMS, may be, in some ways, linked to a common cause.

Final Note

Evaluating and successfully treating someone who has PMS is highly gratifying. This condition can have an adverse impact on family life, the relationship of spouses, and the relationship of the mother to her children. Indeed, for many years it has been thought that little could be accomplished in treating these patients. More recently, various anti-depressants, especially the SSRIs, have been recommended as the main line of treatment in this area. By teaching women how to chart their cycles and to observe the changes in their body that are associated with fertility, by targeting the luteal phase for appropriate progesterone and estrogen production along with β-endorphins and thyroid function, and then by implementing a treatment strategy as outlined in this chapter, *incredible success* in the treatment of this condition can be achieved. This, in turn, can have an enormous impact on the women, their families and their spouses.

For the Doctor

1. The primary luteal-phase support program currently in use is *human chorionic gonadotropin* (HCG) given in a dosage of 2000 units Peak +3, 5, 7 and 9 (Figure 17-3). This stimulates the corpus luteum to increase its production of *both* progesterone and estrogen. It usually is given as an intramuscular injection, but it also can be given subcutaneously.

2. Progesterone also can be used as an oral micronized, sustained-release 200 mg capsule given by mouth every day at bedtime, Peak +3 through P+12. This also can be titrated to a two times a day dosage Peak +3 through P+12 if necessary, and progesterone can be used in addition to HCG if that is thought to be clinically necessary. Progesterone vaginal capsules also can be used; in that case, a 300 mg micronized capsule is used vaginally every day at bedtime from Peak+3 through P+12 (Figure 17-4).

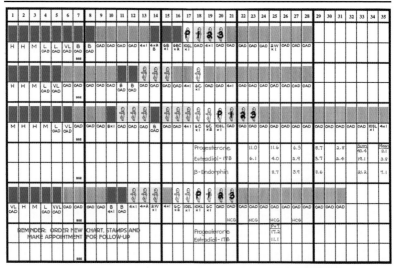

Figure 17-3: A typical patient with her **CrMS** chart during the initial phases of evaluation and treatment. The results of the hormone profile are shown in the third cycle with both progesterone and E$_2$ considered to be decreased. The β-endorphins also were very low. Treatment with HCG luteal phase support, 2000 IU IM on P+3, 5, 7, 9, is shown in the fourth cycle and the corresponding P+7 progesterone and E$_2$ levels have increased (From: Pope Paul VI Institute research, 2004). Refer to page 83 for the VDRS.

3. Naltrexone (Trexan, ReVia) is an opiate receptor antagonist and it is labeled for use in those patients who have heroin addiction or who are alcoholic. It is an extremely good drug for patients who have PMS and decreased β-endorphin levels. In our use of Naltrexone, we have found that the starting dosage of 50 mg per day or 25 mg twice a day produces significant side effects in a patient who is β-endorphin depleted. In fact, that initial dosage is not well tolerated. This can be solved by starting with an *extremely low dosage* of Naltrexone. The standard dosage that we have used begins with 0.25 mg by mouth four times a day (QID) for 10 days and then increases to 0.5 mg QID for 10 days, then 1 mg QID for 10 days and then 2 mg QID for 10 days. The dosage is then increased to 4 mg QID, then 8 mg QID, then 32 mg every day at bedtime (QD hs) and then 50 mg QD hs. These all are cycled on a 10-day program until the highest dose is reached. Then it stays at that dose. With this approach, the overwhelming majority of patients can take Naltrexone without difficulty. On occasion, we see people even at 0.25 mg QID who have difficulty or problems with this drug. In those cases, the dosage has to be started even lower. We would suggest that it start at 0.25 mg by mouth every day for five days, then 0.25 mg two times a day, and so forth, to slowly increase the dosage. It will take longer to get a patient on the Naltrexone using this approach, but the results can be dramatic and it is worth the effort.

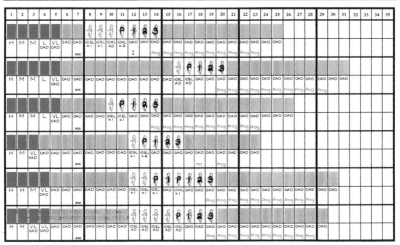

Figure 17-4: In this example, the patient is being treated with progesterone vaginal capsules 300 mg per vagina QD hs P+3 through P+12. In the fourth cycle, the patient decided to discontinue her progesterone. The post-Peak phase shortened and her symptoms recurred. She resumed treatment again in her fifth cycle (From: Pope Paul VI Institute research, 2004). Refer to page 83 for the VDRS.

Real People, Real Problems, Real Solutions

Our **Fertility*Care*™ Practitioner** questioned me about premenstrual syndrome (PMS) on more than one occasion. She had given me a copy of the information on the treatment of PMS from a book and it explained how **NaProTECHNOLOGY** could help me.

I listened and read the information, but still had the mindset that I could deal with this on my own. I had always experienced some form of PMS and recall distinct periods in high school and college when it seemed particularly severe. I had many emotional and physical symptoms that occurred regularly, seven to ten days prior to my period. This included (but was not limited to) irritability, mood swings, crying spells, depressed-type feelings, as well as bloating, breast tenderness, backache, carbohydrate craving and hypoglycemic symptoms. The one to two days prior to my period, I would literally hate the world and everyone in it! After I was married and started to have children, I noticed that the PMS symptoms appeared to intensify after each birth. I did experience some mild to moderate postpartum depression after each of my children's births, but thought I could handle it and never sought treatment… but I couldn't get a handle on the PMS completely.

I contacted my original **Fertility*Care*™ Practitioner** and she gave me the information to submit a referral letter and packet to the Pope Paul VI Institute. She also referred me to another **Fertility*Care*™ Practitioner** who had been treated for PMS by Dr. Hilgers. This "angel" provided me with guidance and talked me through many of my worst days. She truly went above and beyond the call of Christian charity.

I submitted a referral letter to Dr. Hilgers at the Institute and, within a few weeks, I received a response. He was interested in looking more closely at progesterone and other hormones. I did notice, at this time, that my charting pattern had changed with the post-Peak phases becoming shorter. The starting point was the hormonal evaluation. I found a lab manager at a hospital 45 minutes away who was willing to assist me with the evaluation. When the results were analyzed and I contacted the nurses at the Institute, I literally sobbed on the phone. My levels of estrogen and progesterone were very low (I personally like to use the term rock-bottom). I had tried to convince myself that I was either crazy or anxious and that I could make this go away somehow. The nurse explained this was a medical condition that could be treated, and we began to do so. I started with Naltrexone in smaller doses and intramuscular injections of hCG timed with the post-Peak phase of my cycle. In the beginning, a nurse friend gave me the shots, but my husband learned how to do it and became quite proficient at it. The changes began to occur gradually, but the hCG injections tended to have a more immediate effect. My husband and I are still amazed at the effect that this treatment has had on my cycles and my life!

Many people thought I was crazy – trusting some doctor in Nebraska who had never even seen me. I believed he was a man of integrity and I believed he had a great respect for women. I had researched different approaches to PMS treatment before contacting him. I totally put my trust in God at this time and he led me in the direction of the Pope Paul VI Institute. I began the treatment in November 1996 and my quality of life improved gradually over time. I also read a lot of inspirational books, engaged in prayer and bible study, meditation and exercise, as well as trying to surround myself with positive people. I had to also look at such issues as stress management. My personality is such that I tend to be perfectionistic, analytical, etc., qualities that can sometimes make one more prone to anxiety-type disorders. I did a number of self-help measures to help with some of the cognitive aspects of recovery. When I started to feel good again, I couldn't imagine why I had waited so long to pursue treatment. It has made a difference in how I interact with my family. I think I have become a better parent because I am not experiencing the "Jekyll and Hyde" transformations every month.

My message to all women is to be informed and empowered. Learn to respect and appreciate your fertility with the **CREIGHTON MODEL FertilityCare**™ **System**. Have hope that **NaProTECHNOLOGY** will continue to provide answers to reproductive issues that you may deal with in your future. The charting is an excellent medical record and can be a valuable tool in the evaluation and treatment of PMS, among other things.

Susan Loughnane, FCP
Harrison City, Pennsylvania

Postpartum Depression

THE EARLIEST DOCUMENTATION of postpartum mental illness was provided by Hippocrates in 400 B.C.[1] In spite of its evaluation over the millennia, postpartum depression has remained an enigma. Pregnancy, miscarriage or pregnancy loss, infertility, and the postpartum period challenge a woman's mental health. Virtually no life event rivals the hormonal and psychosocial changes associated with pregnancy and childbirth.[2] Because of these depressive episodes, it has been reported that up to 32 percent of women may alter their future childbearing plan by resorting to either adoption, sterilization, or abortion.[3]

Postpartum depression (PPD) is identified in the DSM-IV as *a major depressive disorder with postpartum onset.* It is a major depressive episode that usually begins within the first four weeks following delivery. PPD can be extremely variable in both severity and duration.[4] Symptoms include the following: dysphoric mood, loss of interest in usually pleasurable activities, psychomotor agitation or retaliation, fatigue, changes in appetite or sleep, recurrent thoughts of death/suicide, feelings of worthlessness or guilt (especially failure at motherhood), and excessive anxiety over the child's health.[3]

Postpartum psychosis (PPP) is a *more severe* postpartum syndrome. Its onset usually is within the first three weeks following delivery and often within just a few days.[5] Most episodes are related to a psychotic condition of bipolar disorder or major depression.[6] The symptoms of PPP may include delusions, hallucinations, rapid mood swings ranging from depression and irritability to euphoria, sleep disturbances, and obsessive ruminations about the baby. The risk of suicide in PPP is high (five percent), and up to four percent of women with PPP may attempt infanticide.[7]

PPP is a *psychiatric emergency* that often warrants hospitalization. The prognostic implications for PPP are different from PPD. Nearly two-thirds of these patients will suffer subsequent non-pregnancy-related psychotic episodes.[8-10]

Postpartum mood disorders are common with nearly 40 percent (or more) of women experiencing them. The risk of psychiatric hospitalization within the first three months postpartum is seven times more common than at other periods in a woman's life. The risk of psychosis in the postpartum period is 22 times higher than in the pre-pregnancy state and the relative risk of developing psychosis following childbirth is 16:1. The incidence of puerperal psychosis is 0.1 to 0.2 percent, which is 12 to 14.5 times the prenatal incidence of psychosis.[3]

The incidence of PPD ranges from 12 to 16 percent or up to 25 percent in women with a history of depression. Adolescent pregnancies carry the highest risk for PPD (26 to 32 percent).[11-13] Risk factors that have been identified for PPD include lower occupational status, prenatal depression level, personal psychiatric history, a history of premenstrual syndrome (PMS) or previous postpartum depression, a history of mood disorder (bipolar or major depression), and a genetic vulnerability.[12,14-16]

Cause

Direct evidence supports the involvement of the reproductive hormones estrogen and progesterone in the development of PPD. Studies have shown that maternal mood in the days immediately following delivery is related to the withdrawal of naturally-occurring progesterone.[17]

In an evaluation of serum progesterone levels at the **NaProTECHNOLOGY** research center, women with PPD had higher levels of progesterone during their pregnancies than the normal controls although this was statistically significant only during the first 12 weeks of pregnancy. If the progesterone levels are higher during pregnancy, the larger decrease in progesterone and its metabolites at the time following delivery could be a contributing factor in PPD. Abnormalities in the function of the adrenal gland also play a role.[18]

The Usual Approach to Treatment

Some have recommended psychotherapy as the first line of treatment for PPD.[19] While cognitive behavioral or individual psychotherapy has been effective with and without medication, such therapy often is unavailable, too expensive, or inaccessible because of childcare difficulties. As a result, many women opt for some type of antidepressant therapy.[20]

Antidepressant therapy can be prescribed during the postpartum period except when breast feeding. Response to any available antidepressant requires at least four to six weeks, assuming the patient is taking an appropriate dose. The likelihood of success in the patient who completes the first three weeks of treatment (the initial drop-out rate from side effects is approximately 15 percent) can reach as high as 60 to 70 percent.[21] It is usually recommended that, following full remission of symptoms, medication should be continued for an additional 16 to 20 weeks. At that time, a maintenance dosage may be established. During breast feeding, the safe use of the selective serotonin re-uptake inhibitors (SSRIs) has not been established clearly.

Most recently, estrogen support has been used in the treatment of PPD.[22] It has been hypothesized that the rapid rate of change in estrogen following delivery creates an "estrogen withdrawal state." The use of estrogen has been shown to have a positive effect on PPD,[22-24] but its usage by breast feeding women has been questioned.[23]

In 1956, it was reported that a "striking benefit" could be achieved through the use of progesterone in women with PPD.[25] In this treatment program, 100 mg of progesterone by injection was given every day for about 10 days. It then was given orally in doses of 150 mg per day. Following this, in 1980, Dr. Katharina Dalton[26] advocated the use of progesterone for the treatment of PPD.

In 1988, Dr. Dalton visited our program because of my interest in PMS. During the course of that visit, she commented on her long experience with the use of progesterone in the treatment of PPD. In addition, she seemed to think PPD was a very common problem. In our own clinical experience, this condition was rare — the incidence of PPD in our program was only 2.1 percent. At the time, we thought that because progesterone support during pregnancy in our high-risk pregnancy population was common, it may have had an impact on the overall incidence of PPD in our patient population.

These discussions prompted an interest in the use of progesterone support for the treatment of PPD. Studies then were undertaken to understand the role of progesterone therapy for women with PPD. These were undertaken in two phases.

The Phase I Progesterone Support Study

In the first phase, patients were enrolled from our patient population, along with patients who contacted us from the **Fertility***Care***™ Centers** throughout the United States and were treated by long distance. These patients contacted us because of their symptoms of postpartum depression. These symptoms then were evaluated and documented to the extent possible and progesterone therapy was initiated. No particular protocol for treatment with progesterone was utilized. Rather, an empirical administration of progesterone was utilized to see what might prove to be the most effective means of treating this condition. These patients were followed on a daily to weekly basis until their PPD either resolved itself or needed further psychiatric treatment.

The most common symptoms elicited in this group of patients were *depression, anxiety/panic, uncontrollable crying, fatigue, insomnia, poor appetite, a shaky feeling, and suicidal thoughts.* In addition, other symptoms that were conveyed to us included *helplessness, feeling wired, having strange thoughts, hot flashes, night sweats, a rapid heartbeat, and nausea.*

These patients were treated with progesterone using different programs of treatment. This was an open-ended study program because the best dosages and roots of administration were not known at this time. A few patients also were treated during pregnancy with progesterone along with being treated during the postpartum period. Intramuscular, oral and/or vaginal progesterone (bio-identical progesterone) were used at various doses. From this, *the basic effect of progesterone could be observed* and a program for management could be developed. In 20 of the 23 patients (86.9 percent), either an excellent (73.7 percent) or very good (13 percent) outcome was obtained. Three episodes had poor outcomes (13 percent). In each of the three cases in which the outcome was poor, the patients previously had suffered from severe episodes of PPP and/or the use of progesterone began several weeks or months after the beginning of symptoms. *In cases where treatment was initiated early and aggressively, the symptoms were alleviated with excellent or very good results in all cases (20 out of 20).*

In studying these cases, there were a number of treatment factors that could be identified. First of all, the use of progesterone for the treatment of PPD and anxiety often was *dramatic* when used early in the symptom complex. Patients would tell us such things as, *"This is a miracle," "I am feeling great," "I feel considerably better," "I cannot believe how good I feel within two hours of the progesterone injection,"* and *"The difference is between day and night."*

The results with progesterone treatment were *most dramatic* with the use of *intramuscular injections of progesterone.* I needed to be willing to titrate the dose against the occurrence of a patient's symptoms. On many occasions, we had patients tell us that the symptoms disappeared within minutes or hours following the injection of progesterone. In some cases, oral or vaginal progesterone also had a role to play, but in those cases it was mostly as a supplement to the intramuscular progesterone. As a result of this first phase evaluation of progesterone support, a prospective program for evaluation and treatment was implemented to begin a Phase II evaluation of progesterone support.

The Phase II Progesterone Support Study

In the second phase of this study, 30 patients with PPD were enrolled in a similar fashion as in the first phase study. In each of these cases, the clinical data was accumulated prospectively by the nurses who were interacting with these patients. A list of symptoms was obtained in an objective fashion prior to and after treatment. In addition, the exact treatment dosages and dates could be identified.

The response in the improvement of symptoms was considered to be marked in 26 of the 30 patients (86.7 percent). Three of the 30 patients (10 percent) had moderate improvement while only one had no improvement at all (3.3 percent).

An analysis of the symptom complex both before and after treatment was conducted for all 30 patients. The most common symptoms were *depression, fatigue, crying, anxiety, helplessness, strange thoughts, poor appetite, and night sweats.* Treatment with progesterone provided a statistically significant improvement in all of them. In all other categories, an improvement was identified, but the numbers were too small to identify statistical significance. It should be noted that in the two patients who had suicidal thoughts, however, the symptom disappeared after progesterone therapy.

In this same group of patients, the average number of symptoms both before and after progesterone therapy also was evaluated. The average number of symptoms prior to therapy was 7.57 and following therapy with progesterone treatment it decreased to 2.1. This was statistically very significant.

Because the treatment in both the Phase I and Phase II populations of this study were very similar, cumulative results of both phases were combined. In this group of 53 episodes of PPD in 50 patients, marked improvement was identified in 43 of the 53 episodes (81.1 percent) and moderate improvement was observed in another six episodes (11.3 percent). This resulted in a marked or moderate improvement in 92.4 percent of the episodes treated. Treatment resulted in no improvement in only four of the 53 episodes (7.5 percent). This group decreased in the second phase of the study to only 3.3 percent. The current treatment protocol using progesterone to treat postpartum depression is shown in the action item at the end of this chapter.

While this is an open-ended study without a control population, previous studies conducted with placebo control groups have found that 65 to 74 percent of patients *remain depressed over a four-month period* of time when given placebo.[27] Clearly, there is room for more study to be done in this area and studies to be designed in such a fashion as to take into consideration a randomized, double-blind approach. When results are this dramatic, they cannot be ignored.

In the current literature, progesterone therapy is for the most part not mentioned. The first line of therapy often is considered to be psychotherapy followed by antidepressant agents or antidepressants from the start. Everyone agrees, however, that the prompt recognition and efficacious treatment of postpartum mood disorders are essential to avoid adverse outcomes for both mother and infant.[27] The use of progesterone in these cases falls clearly into that concept.

Progesterone for Depression

One case history that I have treated because of our interest in PMS and PPD is worth reporting. This 50-year-old woman had had a total abdominal hysterectomy with removal of both tubes and ovaries four years earlier (by other physicians). She also had suffered from both PMS and PPD in the past. Her husband called us to see whether we had ever treated depression with progesterone. This postmenopausal woman was about to be released from psychiatric hospitalization and was on multiple psychiatric medications, but still not feeling well. We informed him that we had never treated such a condition with progesterone before, but we would be willing to try, seeing no harm in adding progesterone to her regimen.

After receiving progesterone, she began to feel better. When the progesterone was discontinued, however, she immediately would get worse again. Only intramuscular (IM) progesterone worked. While multiple attempts were made to discontinue her supplemental IM progesterone without success, she has now been on this treatment for over four consecutive years. She is feeling very well, and is off her antidepressants. To date, she has tolerated the injections of progesterone very well and is motivated to continue them because of how well she feels. All of her family members and clinical observation, have documented her improvement.

While IM progesterone is not being advocated here for the primary treatment of depression (unrelated to childbirth), this case report shows such significant improvement that further research needs to be done.

For the Doctor

1. Treatment Protocol for Postpartum Depression with the Use of Progesterone

    A. When symptoms start, give 200 mg progesterone in sesame oil IM and have patient call in 24 hours.

    B. If marked improvement, no need to treat further, but do follow.

    C. If symptoms are improved but have recurred or are still somewhat present:
        ↳ 100 mg progesterone IM QOD x 5 days
        ↳ If markedly improved, no need to treat further but have patient call if symptoms return.
        ↳ If symptoms recur or are persistent, then repeat progesterone 100 mg IM QOD x 5 doses
        ↳ If continues to improve but symptoms persist, repeat the above series and add 200 mg SR progesterone PO BID x 10 days for two months

    D. In about one in 20 cases, IM progesterone may be necessary for up to two months.

Infertility: What Progress Over 50 Years?

NFERTILITY USUALLY IS defined as the inability of a couple to achieve pregnancy when not using contraceptives, but engaging in random intercourse over the course of at least one year. This definition is based upon the original 1950 investigations of Christopher Tietze who reported that 90 percent of 1727 couples, followed for one year, became pregnant.[1] This leaves 10 percent of couples as a group that could be classified, by subtraction, as infertile.

According to the 2002 National Survey of Family Growth (NSFG), the only source of current, nationally representative infertility data, it has been estimated that there are 9.5 million women of reproductive age in the United States who have impaired fertility.[2] The incidence has increased significantly from 10.8 percent of married women in 1982 to 12.9 percent in 1995 and an estimated 15.3 percent in 2002.

Infertility is divided further into primary and secondary. *Primary infertility* is the inability to achieve any pregnancy while *secondary infertility* presupposes the existence of at least one previous pregnancy. In most infertility programs, about 40 percent of the patients coming for medical assistance will be in the secondary infertility category.

Over the last 32 years, the evaluation and treatment of the patient with infertility has undergone significant change. This was influenced most dramatically by the birth of the first baby conceived through *in vitro* fertilization in 1978. Since that time, the trend in the treatment of infertility has been in the development of various means to artificially replace the natural procreative system. This has had an enormous and, one could argue, significantly deleterious effect on the medical care of this group of women and on the practice of medicine itself.

Evaluation of Infertility

The evaluation of infertility has undergone a significant change over the last several decades. *An interest in identifying the underlying causes of the infertility problem has diminished significantly!* As a result, few diagnostic tests are being performed and some of those that are selected are less meaningful.

While almost everyone would recommend that the patient undergo a history and physical examination, there is not always agreement with regard to the other tests to be performed. Ovulation assessment needs to be carried out, but techniques such as basal body temperatures, mid-luteal phase progesterone levels and endometrial biopsy, which in some ways can be considered "medieval," often are recommended. The LH predictor kits (ovulation home test kits) that often are recommended have significant drawbacks.

Programs also want to test for tubal patency (to see if the fallopian tubes are open) and the integrity of the uterine cavity. This often is undertaken with the use of hysterosalpingography (an x-ray of the uterus and tubes). Hormonal integrity is tested with a day-3 FSH level and, of course, the male is tested with a seminal fluid analysis.

In addition to the above, such tests as a clomiphene challenge test, pelvic ultrasound examination, post-coital test and hysteroscopy are used, but only sparingly. Laparoscopy often is considered an *optional* examination and not one that would be used routinely.

There are other tests that are recommended in varying degrees by different programs. These would include such things as rubella and hepatitis screening, HIV testing, Chlamydia serology, evaluation for sperm antibodies and sperm penetration tests.[3-6]

Unfortunately, tests such as the basal body temperature, mid-luteal phase progesterone, endometrial biopsy and LH testing kits *are not definitive tests for ovulation* and definitely not adequate for identifying the various defects of ovulation. The first three will test for the production of progesterone by the ovary (but not abnormal progesterone production). In most of the ovulation defects, however, a corpus luteum is formed (even if ovulation has not occurred) and progesterone is produced causing presumptive signs of ovulation when, in fact, ovulation has *not* occurred or is *defective*. In addition, one can have a perfectly normal LH surge (which will show up in the LH test kits) in cycles where an unruptured follicle is present and ovulation has not occurred. Unfortunately, concepts such as "if a woman is having regular menstrual cycles that are 23 to 39 days in length, then she is ovulating,"[7] while erroneous, continue to be persistent.[8]

Hysterosalpingography, while having its own value, also has its limitations. In the presence of a normal hysterosalpingogram, laparoscopy may identify other pelvic disease in about half of the patients.[9]

Causes of Infertility

In reviewing the medical literature and seeing patients who have been evaluated elsewhere, it is very difficult to get an accurate view of the underlying causes of infertility. Representative authorities each have a different view of what might be significant.[2, 10-12] While it is generally stated that 30 percent of infertility problems will be related to a male factor problem, 30 percent to a female factor problem and 40 percent to a combination of the two, documentation of that is difficult to find and it appears to be mostly wishful politically-correct rhetoric.

In a review of the causes of infertility identified by various authorities, infertility was thought to be due to the male factor in a range of 6.2 to 30 percent. There were a multitude of causes found in women, including tubal factor, tubal/peritoneal factor, ovulatory dysfunction, endometriosis, diminished ovarian reserve, uterine/cervical factors, immunological factors, and unexplained reasons. But in some cases, ovulatory dysfunction was not identified as a cause and in other cases endometriosis was not identified. In most cases, endometriosis was seen to be a relatively infrequent cause of infertility.

In this same review, endometriosis was identified as the causative factor in 5, 5.6 and 25.8 percent of the patients, but endometriosis is extremely difficult to diagnose *without* laparoscopy. Laparoscopic evaluation in the infertile woman has been known for many years to provide a high yield of significant pelvic disease.[13] Cervical factor was identified in a very small percentage of patients. Dr. M. Hull, in 1998, pointed out that cervical mucus defects and disorders are infrequent causes of infertility (three percent) and are difficult to diagnose with certainty. Furthermore, he pointed out that the most obvious defects result from cervical surgery, particularly conization of the lower cervical canal.[3] This was echoed by the Boston IVF group[7] who went on to say that "some women notice this change in the cervical mucus, whereas others do not," implying that this information is not reliable or helpful. In this regard, the obvious following question would be: Why do some women not notice this change in the cervical mucus?

Approaches to Treatment

A staircase approach to the current evaluation and treatment of infertility is shown in Figure 19-1. Many programs have developed complex protocols for the implementation of a treatment program for the infertile patient.[3-5,7] These protocols involve almost invariably an artificial approach to reproduction. The approaches tend to replace the normal sexual procreative union with a physician substitute. While in most textbooks this is referred to as "assisted reproductive technology" (ART), in this book it is referred to as "*artificial* reproductive technology" because it is an artificial substitute for human procreation.

Treatment usually begins with some type of ovulation induction protocol often employing "super-ovulation strategies."[14] "Super-ovulation" means that the ovaries are over-stimulated by hormones so as to develop multiple follicles in each ovary. This is often in the range of 10 follicles per ovary. Usually some form of artificial insemination, either with the husband's sperm or a donor sperm, also is implemented.

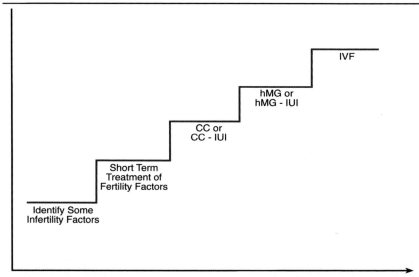

Figure 19-1: A staircase approach to current evaluation and treatment of infertility. It is recommended that for women older than 35 years, the first two steps should be rapidly completed. For women younger than 30 years of age, more time can be spent on these steps. CC = clomiphene citrate; IUI = intrauterine insemination; hMG = human menopausal gonadotropin; IVF = in vitro fertilization.

When these do not work effectively, then *in vitro* fertilization usually is recommended. On occasion, reconstructive pelvic surgery, either by open incision or, most likely by operative laparoscopy, is still used. But over the last 15 years it has been utilized less and less. In fact, there is great concern at this time as to the overall surgical skill of the reproductive specialist in providing these types of therapies.

Artificial Insemination

One of the main techniques used in the current practice of reproductive medicine to help women become pregnant is *artificial insemination.* This is a technique where the physician usurps the role of the husband or father by performing an insemination procedure. This procedure can be done with either fresh or frozen sperm from either the husband or a donor by placing the sperm within the cervix or bypassing the cervix through direct injection of the sperm into the uterine cavity (intrauterine insemination). The procedure usually is combined with the stimulation of ovulation with either clomiphene citrate or FSH. The insemination usually is timed with the use of ultrasound observation of ovulation or the use of the urinary LH test kits.

Success rates for non-medicated intrauterine insemination (IUI) is not much different than for normal intercourse (Table 19-1). With either clomiphene citrate or FSH stimulation combined with IUI, the per-cycle success rate does go up, but so does the multiple pregnancy rate (including high-order multiples, for example, triplets, quadruplets and so forth).

It is well accepted that artificial insemination with donor sperm (AID) is more effective in achieving pregnancy than artificial insemination with husband's sperm (AIH) when used in women whose

Treatment	Success Rate (per cycle) (%)	Multiple Pregnancy Rate (%)
Normal intercourse	3-4	1
Non-medicated IUI[2]	4	1
Clomiphene citrate-IUI	8-10	10
FSH-IUI	15-18	20-25

Table 19-1: Success Rates of Artificial Insemination[1]

1. From: Bayar SR, Alper MM, Penzias AS: The Boston IVF Handbook of Infertility. Parthenon Publishing Group, Boca Raton, 2002.
2. IUI = intrauterine insemination.

husbands have severe oligospermia (low sperm count).[15-18] But the procedure presumes the acceptance of an unidentified biological father. This poses significant and legitimate moral and ethical problems for many patients.

In reviewing the studies on AIH, control subjects who are of similar medical background, and who have fertility-focused intercourse (FFI), are never used as controls. As a result, an artificial approach to insemination is used as a replacement for natural insemination with little or no evidence that it is superior.

This approach to the care of fertility-related problems also has led to a denigration of the integrity of both marriage and parenthood. It has been used to impregnate single women[19,20] and lesbians.[21] The role of the father in the healthy parenting of children has been discarded by many physicians. This is irresponsible and purposely puts children in danger.

Artificial Reproductive Technologies

The artificial reproductive technologies (ART) involve surgically removing eggs from a woman's ovaries, combining them with sperm in the laboratory and returning them to the woman's body or donating them to another woman (this is sometimes referred to as a "test tube baby"). They do not include treatments in which only sperm are handled (for example, intrauterine or artificial insemination) or procedures in which a woman takes drugs only to stimulate egg production without the intention of having eggs retrieved.

The types of ART include the following:[2]

IVF (in vitro fertilization): This involves extracting a woman's eggs, fertilizing the eggs in the laboratory and then transferring all or some of the resulting embryos into the woman's uterus through the cervix. For some IVF procedures, fertilization involves a specialized technique known as intracytoplasmic sperm injection (ICSI). In ICSI, a single sperm is injected directly into the woman's egg. The IVF procedures represent 99.7 percent of all ART performed with 59.6 percent being ICSI procedures.

GIFT (gamete intrafallopian transfer): This involves the use of a laparoscope to guide the transfer of unfertilized eggs and sperm (gametes) into the woman's fallopian tubes through small incisions in her abdomen. This represents 0.1 percent of all ART procedures.

ZIFT (zygote intrafallopian transfer): This involves fertilizing a woman's eggs in the laboratory and then using a laparoscope to guide the transfer of the fertilized eggs (zygotes) into her fallopian tubes. This represents 0.2 percent of all ART procedures.

In addition, the ART procedures often are categorized according to whether the procedure used a woman's own eggs (*non-donor*) or eggs from another woman (*donor*) and according to whether the embryos used were newly fertilized (*fresh*) or previously fertilized (*frozen and then thawed*). The ART procedure includes several steps and typically is referred to as *a cycle of treatment.*

In 1992, the U.S. Congress passed the Fertility Clinic Success Rate and Certification Act (FCSRCA). This required that all clinics performing ART in the United States annually report their success rate data to the Center for Disease Control (CDC). The CDC uses the data to publish an annual report detailing the ART success rates for each of these clinics. One of the *inherent drawbacks* to this reporting requirement is the fact that the CDC contracts with a professional society (The Society of Assisted Reproductive Technology – SART) to obtain the data published each year in the ART success rate's report. SART is an organization of ART providers affiliated with the American Society for Reproductive Medicine (ASRM). While cooperation of the ART clinics is important to conduct such a data analysis, it does produce a potential *conflict of interest* with regard to the type of data reported. Nonetheless, the report provides the only national data available for the United States on the ART programs. The data provided in the November 2008 report (2006 National Summary) now is reviewed.

The success of ART is presented in a variety of ways. The three major ways include the number of "live births per cycle started," the "live births per retrieval," and the "live births per transfer." The most important statistic *from an infertility patient's point of view* is the "live births per cycle started" because this provides that couple with information on success at the point of entry. The national summary statistics most often quote success rates based upon "live births per transfer," which overstates the success rates.

In Table 19-2, the live birth rate per cycle started and cancellation rates in the National Summary are presented. The live birth rate per cycle started was 28.6 percent. The singleton live birth rate per cycle

Table 19-2: Live Birth Rates per Cycle Started and Cancellation Rates: ART 2005 National Summary[1]

Item	Percent
Live birth rate per cycle started	28.6
Singleton live birth rates per cycle started	22.4
Cancellation of cycles started	11

1. From: 2006 Assisted Reproductive Technology Success Rates: National Summary and Fertility Clinic Reports. Centers of Disease Control and Prevention. National Center for Chronic Disease Prevention and Health Promotion. Division of Reproductive Health. Atlanta, Georgia, November 2008.

started was 22.4 percent and the cancellation rate of cycles started was "about 11 percent" (with some centers having much higher cancellation rates). The latter information indicates that of 100 cycles started, only about 89 could move to either the retrieval or transfer stage. Thus, one out of nine patients automatically cannot move into a more advanced phase of treatment because of the cancellation.

There is considerable variation in the live birth rate per cycle started (LBRPCS) when looking at the woman's age upon entry into the program. The success rate is higher for those women less than 35 years of age and significantly lower for those women 38 years of age or older. While the initial live birth rate per cycle started at age <35 years is 39 percent, it decreases to 4 percent for women greater than 42 years of age (Table 19-3). When reporting LBRPCS, one could get the impression that if enough cycles were tried, the pregnancy rate would be very high. While it is impossible to say because of the way the data is presented just how many cycles the average woman actually goes

Table 19-3: Live Birth Rates per Cycle Started by Woman's Age (No Previous Pregnancies) Fresh Non-donor Eggs or Embryos 2006 National Summary[1]

Woman's Age	Percent
<35	39
35-37	30
38-40	21
41-42	11
>42	4

1. From: 2006 Assisted Reproductive Technology Success Rates: National Summary and Fertility Clinic Reports. Centers of Disease Control and Prevention. National Center for Chronic Disease Prevention and Health Promotion. Division of Reproductive Health. Atlanta, Georgia, November 2008.

through, it can be said that the average number of cycles started is almost for sure *less than two cycles.*

One of the *major methodological flaws* in the national data set is that *pregnancy rates are not calculated on a "per woman" basis.* The stated reason for this is that "success rates cannot be calculated on a 'per woman' basis because women's names are not reported to SART and CDC."[2] This is an incredibly weak and inadequate reason for not performing this calculation. There are many ways in which a patient's confidentiality and anonymity can be maintained and protected in such a reporting system. Unfortunately, this leaves one with the mistaken notion that if one undergoes an ART treatment cycle, it will produce an approximately 28.6 percent success rate per cycle started and if one undergoes enough treatment cycles, one should almost be guaranteed a pregnancy. The *drop-out rate* after the first cycle, however, is *extremely high.* Because of duplication with some patients receiving multiple cycles, it is impossible to calculate how many women actually have had access to this form of treatment. What is known is that in the year 2006, 41,343 live births resulting in 54,656 babies resulted from the ART (IVF) programs in the United States.[2] This amounts to ***0.44 percent of all women with impaired fertility*** who are successfully treated in the ART (IVF) programs in the United States. The percentage of women undergoing a subsequent ART cycle (from the 2006 National Summary) shows a sharp drop-out rate after the first cycle with only 42.5 percent entering a second cycle and 12.4 percent going four or more cycles.

The different clinics around the United States provide a number of different services and these also are identified in the 2006 National Summary. Almost all of the clinics provide *cryopreservation* (frozen embryo) services. This allows for the freezing of embryos and often the freezing of gametes (both sperm and ova). *Donor egg* services are provided by 93 percent of the clinics and *single women* are served by 90 percent. In addition, *surrogates* (now referred to as "*gestational carriers*") are provided by 81 percent of clinics and *donor embryos* by 65 percent.[2] This strengthens the notion that *these clinics are not interested* in programs that support biological parenthood with both a mother and a father.

When these procedures are undertaken, more than one embryo almost always is placed (89.3 percent). In fact, *the average number of* *embryos transferred per ART cycle is **2.6***. It is known that the success rate for even a singleton pregnancy increases somewhat by placing more than one embryo. But this also means that the embryo wastage increases significantly. In fact, ***5.88 embryos are placed for every single live birth*** (Table 19-4). The technology is built upon the principle of ***creating life through destroying life***. In order to obtain the 54,656 live babies born from ART cycles (included in this number are the multiple births), an estimated ***266,730 embryos had to be wasted***. It does not count the embryos that were created in the process and stored in freezers, most of whom are terminal.

As a result of this approach to treatment, a large number of successes result in *multiple pregnancies*. In a group of pregnancies from ART cycles in which fresh non-donor cycles were used, 31.8 percent were multiple pregnancies with 28.0 percent being twins and 3.8 percent triplets or greater (Table 19-5).

In comparing the trend over a five-year period of time, the National Summary showed that there has been a decrease in the multiple pregnancy rate during this period of time from 38.4 in 1996 to 31.8 in 2006. There has been a significant commentary on this to see that this happens.[22-27] Compared with women with naturally-conceived pregnancies, however, a 29-fold increase in multiple births among women exposed to these treatments is achieved. By comparison, the multiple pregnancy rate with **NaProTECHNOLOGY** is *only 3.2 percent (**10 times less than with ART**)*.

Table 19-4: Number of Embryos Wasted for Every Live Birth using ART Approaches 2006 National Summary[1]

Type of Cycle	Total Number of Embryos Transferred
Fresh embryos from non-donor eggs	240,843
Frozen embryos from non-donor eggs	45,790
Embryos from donor eggs	36,753
Total embryos transferred	321,386
Number of live babies born from ART cycles	54,656
Embryos: Live Birth Ratio	**5.88:1**

1. From: 2006 Assisted Reproductive Technology Success Rates: National Summary and Fertility Clinic Reports. Centers of Disease Control and Prevention. National Center for Chronic Disease Prevention and Health Promotion. Division of Reproductive Health. Atlanta, Georgia, November 2008.

**Table 19-5: Distribution of 34,719 Pregnancies
from ART Fresh Non-donor Cycles
2006 National Summery[1]**

Outcome of Pregnancy	Percent
Singleton birth	61.6
Twin birth	28.0
Triplets or more	3.8

1. From: 2006 Assisted Reproductive Technology Success Rates: National Summary and Fertility Clinic Reports. Centers of Disease Control and Prevention. National Center for Chronic Disease Prevention and Health Promotion. Division of Reproductive Health. Atlanta, Georgia, November 2008.

The increase in the number of multiple births because of the ART approach has increased significantly the rates of triplet and high order multiple births in the United States. A comparison study between 1980 and 1997 has shown that, on a national scale, there has been a 4.7-fold increase in the number of triplet and high order multiple births.[28] It is well recognized that these multiple pregnancies are at increased risk to deliver prematurely. *Prematurity poses a great risk to the neonates and places an inordinate demand on health care resources!*

There also are maternal complications to the super-ovulated ART procedures. The *ovarian hyperstimulation syndrome* (OHSS) is an exaggerated response to ovulation induction therapy. While it is not limited to the ART procedures, and may theoretically occur with any ovulation-induction protocol, it is clearly more common in those women who undergo super-ovulation techniques. This condition can occur in one to two percent of ovulation induction cycles and ART procedures and *it can be life threatening!* The OHSS is typically associated with gonadotropin stimulation and rarely is observed with the use of other agents (clomiphene citrate and gonadotropin-releasing hormone). It tends to be self-limiting and resolves spontaneously within several days, but it can persist for longer periods of time, particularly in conception cycles. The syndrome has a broad spectrum of clinical manifestations ranging from a mild illness needing only careful observation to severe disease requiring hospitalization and even intensive care.[29] *By contrast, I have never seen a patient with OHSS in 30 years of treating infertility with* **NaProTECHNOLOGY.**

With the ART procedures, there is an increased emphasis on prenatal diagnosis and selective abortion. Many patients are advised that a healthy baby cannot be "guaranteed" and thus, it should be decided *in advance* that prenatal diagnosis be undertaken so that if an abnormal baby is identified it can be aborted. This prenatal diagnosis is accomplished either with genetic amniocentesis or, more and more, with early blastomere diagnosis. This is one of the reasons why women who have suffered from infertility and who desperately want the pregnancy they are working towards actually undergo an induced abortion. These are women who normally would not seek abortion but feel trapped by the *"new abortion" technologies.* For other women, they feel *abandoned by the medical profession* because they would never be willing to participate in such abortion technologies.

What Progress Over 50 Years

An enormous amount of attention has been paid to the artificial reproductive technologies over the last 30 years. National television programs continue to   play a special interest in those parents who conceive sextuplets or septuplets and give birth as a result of these technologies. *The public is led to think that this is really the only approach available to the solution to their problem.* One must begin to realistically question whether or not any real progress has been made.

In 1950, Dr. Meaker[30] reported a series of 65 patients who underwent ovarian wedge resection for polycystic ovarian disease. Of this group, 77 percent with irregular bleeding developed normal cycles and 66 percent of the infertile women became pregnant. In the 1960s, clomiphene citrate became available and polycystic ovaries could be treated medically. But the pregnancy rate decreased to about 30 percent[31] and it was hailed as a success. More recently, *in vitro* fertilization also has been promoted for treating polycystic ovaries with success rates of about 23 to 25 percent per cycle.[32,33] *There is no question that the "per woman" pregnancy rate has declined over the last five decades of treatment of polycystic ovarian disease* (Figure 19-2).

In women with endometriosis, it was not uncommon 25 years ago to get "per woman" pregnancy rates in the 50 to 60 percent range (over a course of 36 months of treatment)[34] while the 2006 National Summary for the treatment of endometriosis claims a 33.1 percent live birth rate per cycle started.[2] The data from the National Summary is interesting in that it has been noted specifically by others that patients with endometriosis-associated infertility who undergo IVF respond with a pregnancy rate that is almost one-half that of women with other indications for IVF.[35] On a "per-woman basis," the pregnancy rates with the standard conservative surgery for endometriosis management were higher two decades ago than they are currently with ART approaches (Figure 19-3).

In 1978, an intrauterine pregnancy rate of 29 percent could be expected in patients who underwent microsurgical salpingostomy (surgically correcting the tubal obstruction)[36] while the National Summary for IVF reported a pregnancy rate per cycle started of 29.1 percent for patients with tubal factor infertility[2] (Figure 19-4).

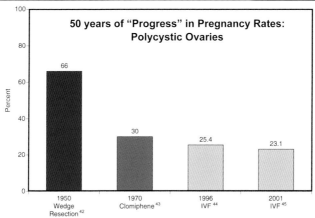

Figure 19-2: Fifty years of "progress" in pregnancy rates in patients with polycystic ovarian disease. In 1950, the pregnancy rate from wedge resection was 66 percent. In 2001, the pregnancy rate per cycle started with IVF was 23.1.

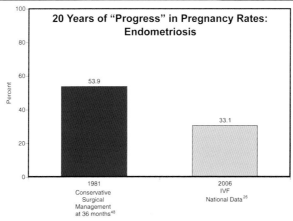

Figure 19-3: "Progress" in the development of pregnancies over 24 years in patients with endometriosis. In 1981, 53.9 percent of patients achieved pregnancy over 36 months ("per woman") with conservative surgical management. In 2006, the pregnancy rate per cycle started with IVF was 33.1.

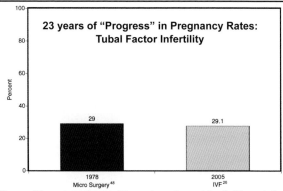

Figure 19-4: "Progress" in pregnancies over 27 years in patients with tubal factor infertility. In 1978, microsurgical correction of tubal adhesions resulted in a 29 percent "per woman" pregnancy rate. In 2005, the live birth per cycle started with IVF was 29.1.

When I discuss these changes in effectiveness of treatment with medical students I tell them that if such a trend were observed in the treatment of HIV/AIDS "all hell would break loose!" But because these are women seeking pregnancy in a culture that spends most of its efforts suppressing or destroying fertility, they are especially powerless. As far as it can be determined, this is the only place in medicine where a decline in success rate has been promoted as an advance in therapy.

The Outcome of Pregnancies

In 1974, Drs. S.R. Stewart and I.D. Cooke[37] made the important observation that "Once the infertile patient becomes pregnant, it does not follow that her management has been successfully completed. The only confirmation of success should be the delivery of a healthy child and so the management of her pregnancy should be as important as the management of her infertility." And yet, the current approach to infertility in the United States and much of the Western world views infertility as an isolated circumstance and once the patient becomes pregnant, she is referred back to her local physician (either an obstetrician or a family physician) for the care of her pregnancy. In actuality, these pregnancies can be highly complicated.

It has been known for a long time that pregnancies achieved with the use of ovulation-induction protocols carry with them an increased risk of pregnancy-related complications. These complications would include such things as *prematurity associated with multiple births*,[38] and the high incidence of *toxemia of pregnancy*.[39] Along with toxemia in pregnancy, which also is seen more commonly in women who have been treated with donor insemination,[40] other problems such as *ectopic pregnancy, gestational diabetes, operative deliveries, fetal distress, low Apgar scores,* and *low birth weight babies* are observed more frequently.[41-43]

More recently, an increased risk of toxemia of pregnancy associated with intrauterine insemination,[44] donor insemination,[45] and donated gametes[46] has been reported. In addition, over and over again complications associated with an increased incidence of preterm labor, low birth weight and very low birth weight have been documented.[47-54] A more complicated issue is the eventual outcome of infants who survive birth after having been conceived by ART. A recent study has shown that children who are born after IVF have an increased risk of developing neurological problems, especially cerebral palsy. These risks are thought to be largely due to the high frequency of multiple births, low birth weight and prematurity.[55]

Intracytoplasmic sperm injection (ICSI) has received a good deal of attention. Several studies have shown evidence of a higher incidence of chromosome anomalies after ICSI[56,57] and a two-fold increase in major birth defects compared to naturally-conceived infants.[58]

Empty Deficiencies of "Modern" Reproductive Technologies

Since the birth of the first IVF baby, there has been observed an insatiable desire to expand the technological frontiers further and further. This has been observed in a variety of different ways. And yet, it continues to expand its problematic base. Women undergoing IVF show higher levels of anxiety and emotional tension than do control patients.[59] Large numbers of multiple pregnancies have been created with all of their attendant problems. These babies are often born prematurely, they are of both low birth weight and very low birth weight and are endangered by their birth status. I have observed at a monthly meeting of the OB-GYN department a doubling of the incidence of low-birth-weight babies born during one year. When inquiring as to the cause (perhaps somewhat naively), one of the members of the OB-GYN staff said rather cavalierly and with complete acceptance, "That's just the ART factor." In any other area of medicine the following questions would be asked: "Why? What can be done about it? How can we reverse the trend?" And ultimately, "How can we stop endangering these children?"

So there has developed a technology that *creates life by destroying it.* Multiple embryos are placed within the uterus in order to obtain one to 5.88 embryos for every one that is successful—resulting in huge mortality risks for the embryo.

Once the woman becomes pregnant, she is asked to undergo genetic amniocentesis or prenatal genetic diagnosis using a blastomere and once more putting her pregnancy and her baby at risk, all for the sake of a "guaranteed" healthy baby. Some very wanted pregnancies end in abortion. *The technology creates life by destroying it.* If the woman achieves a multiple pregnancy, she is challenged to "selectively reduce" the number of fetuses. This euphemistic term for aborting some of her fetuses is *creating life by destroying it.* This has, in fact, become so common that many reproductive endocrinologists in their super-ovulation programs have been virtually unconcerned with the multiple pregnancy rate knowing full well that the perinatologists will "save them" with their selective reduction programs. This goes well for them until they come across a patient who, for strong moral reasons, will *not* create life by destroying it.

This all comes from a profession that has focused all of its energies over the last 30 years on the *micromanagement of human fertility.* As was pointed out earlier, the Boston IVF group recognizes that on the day prior to ovulation there is a "thin, watery mucus that spills out of the cervical canal and covers the portion of the cervix and upper vagina." But then they dismiss it by saying "some women notice this change in the cervical mucus, whereas others do not"[7] (which is all that is to be said about one of the most important biomarkers of human fertility).

This is a profession that has fostered masturbation for the evaluation of the seminal fluid for the male to identify male factor infertility. This has been done without any concern or sensitivity to the aesthetic, ethics or morals of the person. *This is a profession* that has accepted cross-species fertilization with the use of *hamster* egg and *human* sperm penetration assays without any concern for the potential ethical or moral problems that it poses.[60-62] One has to wonder why the majority of women do not seek infertility care when their fertility is impaired. *This is a profession* that has redefined the embryo and introduced the term "pre-embryo: the developing cells produced by the division of the zygote until the formation of the embryo proper at the appearance of the primitive streak about 14 days after fertilization."[63] I learned many years ago that a *definition is not a substitute for knowledge.*

There are estimated to be over 400,000 frozen embryos stored in the United States.[64] It is recognized that these excess embryos result from our imperfection in trying to duplicate natural reproductive processes.[65]

The presence of these embryos provides further motivation for the development of continuing experiments on human embryos and the further development of embryonic stem cells. Harvard University recently ventured into the area of embryonic stem cells and are making available these stem cells to others for research purposes. Why couldn't Harvard University provide funding for further research into the stem cells that are lost day in and day out in the delivery rooms of American hospitals. Umbilical cord and placental stem cells may very well be the hope for the future in this area of research, but because of the politics, not so much the science, there seems to be a "protect at all costs" mentality for the continued research in areas that are unnecessary.

Women have become involved in donating ova so that others might give birth. Large sums of money have been proposed for purchasing such donated ova suggesting that greed has entered into the profession. Some physicians have spoken eloquently against this[66] but often to "deaf ears."

One picks up the newspaper and reads something nearly every day, i.e., "Babies from Thawed Ovarian Tissue by 2009 - Experts,"[67] "Pregnancy Created with Egg Nucleus of Infertile Woman,"[68] "Ethics Expert Supports Sex-Selection in IVF,"[69] or how about the "Successful Pregnancy in a 63-year-old woman."[70,71] Some have cautioned against this as well.[72]

Then, among other things, there is procreation after death or mental incompetence. Most of these cases have to do with posthumous fatherhood.[73] In reality, the move toward this type of parenthood seems very consistent with a "*philosophy of nothingness.*"[74] Why shouldn't the child be brought into the world without a father? More and more, fathers have been relegated to a position that is nearly insignificant and unimportant. The "*philosophy of nothingness*" perpetuates the notion that the father has no fundamental role in raising his child or that his role is completely insignificant and can be discarded without concern.

Missing Links

It would appear that modern reproductive medicine has several "*missing links*" that have kept it from making progress in ways that are more consistent with foundational ethical and medical principles. Some of these "missing links" would be:

1. For most patients seeking evaluation for a reproductive abnormality, *an adequate diagnosis of their underlying disease is not made.*

2. Since an adequate medical diagnosis is not made, an appropriate therapy for that medical condition cannot be implemented.

3. The major "missing link" from a biological perspective is the completely inadequate study of the effects of the endocrine and immune systems on the target organs of reproduction. The lack of sound procreative education and an objective analysis of the biomarkers of human fertility have led investigators down paths that have missed the presence of signs that herald the underlying cause of reproductive abnormalities.

4. Combine this with the apparent lack of appreciation for the notion that infertility and other reproductive abnormalities are *multi-factorial* in their cause and effective treatment can be obtained only when it is implemented in a multi-factorial way.

5. There appears to be a lack of concern for the health care of women who suffer from the various medical diseases that are associated with infertility (see Internet Appendix).

Some would argue that an adequate diagnosis is being made. It is clear, however, that many view "effective, affordable treatments that produce pregnancy" as "more important to infertile couples than reaching a diagnosis."[75] A highly-technological, extremely expensive approach to the treatment of reproductive abnormalities has been developed and is out of the financial reach of most people (it is a *rich man's treatment*). Furthermore, this approach *rarely improves health while often threatening it.* In addition, *we actually have decreased overall pregnancy rates with this surge in technology.*

In any other area of medicine, if the success rate was decreasing and the morbidity and mortality (neonatal morbidity and neonatal mortality) were increasing, hospital committees, professional affairs committees, and other programs of professional involvement would be deeply concerned in working towards its correction. Let us all hope that "modern" reproductive technology has not been canonized to such an extent that its "progress" cannot be reversed and real progress introduced.

Final Note

Some have issued concerns about the potential health problems arising out of human ART programs.[76] Others have pondered whether the move for more choices actually has closed opportunities and exhibited no boundaries.[77] Has the terminology of "rights" become meaningless? R. Rowland, a former research coordinator with the IVF program directed at the time by Dr. Carl Wood at Monash University in Melbourne, Australia, suggested that the stress on choice may give the medical profession more, not less, control in reproductive issues. In the movement toward choosing the sex of your child, using donor ova, utilizing surrogates, promoting embryo experimentation and embryonic stem cell research, eliminating or diminishing the role of fathers, and the movement toward cloning, it would appear that *only those with expanded knowledge of the biology of human reproduction are the ones who are in control.* We have chosen the path of viewing the child as a commodity. It seems that a similar approach was previously used, and it failed miserably, and we have been suffering the consequences ever since.

Action Item: Abandonment

In interviews with women experiencing infertility and seen at the Pope Paul VI Institute's National Center for Women's Health, they were asked to respond to the following question, "Have you ever felt abandoned by your obstetrician or gynecologist?" A number of their responses are recorded here.

Patient A
"Yes. All I ever get are dead ends. It's as if they know nothing of how a woman's body truly functions. They don't know how to get to the root of the problem. They offer no hope."

Patient B
"Yes. As I was being wheeled into the operating room, I truly felt that I could not trust my physician. I was worried that he would take one of my ovaries or both or, worse yet, my uterus."

Patient C
"Yes. Actually, it was the feeling that I was just a number among other thousands of patients. So, my problems were not important

enough to warrant extra attention. They just referred me to a reproductive endocrinologist."

Patient D

"Yes. I felt he was giving me a one-size-fits-all course of action that was not specific to my situation."

Patient E

"Yes. We tried to get pregnant for over six years and went to three different doctors, all of whom I felt abandoned me in my efforts to get pregnant without crossing the morality line. The [Pope Paul VI Institute] was the only [place] that truly helped."

These comments are not isolated. In 58 questionnaires completed by patients who answered this question, 58.6 percent of the answered "yes."

NaProTECHNOLOGY and Infertility

INFERTILITY IS A symptom of underlying disease.[1] The diseases that cause infertility have a "two-pronged effect." They not only hinder the functioning of fertility, but also cause both short and long-term health problems (see Internet Appendix). The persistent unwillingness to address infertility problems from this point of view is one of the *major flaws* in the current approach to the treatment of infertility.

Fertility problems also carry with them significant emotional effects.[2] This is fairly well recognized by those who work in this field, and the psychosocial distress can contribute significantly to the cause of some forms of infertility.

Up until 1978, most of the effort in medicine in evaluating and treating women with infertility was placed into trying to identify and treat its underlying causes. In 1978, *in vitro* fertilization produced a paradigm shift. It led to a "skipping over" of the causes and this continues up to the present time to be the foundational approach to medical care for couples who suffer from infertility. In essence, this is a *symptomatic or "Band-Aid" approach* to treatment and not one that gets to the root causes. When the artificial reproductive technologies began to take hold, now 30 years ago, *diagnostic laparoscopy was in its infancy. Hormone assessment*, while available, *was not readily accessible.* Ultrasound technology still was mired in bulky technology and *real-time ultrasonography was in its infancy. Selective hysterosalpingography had not been developed* and the fallopian tubes could not be catheterized. The **CREIGHTON MODEL FertilityCare™ System** (CrMS) began its first allied health education program for **Fertility***Care*™ **Practitioners** (**FCP**) in 1978. This means of objectively monitoring the biomarkers of the menstrual and fertility cycle was only in its beginning stages.

It is legitimate to ask why there was such a quick and rapid move toward the artificial reproductive technologies. One can only speculate as to why this occurred. It definitely could be stated that it was difficult, if not impossible at times, to actually determine the underlying causes of an infertility problem. Frustration with this approach made ART appealing. We live in a society where there is a perceived need for a quick solution, the so-called "instant gratification" society. The patients have an emotional intensity to them that is somewhat unique and this is related to the importance of human fertility. Physicians, at times, have been emotionally unable to deal with this intensity and the virtue of patience has sometimes been non-existent.

There are perhaps other reasons as well. Some of these are economic. Training in infertility evaluation and treatment over the years has been exceptionally poor (both medically and surgically). Third-party reimbursement has long held a policy against reimbursing for "fertility testing and treatment," which is a throw-back to the notion that infertility is "all in your head." If the physician is not going to be adequately reimbursed for his time and efforts, there is no incentive to become involved with these patients. And, of course, physicians can financially profit enormously from the artificial reproductive technologies.

The Missing Link

In the mid-1970s, Doctors John and Lyn Billings published a series of cycles in their "Atlas of the Ovulation Method"[3] from a woman who had been unable to achieve pregnancy. This series of cycles was from a woman who had had difficulty achieving pregnancy over a seven-year period of time. She indicated that she had noticed clear, stretchy mucus once or twice in the past, but not in recent years. In the cycles shown, complete dryness was recorded except for the day following intercourse (a seminal fluid discharge). Ovarian hormone levels were measured and provided indirect evidence that ovulation was occurring. But acts of intercourse close to the time of ovulation did not result in conception.

When the **CREIGHTON MODEL** program first began its investigations of the Billings Ovulation Method in April 1976, that chart and set of circumstances were known to us, but the explanation

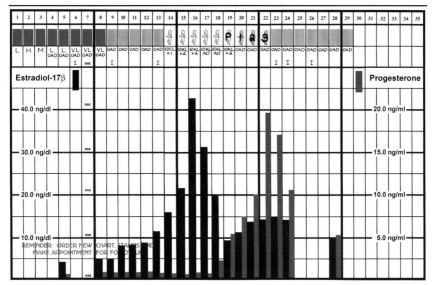

Figure 20-1: A normal CrMS chart with daily levels of estrogen and progesterone. The hormonal profiles are normal. The mucus cycle score is 15.7 (out of 16) and post-Peak phase is 10 days (From: Pope Paul VI Institute research, 2004). Refer to page 83 for the Vaginal Discharge Recording System (VDRS).

was completely unknown. This led us to a series of investigations that have stimulated our research in reproductive health.

In Figure 20-1, a normal cycle is charted with the correlating estrogen (black bars) and progesterone levels (red bars) shown. Both profiles are completely normal. When a completely dry cycle was evaluated (Figure 20-2), a decreased preovulatory E_2 profile and a decreased luteal phase progesterone and E_2 profile were observed. This hormone combination is consistent with *abnormal folliculogenesis* (development and function of the follicle) followed by *abnormal luteogenesis* (development and function of the corpus luteum).

Another dry cycle evaluation with three days of premenstrual brown bleeding is shown in Figure 20-3. While this hormone profile is not as severely blunted as that in Figure 20-2, it still is significantly suppressed when compared to Figure 20-1.

In Figure 20-4, a woman with a limited mucus cycle was studied. In this cycle, the preovulatory E_2 profile is decreased as is the postovulatory P and E_2 profile. In addition, the post-Peak phase of the cycle was 19 days in duration and with studies that came later, this was found to be consistent with the ultrasound finding of a luteinized unruptured follicle (one of the ovulation defects).

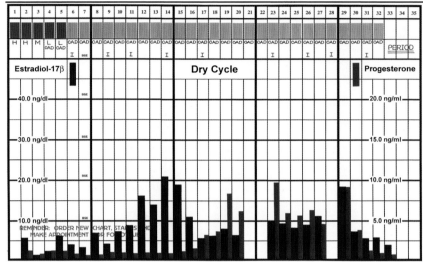

Figure 20-2: An infertility patient with a dry cycle and daily levels of estrogen and progesterone. Both the preovulatory and the postovulatory profiles are decreased revealing very poor follicular development followed by abnormal luteal function (From: Pope Paul VI Institute research, 2004).

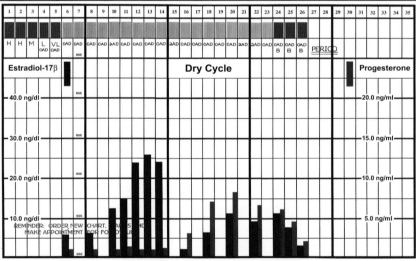

Figure 20-3: Another dry cycle with decreased hormone parameters. Premenstrual spotting also is observed in this cycle (From: Pope Paul VI Institute research, 2004). Refer to page 83 for the VDRS.

In Figure 20-5, another cycle is shown with the hormone profile. In this case, there was a significant drop (greater than 50 percent) in the production of progesterone over a 24-hour period between Peak +5 and Peak +6 of this cycle. This cycle was one of the first where we were able to identify the presence of a late luteal defect (Type III luteal phase defect), which often is associated with a fairly normal preovulatory estrogen profile.

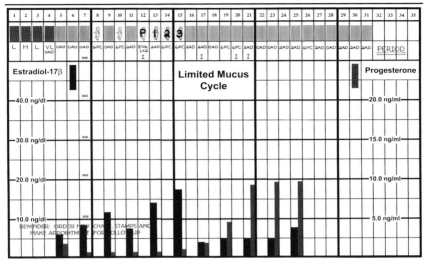

Figure 20-4: A very limited mucus cycle (mucus cycle score = 3.0) and prolonged post-Peak phase (19 days) with a preovulatory and postovulatory hormone profile. The hormone profile is significantly abnormal and the prolonged post-Peak phase strongly suggestive of the luteinized unruptured follicle (From: Pope Paul VI Insitute research, 2004). Refer to page 83 for the VDRS.

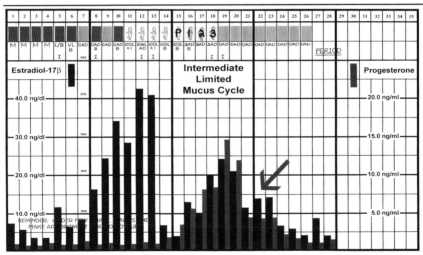

Figure 20-5: A CrMS chart in a patient with infertility. The estrogen and progesterone levels are completely normal up to Peak +6 when the progesterone level shows a significant decrease (at arrow) (Type III luteal phase deficiency) (From: Pope Paul VI Institute research, 2004).

In Figure 20-6, a chart from a woman who had four consecutive miscarriages is shown. As she began charting, it became apparent that she had significant premenstrual spotting. When her hormone profile was drawn, the estrogen levels were blunted, but most prominent was the significant suppression of her luteal phase progesterone production. The premenstrual spotting was thought to be due to inadequate

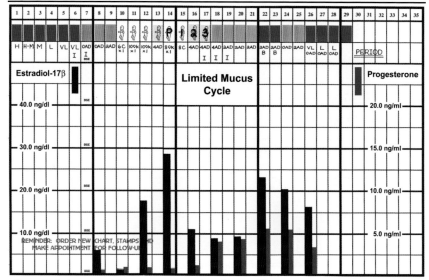

Figure 20-6: A woman with premenstrual spotting, a history of four consecutive spontaneous abortions and a preovulatory and postovulatory hormone profile. The periovulatory estradiol levels are decreased, but what is most remarkable is the significant decrease in postovulatory progesterone (From: Pope Paul VI Institute research, 2004). Refer to page 83 for the Vaginal Discharge Recording System (VDRS).

hormone support for the endometrium and was at least one of the underlying causes of her multiple miscarriages. Premenstrual spotting has been observed in about 15 percent of patients with regular cycles who are experiencing infertility.

While on occasion there is a glimpse of interest shown in the medical literature with regard to abnormal menstrual cycle patterns,[4] vulvar discharge patterns such as these illustrated have been *virtually ignored* by the reproductive medicine community. The lack of procreative education and focus on the naturally-occurring fertility cycle is ultimately the *missing link* in current reproductive medicine.

Philosophy of NaProTECHNOLOGY

As one looks at the evaluation and treatment approaches in **NaProTECHNOLOGY** it becomes striking that there is a significantly different philosophical approach that is taken to the care of these patients. To begin with, the child is viewed differently.

In **NaProTECHNOLOGY**, *the child is viewed as a gift as opposed to a right.* This is defended in the Vatican instruction on the Respect for Human Life (*Donum Vitae*), which is the instruction on the evaluation and treatment of infertile couples: "A true and proper right to a child would be contrary to the child's dignity and nature. The child is not an object that one has a right nor can he be considered as an object of ownership; rather a child is a gift, 'the supreme gift'… and is a living testimony of the mutual giving of his parents."[5]

Donum Vitae addresses the suffering caused by infertility in marriage by outlining the context to which approaches would be appropriate: "… marriage does not confer upon the spouses the right to have a child, but only the right to perform those natural acts that are per se ordered to procreation."[5]

Donum Vitae recognizes what every physician knows when it comes to the treatment of the infertile couple: It is not possible to be 100-percent effective in their treatment. In most cases, one cannot even come close to 100-percent effectiveness. Thus, *Donum Vitae* highlights other important services to the life of the human person: "Physical sterility, in fact, can be for spouses the occasion for other important services to the life of the human person, for example: adoption, various forms of educational work, assistance to other families, and assistance to poor or handicapped children."[5]

These principles are foundational to the approach of **NaProTECHNOLOGY**. In addition, only married couples are accepted into evaluation and treatment so that if a child results they will have the benefit of both a mother and a father. This is not because we are forced to accept the principles put forward in *Donum Vitae*, but because these principles make sense, they are connected to an overall hierarchy of values, they are integrated and consistent and they allow for an orderly program of development for the evaluation of these most significant and difficult problems. Furthermore, and ultimately what is most important, these principles *protect the dignity of women, the integrity of marriage* and *a respect for the dignity and integrity of the child. They are principles that should be amplified rather than reduced.*

The Goals of NaProTechnology

A **NaProTECHNOLOGY** approach to the infertile couple has the following goals:

1. It works towards *finding the underlying causes* of the reproductive abnormality.

2. It allows for the *treatment of these underlying causes.*

3. It assists the couple in achieving pregnancy while maintaining the *natural acts of procreation.*

4. If the treatment program is unsuccessful, *research* into the unknown causes is undertaken.

5. If medically unsuccessful, the program will assist with successful family building by *being supportive of adoption.*

Figure 20-7 presents a basic version of the staircase approach to the management of patients with infertility using **NaProTECHNOLOGY**. The underlying causes are aggressively sought; then they are aggressively treated for periods of time that are agreeable to the patient and the physician. When pregnancy occurs, the pregnancy is supported. If pregnancy does not occur over a period of time, then adoption is recommended.

As soon as adoption is mentioned as a part of an infertility program, there is a natural tendency to think one of two things: either the program is giving up on the individual couple or the program does not have sufficient confidence in its own approach to think that it will be effective. In actuality, both of these could develop if the program is not careful in how it is approached.

In a legitimate **NaProTECHNOLOGY** program, however, **NaProTECHNOLOGY** is viewed as a realistic approach to family building when, in fact, through proper evaluation and treatment, the

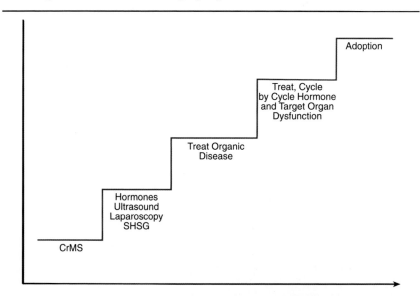

Figure 20-7: A staircase approach outlining the basic principles of a NaProTECHNOLOGY evaluation and treatment protocol for infertility.

woman has not achieved a pregnancy over a period of time that is mutually agreed to by the couple and the physician. In that regard, I have recognized that couples who are involved in infertility treatment have different resources from which to draw on in their search to solve their infertility problem. Some have very little stamina to be involved in a treatment program while others have an incredible amount of stamina to be involved. Thus, it is only when that stamina runs out and the program has not been effective that the couple can legitimately be recommended for adoption. It recognizes only that the program (no matter which one it is anywhere in the world) cannot be 100 percent successful. The program, however, through its support of adoption programs, can assist these couples in achieving their goal of building a family.

Defining Infertility

The standard definition of infertility usually involves the absence of pregnancy in a couple who is engaged with *random* acts of intercourse over a 12-month period of time. This approach to the definition of infertility is one of "subtraction." In other words, it isn't one that truly tests one's fertility, but rather by the absence of expressed fertility, the person is defined as infertile.

With the advent of the Billings Ovulation Method and subsequently the **CrMS**, there has been an emphasis on identifying fertility as well as infertility. For the first time, a family planning system exists that allows the couple to either achieve or avoid pregnancy by selectively having intercourse at a time of fertility or infertility. The achievement of pregnancy is demonstrated in Figure 20-8. With intercourse occurring at the time of fertility *(fertility-focused intercourse: FFI)*, pregnancy is achieved.

The success of such an approach in the achievement of pregnancy was published in 1992[6]. In this group of patients, in couples of normal fertility, 76 percent achieved a pregnancy in the first cycle that they selected the time of fertility for intercourse. By the third cycle, 90 percent were pregnant and by the sixth cycle 98 percent were pregnant.

These data suggest that the definition of infertility can be changed from the principle of "subtraction," which is currently used to a principle of testing one's actual fertility with fertility-focused intercourse. If a couple has not achieved pregnancy within three cycles of FFI, there is a strong suspicion that an infertility problem exists. If

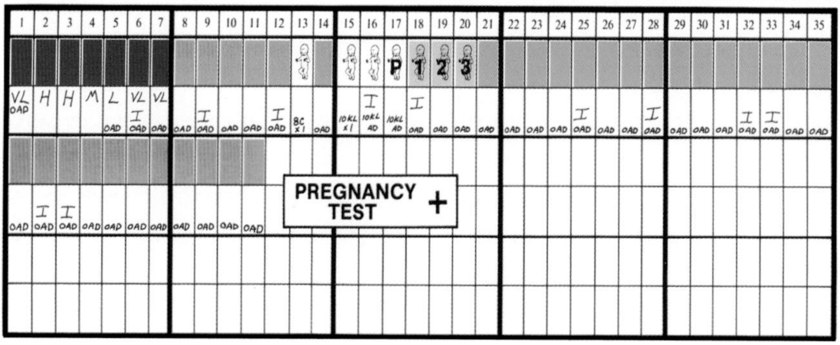

| 1 | 2 | 3 | 4 | 5 | 6 | 7 | 8 | 9 | 10 | 11 | 12 | 13 | 14 | 15 | 16 | 17 | 18 | 19 | 20 | 21 | 22 | 23 | 24 | 25 | 26 | 27 | 28 | 29 | 30 | 31 | 32 | 33 | 34 | 35 |

PREGNANCY TEST +

Figure 20-8: In this cycle, the couple is using the time of fertility (fertility-focused intercourse) and have successfully achieved a pregnancy (From: Pope Paul VI Institute research, 2004). Refer to page 83 for the Vaginal Discharge Recording System (VDRS).

pregnancy has not occurred by the sixth cycle, then testing can begin. In our infertility program almost everyone who comes into the program still meets the standard definition of infertility of one year of random intercourse and still no pregnancy. This is because so few people are yet charting their cycles. In evaluating those cases of individuals who have been charting for a period of six cycles without achieving pregnancy, however, no case has ever been found where some organic and/or underlying abnormality was not identified.

Infertility Evaluation Protocols

Infertility evaluation protocols in **NaProTECHNOLOGY** are basic and direct. They are not overly complex, although a fundamental understanding of the disease process is extremely important, so that the underlying conditions can be properly understood. In-depth reviews of some of these conditions are presented in the chapters that immediately follow.

The approach to investigation begins with the type of menstrual cycle with which the patient presents: *Regular menstrual cycles, long and irregular cycles* or *the absence of menstruation.* At the first visit that information can be easily obtained and an infertility evaluation can begin.

Regular Menstrual Cycles

The most common forms of infertility are observed in women who have regular-length menstrual cycles. The patient's history is taken upon entry in the program; she is instructed to go to an Introductory Session for the CrMS and after two cycles of charting, return for a physical examination and initiation of testing. The tests that are conducted include a seminal fluid analysis on the husband, a full series menstrual cycle hormone profile, a follicular ultrasound series and a diagnostic laparoscopy, hysteroscopy and selective hysterosalpingogram.

Once all of these tests are completed, the patient returns for a *comprehensive management review* in which the videotape of her laparoscopy is shown to her and her husband and all of the tests are reviewed with the idea of **NaProTECHNOLOGY** solutions in mind.

When the patient returns after two months of tracking their fertility cycles using the **CrMS**, the physician reviews it with the idea of paying special attention to the *biomarkers* of the **CrMS**. The basic biomarkers to be reviewed are listed in Table 20-1 and several charting examples illustrating some of these biomarkers are shown in Figure 20-9. The important biomarkers include *the type and intensity of the mucus cycle, the length and stability of the post-Peak phase, the length of the pre-Peak phase, the overall length of the cycle, the presence of premenstrual spotting or tail-end brown bleeding*. These all can be external signs of underlying pathophysiology.

The appearance of *limited mucus cycles* will suggest abnormal reproductive hormone function and an increased risk of ovulatory defect. A *short post-Peak phase* will indicate the presence of an inadequately short luteal phase. A *long post-Peak phase* may suggest the presence of a persistent unruptured follicle. *Premenstrual spotting* and/ or *tail-end brown bleeding* may indicate the possibility of low progesterone levels. These also can be associated with chronic endometritis (an infection of the lining of the uterus).

At the second visit, the *physical examination* is conducted and a *full-series menstrual cycle hormone profile* is ordered. A *follicular ultrasound series* (an ovulation series) also is ordered. These studies

---

Table 20-1: NaProTechnology Assessment–Paying Attention to the Biomarkers

- The type of mucus cycle

- The length and stability of the post-Peak phase

- The length of the pre-Peak phase (and its characteristics)

- The length of the cycle

- Presence of premenstrual spotting

- Presence of tail-end brown bleeding

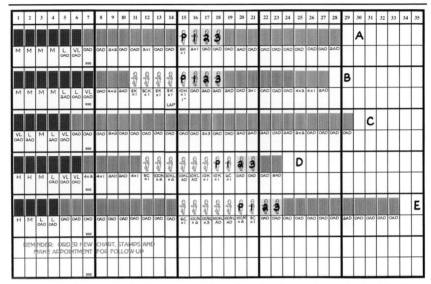

Figure 20-9: Charting examples from women with regular cycles who may be experiencing infertility. Limited mucus cycles are seen in cycles A and B, a dry cycle in cycle C, a short post-Peak phase in cycle D and a normal mucus in cycle E (From: Pope Paul VI Institute). Refer to page 83 for the VDRS.

need to be done by people who are experienced in conducting them. Finally, the diagnostic laparoscopy, hysteroscopy, and selective hysterosalpingogram are discussed in greater detail. This procedure is recommended because its yield is so high. In none of the above tests is one searching for a "needle in the haystack." The results of these tests will uncover the *multi-factorial aspects* of most infertility problems. Each of these will be discussed in greater detail later in this chapter.

Long and Irregular Cycles

In those women who present *long and irregular cycles*, it usually is difficult to do a true ovarian follicular ultrasound series because of the unpredictability of the occurrence of ovulation. Also, because of the nature of the cycle pattern, a different set of hormones are better to evaluate in order to establish the foundation. The initial phases of the protocol are identical to that for women with regular cycles, however, at the time of the physical examination, *an amenorrhea profile* and *a basic pelvic ultrasound* are ordered. The most common problem associated with long and irregular cycles is *polycystic ovarian disease* and these two tests will generally clarify that situation.

It is good to schedule a *two-hour glucose and insulin tolerance test* to see if the patient is insulin resistant. After fasting levels of glucose and

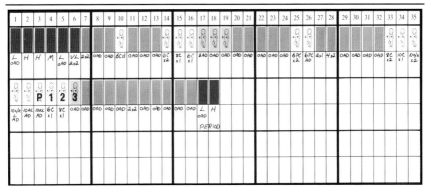

Figure 20-10: An example of a woman with a long menstrual cycle, infertility and polycystic ovarian disease. The cycle is 51 days in duration (From: Pope Paul VI Institute). Refer to page 83 for the VDRS.

insulin have been drawn, the patient is given a 75-gram oral glucose load. Follow-up glucose and insulin levels are drawn at 30, 60, 90 and 120 minutes. This testing process will identify the person who is insulin resistant.

In addition to the above, *a diagnostic laparoscopy, hysteroscopy and selective hysterosalpingogram* also are recommended. Many women with polycystic ovaries (over 50 percent) also will have endometriosis. Thus, a diagnostic laparoscopy will allow for that diagnosis to be made and usually it can be treated with laser at the time of the diagnostic procedure. In addition, a confirmation of the diagnosis can be made by direct observation of the ovaries and an evaluation of the ovary for possible wedge resection sometime in the future also can be undertaken.

When one views a cycle pattern such as that seen in Figure 20-10, it is almost always associated with polycystic ovarian disease. There appears to be, however, a small percentage of these cycle patterns (about 5 percent) that may be of primary hypothalamic origin.

Amenorrhea (Absence of Menstruation)

Patients who come with a history of prolonged amenorrhea should chart only for four to eight weeks prior to coming back for their physical examination. The diagnostic laparoscopy is considered optional in these cases, but can at times be very helpful. The most common cause of amenorrhea is *hypothalamic amenorrhea* and in cases such as that, endometriosis is rare.

The charting sequences that are observed are shown in Figure 20-11. A predominant pattern of dryness or a predominant pattern of mucus (a variable return of peak-type mucus) are the two dominant

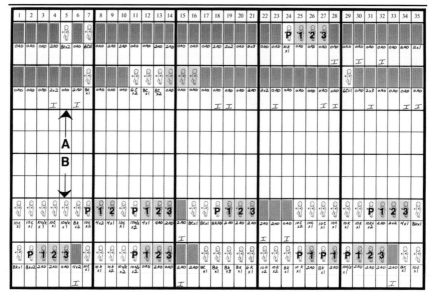

Figure 20-11: A woman with infertility associated with amenorrhea. In example cycle pattern A, the prominent pattern is one of dryness with occasional mucus patches. In cycle pattern B, the pattern is one of a variable return of Peak-type mucus (From: Pope Paul VI Institute).

patterns. The most important feature, however, is the absence of menstruation and, of course, the absence of ovulation. In spite of this being a reasonably ominous-appearing condition, some of the very best success rates are obtained in the treatment of this group of patients.

Timing of Fertility Tests

With the use of the **CrMS**, various fertility tests can be timed much more accurately than previously. It allows for a very simple but reproducible system for the woman to keep so that it will tell the physician and the laboratory where she is in her cycle. The most obvious timing of tests is in the *targeted hormone evaluation,* which becomes common place in **NaProTECHNOLOGY**. Such things as a *postcoital test,* however, will not provide correct information if it is not timed to occur at the time when the good Peak-type mucus is present. Diagnostic laparoscopy is best performed during the preovulatory phase of the cycle so that an interruption of a pregnancy is not a concern and a selective hysterosalpingogram is best performed between day four and eight or ten of the cycle. In this way, the lining of the uterus is still thin and access to the internal opening of the fallopian tube is relatively easy.

Classification of Mucus Cycles

With the use of the *Vaginal Discharge Recording System (VDRS)*, it is possible to objectively classify the mucus cycle. This classification system and the means by which it is obtained is described in the textbook, "The Medical & Surgical Practice of **NaProTECHNOLOGY**."

In a group of patients who came into the program with infertility, their mucus cycle scores were calculated and the mucus cycles classified. In 65.8 percent of this group, the mucus cycles were limited in intensity. This is in contrast to a group of normal fertility controls where the limited mucus cycles were observed in only 21.7 percent of patients.

In another group of patients who had endometriosis (152 patients who underwent conservative surgical excision of endometriosis), 77.6 percent of them either had limited (67.1 percent) or dry (10.5 percent) cycles. It is of further interest to note that in the dry cycle population (n=16) there was only one subsequent pregnancy in that population and that was an ectopic pregnancy.

Ovarian Hormone Dysfunction

It should be pointed out that there often is a significant underlying hormonal abnormality that is observed in women who have infertility and regular cycles. These hormone problems are important because they also are associated with several ovulation-related disorders (see below) and abnormal mucus patterns.

In addition to the above, women with regular cycles and infertility have a very high incidence of *premenstrual symptoms* (Table 20-2). These symptoms are almost as frequent as women who have premenstrual syndrome. The hormonal abnormalities that underlie

Table 20-2: Incidence of Premenstrual Symptoms in Patients with Regular Cycles and Infertility[1,2] (N=252)

Symptom	%	Symptom	%
Irritability	90.5	Depression	74.1
Breast tenderness	85.7	Weight gain	69.4
Bloating	85.3	Fatigue	67.3
Teariness	80.2	Headache	50.8
CHO craving	75.1	Insomnia	29.0

1. Symptoms began at least four days prior to onset of menses.
2. From: Pope Paul VI Institute Research, 2004.
3. CHO=carbohydrate craving

premenstrual syndrome (see chapter on premenstrual syndrome) are very similar to the hormone abnormalities observed in patients with regular cycles who also experience infertility. It is highly likely that there is an underlying hormonal linkage between these different conditions. In other words, there appears to be a link between the underlying problems that exist in premenstrual syndrome and in those that exist in infertility.

Ultrasound Findings

It has been suggested that if a woman has regular menstrual cycles that she can be considered to be ovulating normally.[7] *Nothing could be further from the truth!* In addition, *current approaches* to studying ovulation in infertility programs are *significantly flawed.* Standard tests such as basal body temperature curves, endometrial biopsies, a mid-luteal phase progesterone level and/or urinary LH detector kit simply do not give adequate information about the ovulation process to be considered reliable.

In patients who have infertility problems, the incidence of ovulation-related defects ranges from 56 to 61 percent. This can be determined by the careful conduct of daily follicular ultrasound examination of the ovaries around the timing of ovulation. This technique is described in detail in the textbook, "The Medical & Surgical Practice of **NaProTECHNOLOGY**."

The question often asked in an infertility program is, "Is this woman ovulating?" *That is the incorrect question to be asking.* A better question to ask is, "Is ovulation normal? Or is there a defect in ovulation?"

In actuality, when one studies ovulation closely by daily ultrasound and hormonal parameters, one realizes that there are a number of different *"ovulatory events"* that mimic ovulation but are either completely anovulatory or represent a significant defect in the ovulation mechanism. An example of an ovulatory defect that is anovulatory is the *luteinized unruptured follicle syndrome.* An example of an ovulatory defect in which the ovulation process is significantly defective is the *immature follicle.* While ultrasound is commonly used in the artificial reproductive technology programs to monitor ovulation inducing medications, it is rarely used for studying *spontaneous ovulation patterns and their defects. The latter is extremely important* if one is to design treatment strategies that meet the specific demand of the underlying problem.

Laparoscopy Findings

There are two main problems that confront the current use of laparoscopy in the evaluation of the infertile patient. The first has to do with the current *laissez faire* attitude with regard to its utilization. Because there has been a de-emphasis on making a diagnosis of the underlying problems, the actual use of diagnostic laparoscopy has lagged.

The second problem that exists is the general lack of skill in doing good diagnostic laparoscopy. These skills are outlined in the textbook, "The Medical & Surgical Practice of **NaProTECHNOLOGY**." They apply *"near contact" laparoscopic techniques* and a good every day understanding of the appearance of such conditions as endometriosis, polycystic ovarian disease and pelvic adhesive disease. They are essential to implementing a good diagnostic strategy when using laparoscopy.

Again, it should be emphasized that the implementation of the routine performance of diagnostic laparoscopy in this group of patients is not looking for a "needle in a haystack." In 250 consecutive laparoscopies performed for infertility, the main postoperative diagnosis is shown in Table 20-3. In this group of patients *72.8 percent had endometriosis*. If you were to apply these data to a group of women who had regular menstrual cycles and infertility (excluding those patients who had polycystic ovarian disease and anovulatory patterns),

**Table 20-3: Main Postoperative Diagnosis
Consecutive Laparoscopies for Infertility[1] (N=250)**

Main Postoperative Diagnosis	n	%
Endometriosis	182	72.8
Pelvic adhesions	21	8.4
PCOD	16	6.4
Normal pelvis	**15**	**6.0**
Tubal obstruction	10	4.0
Anovulation	6	2.4
Peri-adnexal adhesions	4	1.6
Totals	**250**	**100.0**

1. From: Pope Paul VI Institute research, 2004.

nearly 80 percent of the patients had endometriosis. This is significantly different than that reported in major medical textbooks ranging from 5 to 25 percent of the infertile patient population. Ultimately, *diagnostic laparoscopy is an under-utilized and an under-skilled procedure* and as a result, *patients are not well served.*

Diagnostic Summary

When one reads in major textbooks of reproductive medicine that there are certain causes for infertility and the listing of these causes suggests that each patient has a single cause for their infertility it is *extremely misleading.* And yet, it is recognized that the cause of infertility is often *multifactorial.*[8,9]

A **NaProTECHNOLOGY** evaluation allows one to elicit the various underlying causes and put together these multiple factors so that a *comprehensive, multifactorial treatment approach* can be implemented. This, along with the CrMS, is what allows **NaProTECHNOLOGY** to be so successful in the treatment of infertility and other reproductive anomalies.

In Table 20-4, a large group of infertility patients evaluated through the **NaProTECHNOLOGY** protocols outlined in this chapter are

Table 20-4: Total Female and Male Diagnosis of Patients with Primary and Secondary Infertility following Complete NaProTechnology Evaluation[1]

Female Diagnosis	%	Male Diagnosis	%
Endometriosis[2]	77.4	Normospermia	45.5
Target organ dysfunction[3]	68.2	Mild oligospermia	26.7
Ovulation disorders (anatomic)[4]	56.5	Moderate oligospermia	18.0
Luteal phase deficiency[5]	53.7	Severe oligospermia	8.1
Pelvic adhesions[2]	38.9	Azoospermia	1.7
Tubal defect[2]	23.9		
PCOD[2]	15.6		
Anovulation[2]	0.9		

1. From: Pope Paul VI Institute Research, 2004.
2. Based upon a complete evaluation of 660 patients with infertility.
3. Based on the mucus cycle score of 289 consecutive patients with regular menstrual cycles and infertility.
4. Based upon the ultrasound evaluation of ovulation disorders in a subgroup of 460 patients with regular cycles.
5. Based upon a targeted hormone evaluation of postovulation progesterone production in a subgroup of 328 separate patients.

shown with the actual incidence of the underlying abnormalities shown. This is split into the female and male diagnostic categories. Furthermore, the classification of the seminal fluid analysis into normospermia, mild, moderate and severe oligospermia, also is shown in Table 20-4 for reference.

It can be seen that in women, the top four associated causes of infertility are endometriosis (77.4 percent), target organ dysfunction (68.2 percent), ovulation-related disorders (56.5 percent) and luteal phase deficiency (53.7 percent). Pelvic adhesive disease (with or without endometriosis) is seen in 38.9 percent, tubal defects in 23.9 percent, polycystic ovaries in 15.6 percent and pure anovulatory infertility in 0.9 percent. The totals add up to more than 100 percent because most patients experience several of these at the same time.

A normospermic male was observed in only 45.5 percent of the patients while severe oligospermia was observed in only 8.1 percent and azoospermia in 1.7 percent.

Infertility is clearly multifactorial in its origin. This can be discovered if good diagnostic testing is conducted and an effort is made to find the underlying causes. Without such efforts, these factors will not be discovered.

Treatment

In a **NaProTECHNOLOGY**-driven program, treatment is designed to address the various underlying causes that are identified. For example, if an underlying hormonal dysfunction is identified, then that hormonal dysfunction is corrected. If the mucus cycle is dry or limited, then mucus-enhancing agents can be used. If an ovulation-related abnormality is identified, then that is corrected. If the mucus cycle is dry or limited, then mucus-enhancing agents can be used. If an organic abnormality (such as endometriosis, pelvic adhesive disease, tubal obstruction, or so forth) is identified, then that too is corrected.

With the use of the **CrMS,** one can implement treatment strategies that properly target the menstrual cycle. For example, the ability to use progesterone in the menstrual and fertility cycle requires definitive knowledge that one is in the postovulatory phase. The **CrMS** routinely provides that information at virtually no charge to the patient. Thus, these treatment protocols can be implemented in a long-term fashion without a great deal of difficulty.

A variety of surgical techniques have been developed to address the various organic abnormalities such as endometriosis and pelvic adhesive disease. These surgical approaches have as their primary goal the correction of the underlying problem while accomplishing surgery in a *"near adhesion-free"* environment. A thorough understanding and knowledge of these approaches are necessary in order to provide the whole spectrum of **NaProTECHNOLOGY** care to the infertile couple.

One of the distinct advantages of the **NaProTECHNOLOGY** approach to the treatment of infertility is its *strikingly low multiple pregnancy rate*. At the Pope Paul VI Institute, this rate is 3.2 percent. In Ireland, this rate is about the same (3.4 percent).[10] With the national IVF multiple pregnancy rate averaging 31.8 percent, *this represents a nearly 10-fold decrease* with its subsequent benefits to the family and the babies.

Case Presentations

In Figure 20-12, a 29-year-old woman who had been trying for seven years to achieve pregnancy without success began charting the **CrMS**. The teaching of this client was done by long distance and the

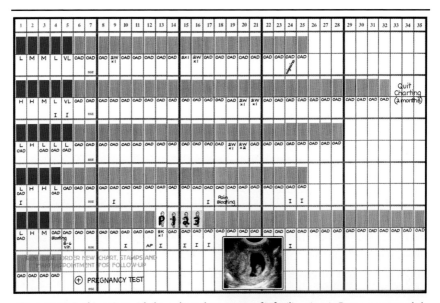

Figure 20-12: In this patient with dry cycles and seven years of infertility, vitamin B$_6$ was recommended as a mucus-enhancing supplement. In the last cycle, limited mucus was observed and pregnancy achieved without any additional assistance except fertility-focused intercourse (From: Pope Paul VI Institute research, 2004). Refer to page 83 for the Vaginal Discharge Recording System (VDRS).

client was never seen directly. But she had undergone extensive infertility evaluation including basal body temperature curves, seminal fluid analysis, hysterosalpingography and diagnostic laparoscopy. She also underwent ovulation induction with clomiphene citrate (Clomid) and artificial insemination all without success.

She had heard of the work of the Pope Paul VI Institute and called the **Fertility***Care*™ **Center** at the institute. She was assigned one of the FCPs who taught her how to track her cycles. No pregnancy occurred in the first several cycles so the teacher implemented a "vitamin B_6 protocol." This protocol allows for the patient to take vitamin B_6 as a *mucus-enhancing agent*. In the very first cycle in which she took vitamin B_6, she had a mucus discharge that she had never seen before. The couple had intercourse and achieved a pregnancy. The chart not only shows the pregnancy cycle, but also the ultrasound photograph showing the intrauterine pregnancy. She went on to deliver a full term, healthy baby.

In Figure 20-13, a patient who failed *in vitro* fertilization on two previous occasions is shown. She came to us for further evaluation and instruction. During the course of the evaluation, it was found that she

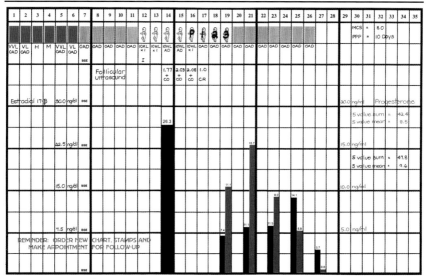

Figure 20-13: Limited mucus cycles, endometriosis, ovarian dysfunction and a husband with a very low sperm count were identified in this patient who failed two previous IVF procedures. In spite of these abnormalities with proper NaProTECHNOLOGY treatment, she achieved a pregnancy and had a normal healthy baby (From: Pope Paul VI Institute). Refer to page 83 for the Vaginal Discharge Recording System (VDRS).

had limited mucus cycles, decreased progesterone production and endometriosis. The endometriosis was treated with laser laparoscopy and this 42-year-old woman was treated prospectively with clomiphene to induce ovulation and to help correct the underlying hormonal dysfunction. Her husband's sperm count was 1.4 million with 15 percent motility. After undergoing a varicocele repair (prior to coming to our program) and then took clomiphene to improve his count. In the eighth cycle of treatment she achieved a pregnancy that eventually resulted in a healthy live-born baby girl.

Effectiveness of NaProTECHNOLOGY in Infertility

Data on a total of 1,045 patients who have been treated for infertility by way of **NaProTECHNOLOGY** is presented here. This population represents patients who have been treated and have, as organic causes of infertility, endometriosis, tubal occlusion, polycystic ovarian disease, pelvic adhesive disease, anovulation (amenorrhea), azoospermia, or in some cases, unknown causes.

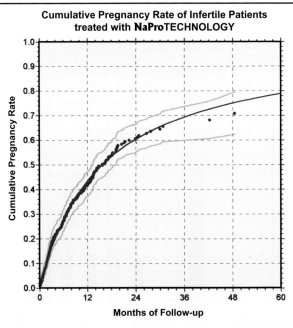

Figure 20-14: The cumulative pregnancy rate of a large group of infertility patients treated with NaProTECHNOLOGY (From: Pope Paul VI Institute research, 2004). The light blue lines represent 95-percent confidence intervals.

This study population had an average age of 30.4 years and an average length of time trying to achieve a pregnancy of 3.42 years. Many of them had previous infertility testing prior to being seen and many of them also had previous unsuccessful infertility treatment.

In Figure 20-14, the cumulative pregnancy rate for this infertility population treated with **NaProTECHNOLOGY** is shown. In this analysis, over 60 percent of patients became pregnant by 24 months and nearly 70 percent by 36 months. This includes pregnancies from most causes of infertility including those who had severe oligospermia, various stages of endometriosis, tubal occlusion, etc. It does not, however, include those patients whose husbands were azoospermic. In the **NaProTECHNOLOGY** model of infertility evaluation and treatment, azoospermic couples are encouraged to look seriously at adoption as the solution to their family building.

Early in the work of the **CrMS**, we found that some patients would become pregnant over a period of time if the only treatment they received was from the application of the **CrMS** itself. Furthermore, it was learned that the type of mucus cycle mattered with regard to overall pregnancy rates. In 40 patients who had limited mucus cycles and an average length of infertility of 3.2 years, 16 achieved pregnancy in an average of 5.4 months. Those patients who entered with dry cycles, however, had significantly lower pregnancy rates with only 20 percent (n = 10) over a period of 12 months. This was the first indication that there was a distinction between the capability of achieving pregnancy in women with different types of vulvar mucus cycle patterns. The only treatment that this group of patients received was supplementation with vitamin B$_6$ and fertility-focused intercourse.

In evaluating the success of **NaProTECHNOLOGY** in patients with infertility and endometriosis, the first presentation of data is a comparison between the results of treatment with **NaProTECHNOLOGY** to the classic study published by Dr. John Rock and others in 1981[11] (Figure 20-15). This latter study of the effectiveness of conservative surgery for endometriosis has been used as the gold standard for pregnancy rates associated with the surgical treatment of endometriosis over many years. While the curve for success in **NaProTECHNOLOGY** would appear to be significantly higher, statistical significance could not be calculated because the raw data from the original Johns Hopkins study no longer was available for comparison. In both groups, only normospermic husbands were included.

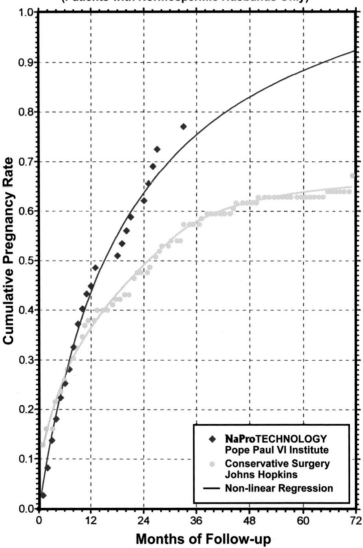

Figure 20-15: Cumulative pregnancy rate of patients with endometriosis treated with NaProTECHNOLOGY compared to conservative surgery only. Patients with normospermic husbands only (From: Pope Paul VI Institute research, 2004 and Rock JA, Guzick DS, Sengos C, et al: The Conservative Surgical Treatment of Endometriosis: Evaluation of Pregnancy Success with Respect to the Extent of Disease as Categorized Using Contemporary Classification Systems. Fertil Steril 35:131-137, 1981).

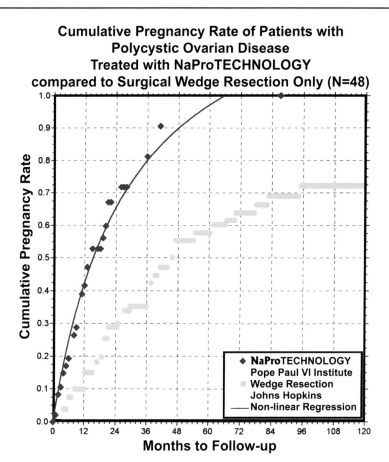

Figure 20-16: Cumulative pregnancy rate for patients with polycystic ovarian disease treated with NaProTECHNOLOGY compared to surgical wedge resection only. (From: Pope Paul VI Institute research, 2004 and Adashi EY, Rock JA, Guzick D, et al: Fertility Following Bilateral Ovarian Wedge Resection: A Critical Analysis of 90 Consecutive Cases of the Polycystic Ovary Syndrome. Fertil Steril 36:320-325, 1981).

In Figure 20-16, the approach of **NaProTECHNOLOGY** is compared to the classic description for ovarian wedge resection in polycystic ovarian disease by Drs. Adashi and Rock[12] published in 1981. Cumulative pregnancy rates to just above 80 percent were seen in **NaProTECHNOLOGY** by the 36th month post ovarian wedge resection. A statistical comparison could not be made because data from the original Johns Hopkins study were no longer available. Nonetheless, the approach of **NaProTECHNOLOGY** clearly improved our ability to be successful in patients with polycystic ovarian disease.

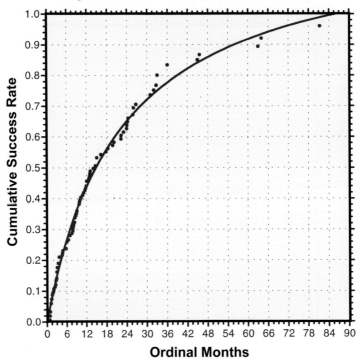

Figure 20-17: The combined cumulative pregnancy rate and adoption rate for endometriosis patients treated with NaProTECHNOLOGY. This graph indicates the overall family-building rate associated with NaProTECHNOLOGY (From: Pope Paul VI Institute research, 2004).

In **NaProTECHNOLOGY**, if medical treatment is not successful, then support for adoption as a *family-building technique* is incorporated into the overall plan of action. Adoption is not seen as a "failure" of **NaProTECHNOLOGY** or a failure of medical treatment. It is recognized as a realistic means of building one's family when medical and surgical treatment fails, keeping in mind that there is no system of infertility evaluation and treatment that comes close to approaching 100-percent success rates at the present time. Evaluation of a large group of patients who were treated for endometriosis, looking at both the cumulative pregnancy and adoption rates, is identified in Figure 20-17. *Assisting couples in achieving such a high rate of family building is acknowledged as a very significant accomplishment of the work in* **NaProTECHNOLOGY**.

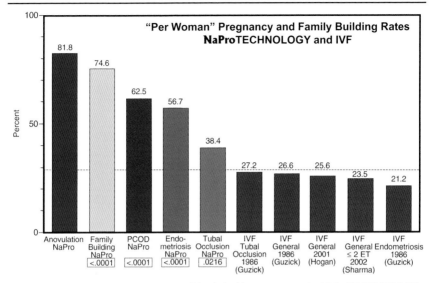

Figure 20-18: The "per woman" pregnancy and family-building rates comparing NaProTECHNOLOGY and in vitro fertilization (From: Pope Paul VI Institute research, 2004 and the listed references).

In Figure 20-18, the "per woman" pregnancy and family-building rates by different organic causes of infertility treated with a **NaProTECHNOLOGY** approach are compared to the results of several different evaluations of *in vitro* fertilization. It is difficult to make these comparisons because so few studies in IVF allow for the calculation of "per woman" success rates. Thus, the studies quoted range from the year 1986 through 2002. In five categories of application in **NaProTECHNOLOGY**, however, the "per woman" pregnancy rates and family-building rates are statistically higher than the comparable "per woman" pregnancy rates in IVF.[13-15] In the case of the study by Sharma, et al.,[14] different "per woman" success rates can be identified. These range from a high of 47.2 percent to a low of 23.5 percent. The upper range is obtained, however, by transferring more than two embryos. When ≤ 2 embryos are transferred, then the rate decreases to 23.5 percent. This latter statistic is more comparable to the overall outcome of **NaProTECHNOLOGY** when looking at such factors as the multiple gestation rate and is consistent with the current effort to promote ≤ 2 embryos per transfer.[16-18]

This should not be considered terribly surprising. A randomized-controlled trial of either IVF or a standard infertility treatment program was published in 1999.[19] In this case, the use of a standard infertility treatment program resulted in a higher pregnancy rate and lower cost than IVF. A similar comparison was made in 1995.[20] Again, traditional forms of treatment for endometriosis-related infertility revealed higher pregnancy rates than the artificial reproductive technologies. These treatment approaches are more comparable (although not identical to) **NaProTECHNOLOGY**.

Conclusions

The ability to evaluate success rates in infertility treatment can be very complex and difficult. In fact, some have wondered whether or not some authors understand their own data.[21] Survival curve analysis, "per woman" pregnancy rates and fecundability rates can be used to conduct this type of an evaluation. In addition, cycle-by-cycle pregnancy rates can be utilized as well and have been used almost exclusively by the advocates of the artificial reproductive technologies. What often is overlooked is the decreasing, cycle-by-cycle fertility rate and the high discontinuation rate that ultimately lowers the overall "per woman" pregnancy rate.

This analysis shows that **NaProTECHNOLOGY** *exceeds* the conventional means of treating infertility by survival curve analysis, "per woman" pregnancy rates and fecundability rates. In addition, it exceeds the artificial reproductive technologies in treating infertility when evaluated by survival curve analysis and "per woman" pregnancy rates.

There are several important points that need to be kept in mind relative to this assessment. First of all, in **NaProTECHNOLOGY** *the number of women who eventually will achieve a pregnancy is higher than the number of women who will achieve a pregnancy with the artificial reproductive technologies.* While it is true that it may take longer to achieve that pregnancy, the actual goal of achieving a pregnancy is higher and significantly higher with **NaProTECHNOLOGY**.

Secondly, in **NaProTECHNOLOGY** the underlying causes of infertility are investigated and, in many cases, identified and treated. In ART, these are neither investigated adequately nor treated.

Thirdly, the success rates cited here for **NaProTECHNOLOGY** are expected to improve even further in the years ahead as surgical techniques advance and our ability to treat the various other dysfunctions progressively improves.

Finally, in **NaProTECHNOLOGY** the multiple pregnancy rate is only 3.2 percent, which is *more than 10 times less* than what is seen in most ART programs. So while the speed to pregnancy may be higher for those women who actually achieve a pregnancy in the ART programs, the pregnancies are much more complicated, fewer women actually become pregnant and the disease or diseases they have are not found and treated.

What Does NaProTECHNOLOGY Accomplish?

NaProTECHNOLOGY allows for the diagnosis of the underlying problem and the treatment of the underlying causes. It has excellent pregnancy rates and, with appropriate evaluation and treatment, it fosters a natural acceptance of the underlying condition because the underlying causes are understood. In some ways, if the woman does not become pregnant, she reaches an acceptance level of the condition that has led her to this dilemma. In many ways it is similar to a death and dying situation where an individual will go through various stages of anger and denial. But once the individual reaches acceptance, then she can move on with her life. In **NaProTECHNOLOGY** this happens all the time. In 30 years only a handful of patients have left the **NaProTECHNOLOGY** approach and gone to artificial reproductive technology. This natural acceptance of the underlying causes is

**Table 20-5: Side-by-side Comparison
NaProTechnology vs. ART**

Comparison Subject	NaProTechnology	ART/IVF
Diseases are identified	Yes	No
Disease are treated	Yes	No
Foundation is laid for future success	Yes	No
More total pregnancies are achieved	Yes	No
Fertility-focused intercourse	Yes	No
Speed to pregnancy is shorter*	—	Yes
Cycle-by-cycle pregnancy rate is greater*	—	Yes
Built on foundation of destroying life	No	Yes
More cost effective	Yes	No

* When successful, but overall much lower "per woman" success.

extremely important in helping these couples resolve their long-standing infertility and their search for rational causes.

In the future, a search for the various causes of infertility that we still do not understand will continue under the auspices of **NaProTECHNOLOGY**. **Only with such an approach can a cure to infertility eventually be found.** Potentially, **NaProTECHNOLOGY** can cause a new paradigm shift in the thinking of a profession.

In Table 20-5, a side-by-side comparison of **NaProTECHNOLOGY** and the artificial reproductive technologies (ART/IVF) is shown. In **NaProTECHNOLOGY**, the *diseases that cause infertility are identified and treated*, a foundation is laid for future success, and more total pregnancies per woman are achieved than with the ART/IVF approaches. It does take longer, however, and therefore the speed to pregnancy is shorter in ART/IVF. The cycle-by-cycle pregnancy rate also is greater, but because so many people discontinue ART/IVF approaches, the actual number of pregnancies achieved or the pregnancy rate "per woman" is lower. In addition, the ART/IVF approaches are built on the foundation of destroying life, which is not present in the **NaProTECHNOLOGY** approach. **NaProTECHNOLOGY** also is more cost effective.

Real People, Real Problems, Real Solutions

On May 29, 2007, my son, Robert Thomas, turned 11 months old. I am so blessed to have Robbie in my life. He is the answer to many prayers. I know that Robbie would not be here today if it were not for The Pope Paul VI Institute and **NaProTECHNOLOGY**. Before learning about Dr. Hilgers, my husband and I had a long journey with infertility and other health problems. In 1999, I had my first miscarriage. My doctor said that it was just bad luck and we could try again in three months. Three months later we were pregnant again. The pregnancy progressed normally until around 26 weeks when I started having contractions. I was put on terbutaline every four hours to control the contractions. Thankfully, the medication worked and I delivered my daughter at 38 weeks. When Diana Rose was born in January 2001, the doctor and nurses were surprised to see the condition of my placenta and umbilical cord. The placenta was calcified and gray and the umbilical cord was very short in length. The doctor had no answers for us when we asked her what caused the placenta to look so unhealthy. We were so blessed to have a healthy baby girl. In 2002, I miscarried a second time. The doctor said they do not do any testing until there are three miscarriages. When I became pregnant for the fourth time, I called the doctor's office immediately. They said that there is nothing they do to save a pregnancy and that they would see me at nine weeks. It was too late. I lost the baby before my first visit. I was devastated. My doctor had no answers as to why I had miscarried three times. She recommended a fertility doctor and genetic testing. I left the office that day and never went back. My husband did some research and came across Dr. Hilgers. We met with a FCP in August 2004 and started charting immediately. I had my blood drawn locally and sent to Omaha. In April 2005, we drove out to Omaha. Dr. Hilgers had answers to my questions about my infertility and other problems. He was so compassionate and caring. He went over my blood work with us. We were amazed at what we learned. I had very low estrogen and progesterone. This explained why I was depressed, anxious, and had insomnia at times. It also explained why I had three miscarriages. He also told us that he would find endometriosis when he performed the laparoscopy the next day. Dr. Hilgers found extensive endometriosis and adhesions. Now I know why I had so much pelvic pain. We went back for major abdominal surgery. Dr. Hilgers removed endometriosis from my uterus, ovaries, bowels and rectum. He also removed three-quarters of one of my ovaries due to the extensive endometriosis. However, Dr. Hilgers gave us 75 percent to 80 percent chance of getting pregnant. We came home with such peace knowing that we had done everything possible to help make me healthy. Now we could focus on getting pregnant. I was started on Clomid, vitamin B$_6$, and mucus-enhancing medicine. Five months after the surgery, I was pregnant. We could not believe it. I called Dr. Hilgers' office immediately and they sent me for a blood draw. My progesterone was low so I started shots of hCG and progesterone immediately. I was monitored regularly with blood draws and Dr. Hilgers adjusted my dose accordingly. I continued the injections until 37 weeks because my body did not maintain a healthy level on its own.

Jeanine Jahaske
Roselle, Illinois

Recurrent Miscarriage

SPONTANEOUS ABORTION is defined as the spontaneous loss of pregnancy prior to the 20th gestational week. Pregnancy losses that occur during this period of time are said to occur in about 15 percent of pregnancies.[1] At the same time, the risk of miscarriage increases proportionately to the number of previous miscarriages experienced.[2] Unfortunately, a definite cause has been difficult to determine.

Over the years, miscarriages have been observed by doctors and the public as a somewhat "normal" finding. Often it has been thought to be "nature's way" of ending a pregnancy that was doomed to fail in any regard. There has developed, however, a somewhat more aggressive approach over the past 5 to 10 years towards evaluation and management of women with miscarriages. It is now well recognized that a definition of recurrent pregnancy loss includes two or more consecutive spontaneous miscarriages[1] and that this warrants a full evaluation.[3] Furthermore, it is becoming more and more recognized that there appears to be an association between infertility and miscarriages.[4-6]

A variety of factors underlie the occurrence of miscarriage. These include genetic, hormonal, anatomic, immunologic and microbiologic variations.[1] One of the well-recognized features of miscarriages is its increased frequency associated with advancing maternal age.[7] *We are slowly coming to recognize that no miscarriage can be considered normal. All miscarriages are the result of an abnormal reproductive event.* It is the current challenge of medicine to find the underlying causes and, in some cases, the underlying causes are common occurrences that are often overlooked.

The CREIGHTON MODEL System

A large number of patients with a history of miscarriage have been followed with the **CREIGHTON MODEL System** (CrMS). With a history of at least one previous miscarriage, the incidence of *limited mucus cycles and dry cycles* totalled 74.5 percent. There is not a large difference in the mucus cycle based on the previous history of one, two, three or more miscarriages. For the whole group, when compared to a group of normal fertility controls, the *mucus cycles were markedly more limited.*

A number of biomarkers have been further evaluated. The mucus cycle score (5.43), menstrual score (5.78), and the length and variability of the post-Peak phase (13.04 +/- 3.52) were all significantly different from the normal fertility controls.

In Figure 21-1, a hormonal correlation during the course of a cycle in which the patient became pregnant and subsequently miscarried is shown in association with the tracking of the fertility cycle with the CrMS and the tracking of the ovarian follicle. The mucus cycle was

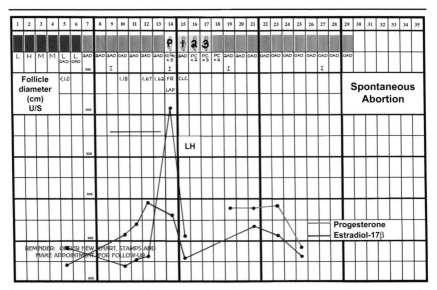

Figure 21-1: Conception in a limited mucus cycle leading to spontaneous abortion. An ultrasound study of the follicle revealed an immature follicle. Preovulatory E_2 levels are suppressed and postovulatory P and E_2 levels are suppressed. The mucus cycle is limited. The LH level is normal (from Pope Paul VI Institute research, 2004). Refer to page 83 for the Vaginal Discharge Recording System (VDRS).

markedly limited (MCS=1.7). In addition, the follicle was immature at the time of rupture (MFD=1.62 cm). This coincided with decreased preovulatory estrogen levels and decreased post-Peak progesterone and estrogen levels. The only hormone that appeared normal during the course of this cycle was the LH surge.

The risk of miscarriage is known to be increased in women who have an inadequately short luteal phase. In Figure 21-2, a woman with a short, five-day post-Peak phase is shown in association with her periovulatory estrogen and postovulatory progesterone and estrogen profiles. This five-day post-Peak phase provides an excellent estimation of what also is an extremely short luteal phase as determined hormonally. The preovulatory estrogen profile is reasonably normal. In a cycle such as this, pregnancy may occur, but the likelihood of sustaining it is extremely low because the hormonal support after ovulation is inadequate.

This condition is perhaps *the first one* that now can be evaluated and treated before a woman even becomes pregnant, *thus eliminating the need altogether for miscarriage.* The evaluation begins with tracking the fertility cycle with the **CrMS**, identifying the short post-Peak phase and obtaining hormonal support through stimulation of the corpus

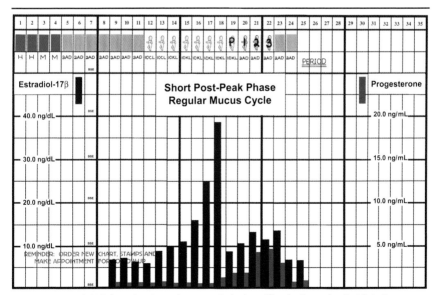

Figure 21-2: A CrMS chart showing a short post-Peak phase (five days) correlated with its hormone profile that shows a very short luteal phase (seven days). Pregnancy in this situation should universally lead to miscarriage (From: Pope Paul VI Institute research, 2004). Refer to page 83 for the VDRS.

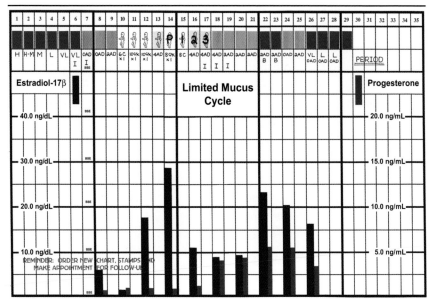

Figure 21-3: A woman with premenstrual spotting, a history of four consecutive miscarriages, her CrMS chart and her hormone profile. Her postovulatory progesterone levels are markedly decreased (From: Pope Paul VI Institute research, 2004). Refer to page 83 for the VDRS.

luteum with HCG (HCG 2000 IU intramuscularly or subcutaneously Peak +3, 5, 7 and 9).

Another biomarker that is very helpful is the presence of *premenstrual spotting*. In Figure 21-3, a woman with four previous miscarriages began tracking her fertility cycle and obtaining her hormone levels. Her premenstrual spotting began seven days prior to the onset of menstruation. She had a decreased luteal phase progesterone and estrogen profile and a moderately depressed periovulatory estrogen profile.

The post-Peak phase in women who eventually miscarry also is *highly variable* in comparison to the relatively stable length of the post-Peak phase in women who do not miscarry. In Table 21-1, the length of the post-Peak phase of the previous 19 cycles prior to a conception that ended in miscarriage are shown. The range in length of the post-Peak phase in this woman was seven to 14 days during the course of that period of observation. This represents a highly *unstable post-Peak phase* (which estimates a highly unstable luteal phase) and is known to be associated with significantly decreased progesterone and estrogen levels. Thus, when she did become pregnant, it was not surprising when she miscarried. This type of variability in the length of the post-

**Table 21-1: Variation in Length of Post-Peak Phase
Prior to Conception Leading to Miscarriage (One Patient's History)**

Length of the post-Peak phase in days

14	11	10	9
13	11	11	8
9	13	11	11
8	7	7	10
11	6	12	

Range = 7 - 14 days (7 days)

Peak phase or instability in its length is *an important biomarker* of decreased progesterone and estrogen production during the luteal phase of the menstrual cycle and its associated long-term medical effects.

Hormonal Parameters

It is well recognized that the production of progesterone in a pregnancy that ends in miscarriage is significantly decreased.[8-10] This has been well documented for pregnancies that miscarry during the first trimester and for pregnancies that miscarry between 12 and 20 weeks of gestation. It has been tempting to suggest (and many treatments take this approach) that it is the decreased progesterone that is the cause of the miscarriage and subsequent support of the pregnancy with progesterone should be therapeutic. Unfortunately, it is much more complex than that.

We have evaluated a large group of women with a history of one, two, three or more miscarriages. This evaluation looked at the periovulatory estrogen levels along with the postovulatory progesterone and estrogen levels.

The *periovulatory estrogen* production by the developing follicle is *significantly decreased* in those women who have had a previous history of miscarriage. It is more suppressed in those women who have had three or more miscarriages. But when evaluated, the periovulatory estrogen profile was suppressed for all categories in patients who had miscarriages as compared to the normal ovulation control group.

The progesterone production by the corpus luteum in this group of patients also was markedly decreased for all categories of patients with miscarriages. The most remarkable decrease in the progesterone production by the corpus luteum was observed, for all categories, on

Peak +7, Peak +9 and Peak +11; although in some categories the decrease started as early as Peak +5.

This hormone pattern strongly suggests that there is an underlying feature of *abnormal folliculogenesis* (the abnormal growth and development of the follicle resulting in abnormal ovulation), which is an underlying feature to the cause of miscarriage. In fact, the finding that mucus cycles are significantly limited in this category of patients and that this finding is secondary to both decreased estrogen production and receptor formation, the prevalence of these hormone findings suggests strongly that *abnormal folliculogenesis* is at the root of many miscarriages. This is a finding that could explain some of the underlying genetic abnormalities that have been promoted as causes to the problem of miscarriage.[11-13]

Premenstrual Symptoms

With abnormal function of the follicle, there usually follows abnormal function of the corpus luteum and this also is seen in women with miscarriage. With this degree of luteal phase dysfunction, one would expect that patients who have miscarriages would have an increased rate of premenstrual symptoms. In fact, that has been studied and the incidence of various premenstrual symptoms was relatively high for this group of patients.

Ovulation Disorders

With these hormone profiles, one also would anticipate an increased risk of ovulation-related abnormality in women who have undergone a miscarriage. The incidence of various types of ovulation-related abnormalities has been studied. Anatomically abnormal ovulation patterns by ultrasound were identified in 40.6 percent of the women who were studied with previous miscarriage. We have been able to show that immature follicles (small follicles) are associated with miscarriage, and this particular defect is the most common abnormality observed in women who have previous miscarriages.

Role of Endometriosis

Endometriosis also has been shown to be a link to miscarriage. Dr. S. Daya has conducted an analysis of studies that showed an increased rate of miscarriage before treatment of endometriosis and a decreased rate of spontaneous abortion following treatment.[14]

Within our own studies of 192 patients with a previous history of spontaneous abortion, *endometriosis was found in 85.4 percent of patients*. This percentage is much higher than usually reported, in part because of the "near contact" laparoscopic approach used in our program. This is a condition, however, that is rarely even looked for. In our program, it is routine to look for it. It is a significant finding and correlates well with the hormone, mucus cycle, and ovulation-related abnormalities seen in endometriosis itself.

It is thought that the peritoneal fluid from patients with endometriosis may have an adverse affect on the reproductive process and be causative to both infertility and miscarriage.[15-17] Surgical treatment is considered the treatment of choice for endometriosis in our program. Most of these patients can be treated by laser laparoscopy with a smaller percentage being treated with excision of their endometriosis via open incision. With endometriosis being so prevalent in this series, laparoscopy is considered an important part of the overall evaluation and treatment for patients with recurrent miscarriage (two or more).

The role of endometriosis and its treatment is demonstrated in Figures 21-4 and 21-5. These laparoscopic photographs are in a patient who had six previous miscarriages. Endometriosis was identified in the crease between the proximal portion of the right fallopian tube and the lateral portion of the right posterior uterus (Figure 21-4). It also was observed as a small superficial lesion on the left ovary (Figure 21-5). In both cases, the surgery was laser vaporization and subsequent pregnancy occurred and went full term with adequate progesterone and HCG support.

Role of Progesterone

It has been shown that progesterone support can correct and maintain the endometrium[18] and that progesterone support can reduce the risk of miscarriage in a subsequent pregnancy.[19-29] On the other hand, other studies have shown progesterone to have no effect.[30-33]

In work done at our center, progesterone levels were followed in subsequent pregnancies in patients who had a previously diagnosed luteal phase defect. The Type I, II and III luteal phase deficiencies were studied. In this group of patients, there was a markedly-decreased progesterone profile in the pregnancies of those patients with a pre-existing Type I luteal phase deficiency. While there were some statistical

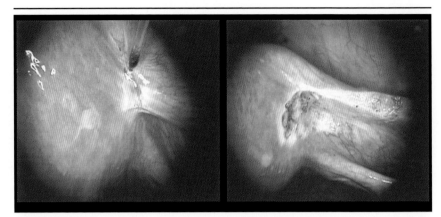

Figure 21-4: This patient with six previous miscarriages has endometriosis between the proximal portion of the right fallopian tube and the posterior surface of the uterus (left). On the right, this is shown following laser vaporization. This patient eventually conceived and had a full-term pregnancy.

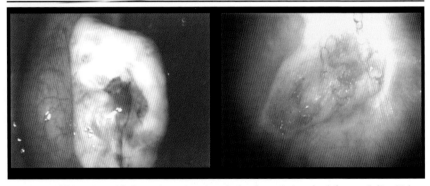

Figure 21-5: This patient with six previous miscarriages had endometriosis on her left ovary (left), which was laser vaporized (right). She subsequently had a normal healthy pregnancy.

differences also observed in the Type II luteal phase deficiency, the Type III luteal phase deficiencies showed no statistical difference from the normal controls. These data may offer some clues as to who might best benefit from progesterone supplementation in pregnancy.

It appears clear that those with a pre-existing Type I luteal phase deficiency not only need progesterone support during the luteal phase of the menstrual cycle (the post-Peak phase), but they also need progesterone support during the course of their pregnancies. In Type II luteal phase deficiency, it is likely that progesterone support also will be necessary; although, in some cases it may prove otherwise. In Type III luteal phase deficiency, it is likely that progesterone support will be unnecessary.

This makes for a reasonably rational approach on which progesterone therapy can be based. In actual implementation, however, it is still somewhat difficult because it is not known in all cases whether or not the woman has a pre-existing luteal phase deficiency to begin with. Secondly, there will be some degree of variation around this rationale; and thus, the only approach that appears to be workable is to provide progesterone supplementation to those patients with a history of previous miscarriage and monitor their progesterone levels during the course of the pregnancy.

Role of HCG

HCG has a well-known effect on the corpus luteum. It will stimulate the production of both progesterone and estrogen. Recent evidence suggests that it also may act as a growth and differentiation factor during pregnancy.

While the reports on HCG use in recurrent miscarriage have been mixed, the weight of the evidence is in the direction of it being of some value. In addition, there are no known side effects to the administration of HCG either to the woman or to her baby (outside of perhaps some local irritation at the site of injection – although, these injections are generally very well tolerated). Thus, it seems reasonable to use HCG as an additional part of the approach to the treatment of women with recurrent spontaneous abortion.

Evaluation and Treatment Protocol

In women with miscarriage, our **NaProTECHNOLOGY** program takes a new approach. First of all, it identifies miscarriage as an abnormality rather than simply a frequently-occurring normal reproductive event. Furthermore, it recognizes that there are underlying causes to each miscarriage even though we may not always know what they are. Finally, it recognizes that there is a significant sense of loss that both the mother and the father may experience as the result of such an event. Spontaneous abortion is not taken lightly as a medical event.

In **Fertility**_Care_™ **Centers** throughout the United States and in other countries, women now are beginning to track their fertility and identifying, in a prospective fashion, certain types of events that are known to be associated with miscarriage. These events include the appearance of *short post-Peak phases, variability in the length of the post-*

Peak phase, and *limited mucus cycles.* Thus, when these events are shown to occur in a prospective identification, it poses a unique challenge to both the **Fertility***Care*™ **Practitioner** as well as the **Fertility***Care*™ Medical Consultant.

If the patient has never experienced a miscarriage before, then these patterns become even more challenging. If the woman also experiences significant premenstrual symptoms or premenstrual spotting, this also increases the potential that a luteal phase progesterone deficiency might occur and an intervention might be necessary.

In the case of a short post-Peak phase, that intervention should definitely be made. In these cases, clinical observation has shown that miscarriage occurs universally in situations such as this. The treatment for this is simple. Administering HCG 2000 units IM (or subcutaneous) on Peak +3, 5, 7 and 9 will appropriately lengthen the post-Peak phase and support the luteal phase progesterone and estrogen production. In this fashion, the pregnancy chances can be significantly enhanced. Once pregnancy is achieved, then progesterone should be monitored and progesterone supplementation begun.

In patients with limited mucus cycles, variable post-Peak phases, premenstrual spotting and/or premenstrual symptoms, the challenge is more complicated. Here it seems reasonable to at least screen the luteal phase (presuming no previous miscarriages have occurred) with a Peak +7 progesterone and estrogen level. If they are low, then implementation of hormonal support with post-Peak HCG seems reasonable. The aim in treatment is to try to reduce and eliminate the potential for miscarriage altogether; although, that is not at all universally possible at the present time.

In a patient who has experienced one miscarriage, she should be asked to begin charting the **CrMS** and observing for the above biomarkers. After charting has begun, then at least a limited hormone profile would be reasonable. In this way, the underlying hormone events can be understood better and appropriate supplementation begun. When two or more miscarriages have occurred, then a more complete evaluation should be undertaken. The patient's history is taken, she tracks her fertility cycle for two cycles and returns for a physical examination. At that time, a full series menstrual cycle hormone profile, follicular ultrasound series, and diagnostic laparoscopy are undertaken. A seminal fluid analysis is considered *optional* depending upon the length of time that the patient has been trying to achieve pregnancy.

This approach will allow the full details of the various hormone parameters of follicular phase and luteal phase deficiency to be identified along with any anatomic ovulation-related abnormalities. In addition, endometriosis will be found and can be appropriately treated.

Testing for chromosome abnormalities and other more complex autoimmune abnormalities are not conducted at this point; if treatment fails, however, then such an evaluation can be considered and undertaken.

Once pregnancy is established, these patients are supported with progesterone. In addition, those patients who have had two or more miscarriages also are supplemented with HCG in the dosage of 5000 IU two times weekly through at least the 16th week of gestation.

Another factor to consider is the presence of a low-grade almost sub-clinical (without symptoms) infection of the lining of the uterus. This can be identified by getting cultures of the lining of the uterus or documenting the persistence of tail-end brown bleeding at the end of menstruation and/or the presence of premenstrual spotting in women who have achieved normal hormone levels and yet these signs persist. Success in treatment demands that these infections be treated.

Results of Treatment

The results of treatment can be evaluated in a number of different ways. First of all, while others have shown that the treatment of endometriosis does decrease the subsequent risk of miscarriage, the data from our program can now be added to that. The treatment of the endometriosis will decrease the risk of miscarriage in a subsequent pregnancy. The pregnancy rate in patients who had either two or three previous miscarriages is nearly 80 percent at 24 months, for both situations. The cause of most miscarriages is related to events that are present prior to conceiving. Thus, to decrease the risk of subsequent miscarriage, each of the causes need to be identified and treated in advance of the next attempt to achieve pregnancy.

Real Persons, Real Problems, Real Solutions

In the 1980s (sometime during either my high school or college years), my mom dragged me to a conference at Creighton University. I'm sure the conference was religious in nature, but I honestly don't remember anything about it other than one speaker I listened to: Dr. Thomas Hilgers. Somehow I stumbled into the room where he was speaking about a woman's cycle and his **CREIGHTON MODEL** of charting the cycle. I remember thinking that it was so logical and wondered why all women weren't taught this method. If all women knew how to read their cycles, it would be so much easier to get pregnant, and there would be far fewer "unwanted" pregnancies. Over the years, whenever the topic of pregnancy or infertility arose, I often told people about this talk I had heard and how it made so much sense medically.

In 2002, while in my mid-30s, my husband and I were preparing for marriage. We were required by the Church to do some form of education. One of the options was to take a natural family planning class. I thought it would be a good time to learn the **CREIGHTON MODEL**, and we signed up at Pope Paul VI Institute never thinking in a million years we would ever have to use Pope Paul VI Institute or Dr. Hilgers. After all, my mom gave birth to seven children and my sisters combined had given birth to a total of 15 (now 19), and none of them ever had any fertility problems, so I assumed I wouldn't either. The classes, taught by Kathy Cherovsky, were surprisingly interesting and immediately drew attention to a couple of things I had not been aware of related to my cycle. Kathy was an excellent teacher and made a very personal topic easy to discuss.

Once we were married, we got pregnant within a few months of trying. I called my doctor to set up an appointment for the 8-week ultrasound. We heard the heartbeat right away, and the doctor told us that once you've heard the heartbeat, at that point, there was only a 3 percent chance that a miscarriage would occur. As it turned out, I was in the 3 percent. At 13 weeks, I went in for another appointment, but there was no heartbeat. We were devastated. The doctor said it was just "bad luck," and since we hadn't had any trouble getting pregnant the first time, we probably wouldn't have any trouble again. That didn't ease the pain any. The next day, I had a D&C. After six months of not being able to get pregnant again, the doctor suggested that because of my age and because it typically takes several months to get an appointment, I should probably contact a specialist.

I immediately called Pope Paul VI [Institute] to set up an appointment. Fortunately, I had been charting for two years, so I didn't have to wait too long to see Dr. Hilgers. When he looked at my charts, he identified several things that were likely causing the problems and he recommended an ultrasound series and blood work including checking the thyroid. He also said that I would probably need surgery to remove endometriosis. It was refreshing to hear an actual diagnosis and not just blame the miscarriage on "bad luck." We appreciated that Dr. Hilgers wanted to fix the problems that existed. After the ultrasound series and blood work, I got pregnant again. This time, I lost the baby after only nine weeks. Once again, we were crushed, but we were optimistic that once the surgery was over, we'd be successful.

After my second miscarriage, I received a notice from my former doctor that it was time for my annual exam. I don't know why, but I decided to go ahead and see him for that exam. When I told him I had had a second miscarriage, he asked if I was seeing a specialist. When I told him it was Dr. Hilgers, he said, "Oh, let me guess. He said your progesterone levels caused it." I couldn't believe his lack of professionalism and attempt to discredit another physician when his only answer was that it was "bad luck." During that exam, the doctor took three phone calls, the last one being someone I knew. I found out later he was calling to discuss their sons' hockey practices. It took all of my strength to stay until the exam was over. I decided right then that would be my last visit to his office.

Finally, in March 2005, I had a laparoscopy and hysteroscopy. Dr. Hilgers lasered off quite a bit of endometriosis, cleared a blocked tube and identified a cyst. In June, I got pregnant again only to have my third miscarriage in July. I was starting to lose hope of carrying a child to full term and wondered how many more miscarriages we could emotionally survive. They were ripping our hearts out and most people didn't understand the pain we were going through. Even after three miscarriages, I still believed we were at the right place (Pope Paul VI Institute) in order to receive the best medical care to treat the problem I had. The staff was so caring and professional. However, we decided to pursue another option and began looking into adoption. We contacted a local adoption agency, as well as a couple of local adoption attorneys. The adoption agency recommended that we pursue all fertility treatments before beginning the adoption process, but we didn't think we should limit ourselves, so we forged ahead with the adoption process and continued treatment at Pope Paul VI Institute.

We got through all of the adoption paperwork and meetings and only had the home study left when I found out I was pregnant for the fourth time. I went to Pope Paul VI Institute for a blood test in the morning. I had planned to go to Mass over the lunch hour because it was my Dad's birthday. Right before I left, I got a call from Pope Paul VI Institute telling me the test was positive and I needed to come in for a progesterone shot. When I got to Mass, the priest was talking about some young Hispanic students who were at the early morning Mass that day to celebrate the feast of Our Lady of Guadalupe. I had been praying to Our Lady of Guadalupe, but didn't realize that it was her feast day. Once I found out, I knew it was a good sign that the positive pregnancy test came on that day.

Except for my feet swelling and getting a kidney stone, my pregnancy went smoothly, and I felt great through it all. I had many ultrasounds, and after each one we sighed a huge sigh of relief. After 14 weeks, I felt some level of comfort because I had never made it that far. Finally, almost four years after we were married, we were blessed with a beautiful little boy, Matthew, on August 13, 2006. He was three days early, but he was a long time coming. We are forever grateful to God for blessing us with our son and to Dr. Hilgers and the staff at the Pope Paul VI Institute for their years of research, their outstanding medical care, and for doing their work using methods that not only follow the Catholic Church's teaching, but medically make so much sense.

Marcia Holbrook
Omaha, Nebraska

Editor's note: After writing the above story and prior to the publication of this book, Mrs. Holbrook had her second full-term delivery of a healthy baby.

For the Doctor

1. *A wide assortment of peritoneal fluid toxins have been investigated.* These would include prostaglandins, complement components, cytokines and growth factors.[15] Interleukin-1 (IL-1) and tumor necrosis factor-alpha (TNF-α) are secreted by activated macrophages. When T-lymphocytes are stimulated by IL-1, they produce IL-2. This continues a cascade of cytokine production by inducing interferon-gamma (IFN-γ) production by other T-lymphocytes and also causes activation of natural killer (NK) cells. These cells have been shown to cause a lysis of trophoblastic cells.[16] In fact, these cytokine levels have been shown to be decreased in peritoneal fluid in women who have endometriosis that has been medically treated.[17] This reduces embryotoxicity. One would anticipate that surgical correction and removal of the endometriosis would produce similar results.

It is thought that the adverse effects of endometriosis may very well occur during follicular development and result in abnormalities in the morphologic development of the embryos.[14] This also would be consistent with the hormone parameters that have been shown to exist in these situations.

2. A number of investigators have studied the effects of HCG administration in the treatment of recurrent miscarriage. These trials have had somewhat mixed results. Initially, a group of women with recurrent miscarriage and low progesterone levels were treated with HCG and a significant decrease in the miscarriage rate was found.[34] In an IVF population, luteal phase support with HCG also seemed to improve pregnancy outcome[35] and a placebo-controlled trial of patients with habitual miscarriage (a history of the three previous pregnancies ending in miscarriage) was published.[36] Only two of the 32 patients miscarried (6.2 percent).

A follow-up to that study failed to confirm the previous placebo-controlled data that allocated the use of HCG in habitual miscarriage.[37] This was followed again by a report in a group of women who had threatened miscarriage (a different population of patients). In this group, the use of HCG was used in a similar fashion, but those with a history of habitual miscarriage were excluded. Only those patients with a history of vaginal bleeding prior to the eighth gestation week of a viable intrauterine pregnancy were included. In this population, the supplementation with HCG was found to be statistically improved over that of bedrest alone.[38] At the same time, it was reported that it would be appropriate to consider the HCG-therapy regimen employed in the study. Other studies also have suggested that it can be used in recurrent pregnancy loss.[39,40]

3. While it often has been recommended that the chromosomes of the biologic

mother and father be studied in cases of habitual miscarriage, such study often is unproductive. It is expensive and most often comes back normal. Thus, it is not a factor unless a basic evaluation and treatment program is unsuccessful.

4. With regard to immunologic factors, this is a very complex area. Antiphospholipid antibodies (lupus anticoagulant and anticardiolipin antibodies) are the only validated immune causes of recurrent miscarriage. The overall role that this plays in the evaluation and treatment of patients with recurrent miscarriage, however, is not yet clear.

Antiphospholipid syndrome (APS) is characterized by the presence of circulating antiphospholipid antibodies in association with specific clinical features, which may include thrombosis (either arterial or venous) or adverse pregnancy outcomes, most often fetal loss. Pregnancies that are affected by APS but do not result in fetal loss can be complicated by severe pregnancy-induced hypertension, fetal growth restriction or placental insufficiency requiring preterm delivery. The term antiphospholipid antibodies describes a family of autoantibodies that likely involve a range of target specificities and affinities, but all of which recognize various combinations of phospholipids and/or phospholipid-binding proteins.[41]

The most commonly detected antiphospholipid antibodies are lupus anticoagulant, anticardiolipin antibodies and anti-β_2-glycoprotein I antibodies. Because there is no definitive association of specific clinical manifestations with a particular antiphospholipid antibody, multiple tests (most commonly lupus anticoagulant and IgG and IgM anticardiolipin) should be used in seeking the APS diagnosis.[41]

The treatment for APS involves supplementing with low-dose aspirin (75 mg per day) and possibly the use of subcutaneous unfractionated heparin (5000 units every 12 hours). In one study, the combination of these two therapeutic agents significantly improved the live birth rate.[42] In that trial, the heparin was used every 12 hours. In a second randomized controlled trial, the addition of low-molecular weight heparin did not significantly improve pregnancy outcome; although, a high success rate was achieved when low-dose aspirin was used for APS. In this study, the heparin was used only 5000 units subcutaneous on a daily basis.[43]

Endometriosis

OT LONG AGO, I received the following letter from a young, single woman with endometriosis:

"I'll start six years ago, before I knew what endometriosis was. I was in college in 2001 when I started having pains. They were not frequent and were about seven to 10 days before my period started. I figured it was ovulation pains, so I ignored them. Before that time, I don't recall ever having pain associated with my cycle (I started when I was 13… in 1994). In early 2001, the pain would be sharp and on one side or the other of the pelvis. It wasn't every cycle – perhaps every fourth or fifth cycle. One of my college roommates had ovarian cysts and I just chalked it up to that and thought nothing more of it.

But the pain got worse. It usually came in the morning. Sometimes it would wake me early. It was so bad I couldn't walk, so I would roll out of bed and crawl to the medicine cabinet and take ibuprofen. Usually after 30-45 minutes or so the pain would subside and return in a few months.

Fast forward to December 2002. I was out of college and working my first job. The pain was constant during the month of December. I was maxing out on ibuprofen. I took the most I could take (as suggested on the bottle), but it didn't cut the pain at all. I went to my family physician and she did a sonogram. She told me I had some small ovarian cysts, but they were small and couldn't be the cause of the stabbing pain I felt. "You are probably just stressed. Try to relax" was her advice to me.

I found her advice unacceptable, so I sought advice in Coffeeville, Kansas (where

275

I lived at the time). The doctor there did several tests, including a CT scan. He said he didn't find anything alarming or out of the ordinary. At that point, I just quit searching for answers. At that time, I had minimal health insurance coverage and was up to my ears in debt from the procedures and tests.

In 2004, I got engaged and as a result of that, began charting my cycles. We broke up before the wedding, but I have been charting ever since. During that time, I decided to start documenting the pain and its location on my charts. My instructors (who are both nurses) reviewed it and told me I needed to look into it further. I delayed because I had little insurance and was still paying off my other medical expenses.

Finally in 2005, I heeded the advice of my teachers and went to the doctor, a CREIGHTON MODEL medical consultant. He diagnosed me with Hashimoto's Thyroiditis. He also sent me to an OB/GYN because he thought I had endometriosis (at this point, my health insurance rocked – and still does). Dr. Brown (the OB/GYN) also thought I had endometriosis and suggested surgery. So I underwent surgery April 7, 2006. He affirmed that I had endometriosis and said it was a small amount and removed a small amount directly behind my uterus with a laser.

I really hoped the surgery would clear things up, but the pain persisted. I kept waiting and after a month and a half, returned to Dr. Brown's office. At that time, he suggested Lupron shots. I wasn't thrilled at that idea, so I held off. The pain wasn't quite as bad as before surgery, but it was still there. Eventually in August 2006, the pain reached the point that it was before the surgery. I was sitting at my desk at work thinking, "Don't cry, don't cry…" because the pain was so intense. At that point, I decided to start Lupron (I was almost despondent and felt I had no other options).

The Lupron shot didn't really help immediately. The fourth and fifth month (of my six-month therapy) offered a big relief, but I had my last shot about three weeks ago and I am back in awful pain. During the six-month shot therapy, I returned to waking up in the middle of the night in pain… one night I had a dream that I was in labor… and I woke up, relieved it was just a dream, only to realize I had the dream because I was in so much pain and woke up because of that pain.

So here I am. It's near the end of my Lupron treatment and I'm still in pain. It's a deep pain. Palpation does not bother me. It feels like someone has an ice pick and is hammering it into my pelvis. Or perhaps that fictional figure of Captain Hook is dissecting me with no anesthesia.

Anyhow, I get the impression from my OB/GYN that he wants to "manage" my cycles with the pill. I am getting tired of "Band-Aid" solutions. I want to have some long-term relief. The thing that puzzles me about this whole endometriosis situation is what I read about it. I have read that people with this condition usually have really heavy, long periods. I have incredibly light periods. Maybe one day of moderate flow, one day light and several spotting days. My entire cycle length is generally long… but not the flow. I just don't understand. Everything I've read about endometriosis doesn't seem to apply to me.

I am not married, nor am I looking to be so anytime soon, but would like to have the option of bearing my own children in the future. In short, I don't know if my fertility is affected, but I would like to keep that option open.

The nurse told me you prefer the CREIGHTON MODEL and I respect that. Here is my struggle with that: I have a weak to non-existent mucus sign. It is either present or not. It doesn't matter if I take vitamins or not, it's just not present. Well, it's there, but the quality and quantity of it do not change. I don't understand it and I can't tell you why it is that way."

Endometriosis is a disease marked by the implantation of endometrial tissue in locations other than the lining of the uterus. The first known description of this disease was by a German physician, Daniel Shroen, in 1690.[1] It is thought to affect about 5 million American women;[2] although that is almost for certain an underestimate. The research registry of the Endometriosis Association, in an analysis of 3,020 case histories, notes the following symptoms associated with endometriosis: dysmenorrhea (menstrual cramps), pelvic pain, dyspareunia (painful intercourse), infertility, heavy or irregular bleeding, nausea at the time of menses, diarrhea and/or painful bowel movements, dizziness, headaches with menses, fatigue, low-grade fever and low resistance to infection.[3]

Diagnosis

Clinical history, physical examination and other nonsurgical attempts to diagnose endometriosis are notoriously in error.[4,5] The "gold standard" for diagnosis is a diagnostic laparoscopy with histological (microscopic examination of the tissue) confirmation.[6,7] Laparoscopy should be performed in the first half of the menstrual cycle (the pre-Peak phase) because laparoscopy often is combined with laparoscopic treatment, and treatment prior to menstruation is associated with a higher recurrence rate with a shorter recurrence-free interval.[8]

Diagnostic laparoscopy requires a "near-contact" technique and a thorough understanding of the various appearances of endometriosis.

This is all *detailed* in "The Medical & Surgical Practice of **NaProTECHNOLOGY**."

Location of Endometriosis

A thorough evaluation of the anatomic distribution of endometriosis has been published. This distribution is very similar to what I have found in my work with this disease. What is most striking is the relative lack of involvement of the fallopian tubes. In addition, the frequency with which the sigmoid colon, anterior rectum, terminal ileum and cecum are involved is striking and must be specifically evaluated at the time of laparoscopy.[9]

Endometriosis also has been found in a variety of other locations. These would include the lung,[10-13] ureter [14-16] (even to the extent of kidney damage[17]), the diaphragm, [18,19] the sciatic nerve, [20,21] the perineum, [22,23] the uterine artery,[24] and the liver.[25] In addition, it can undergo malignant transformation; although this is not common. There are, nonetheless, numerous reported cases of malignancy arising from endometriotic deposits, and there is substantial evidence that endometriosis can be associated with certain cancers of the ovary.[26] It has even been identified in men.[27]

The Development of Endometriosis

Endometriosis is as close to a malignant disease as one can get while still remaining benign. Those aspects of endometriosis that are similar to malignant disease include its ability to metastasize (spread) both locally and distantly, the ability to attach to other tissues and invade and damage them, and an ability to exhibit cellular proliferation, cellular invasion and neoangiogenesis (the formation of new blood vessels).

The development of the disease most likely represents many possible pathways. The classic explanation is one of *retrograde menstruation* (menstrual blood going back through the fallopian tubes). It also can be spread *hematologically* (through the blood) and *lymphatically* (through the lymphatic system). It has a *genetic predisposition,* and there are *omnipotent cells* that may give rise to it. *Impaired cellular immunity* may play a role and it can be *transplanted surgically.*

The most commonly expressed theory is that of *retrograde menstruation.* This was first described by Dr. J.A. Sampson in 1927.[28]

The basic theory is that women, during the course of their menstrual flow, will have endometrial cells that flow backward through the fallopian tubes, land at various sites in the pelvic cavity and implant themselves. The troubling part of this theory has been that nearly all women have retrograde menstruation to some extent, but all women do not get endometriosis.[29,30] Thus, there must be some other aspect to this event that makes the person who gets endometriosis particularly susceptible to it. This may be an impaired cellular immunity. The basic defenses against the formation of endometriosis would be seem to be the immune mechanisms. These mechanisms are clearly suppressed in women who have endometriosis and thus retrograde menstruation (along with an impaired immune response) may become a viable option for the development of this disease.

There is no question that lymphatic and vascular spread also can occur, and this would explain metastases that are distant. In addition, endometriosis has been observed in the pelvic lymph nodes of approximately 30 percent of women with the disease.[31] While lymph node dissection is not generally part of the surgical procedures involved in the treatment of endometriosis, this involvement of the pelvic lymph nodes might be one explanation for why pelvic pain is not eradicated in some women who have surgical treatment of endometriosis.

Endometriosis also has been observed in the abdominal wall after cesarean section and in the periumbilicus. This supports the theory of its ability to be transplanted.

Association with Infertility

In my own population of patients, the most common symptom seen is that of infertility. These women also may have symptoms of dysmenorrhea (menstrual cramps) and pelvic pain. On physical examination, the majority have a normal pelvic exam. While many see pelvic pain, dysmenorrhea, and dyspareunia (painful intercourse) as the three major symptoms associated with endometriosis (along with abnormal bleeding), in the infertility population it is quite common for the severe dysmenorrhea to be absent and for the patient to have a normal pelvic exam. Diagnostic *laparoscopy* becomes the only way the disease can be positively identified. In these same cases, pelvic ultrasound examination is of somewhat limited value unless there are ovarian endometriomas (cysts of endometriosis). Peritoneal endometriosis, for the most part, cannot be detected by ultrasound.

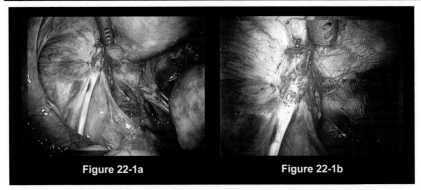

Figure 22-1a   **Figure 22-1b**

Figure 22-1: A red "flame" lesion of endometriosis at the apex of the left uterosacral ligament is shown. (From: Pope Paul VI Institute research, 2004).

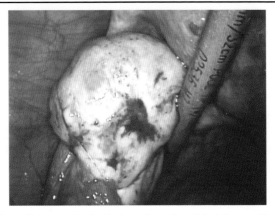

Figure 22-2: A brown lesion associated with the under surface of the left ovary. (From: Pope Paul VI Institute research, 2004).

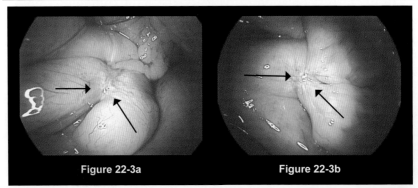

Figure 22-3a   **Figure 22-3b**

Figure 22-3: Endometriosis on the terminal ileum (22-3a) and its mesentery (22-3b). In 22-3a some narrowing of the lumen is present secondary to the scarring that is present. (From: Pope Paul VI Institute research, 2004).

Over the years, there has been a good deal of discussion as to whether or not ovarian and luteal phase dysfunction occur in women who have endometriosis. In our own studies, we have found a very high incidence of both limited mucus cycles and dry cycles in patients with endometriosis who are charting the **CREIGHTON MODEL System** (CrMS). In Table 22-1, a series of 152 patients who underwent a conservative surgery for endometriosis are shown with the category of their mucus cycle identified. Of this group, 67.1 percent had limited mucus cycles and 10.5 percent had dry cycles (77.6 percent either limited or dry). This would compare to about a 20 percent incidence of limited mucus cycles (and only rarely dry cycles) in a normal fertility population. What is additionally interesting about this population is that in the 16 patients who had dry cycles, only one of them became pregnant and she had a tubal pregnancy. An example of this type of pattern with its associated progesterone and estrogen profile is shown in Figure 22-4 in a patient with endometriosis. Her mucus cycle score is 4.7. The average mucus cycle score in a group of patients with infertility and endometriosis is 6.7 and is shown in comparison to normal fertility (average mucus score in normal fertility = 9.3) in Table 22-2.

Table 22-1: The Creighton Model System:
Types of Mucus Cycles in Patients with Endometriosis
treated with Conservative Surgery (N=152)

Type of Mucus Cycle	n	%
Regular	34	22.4
Limited*	102	67.1
Dry*	16	10.5
Total	**152**	**100.0**

* 77.6 percent is limited or dry

Table 22-2: Average Mucus Cycle Score of Patients with Normal
Fertility vs. Patients with Infertility and Endometriosis

Group	n	Average Mucus Cycle Score
Normal fertility controls	62	9.3
Endometriosis	206	6.7[1]

1. From: Pope Paul VI Institute research, 2004.

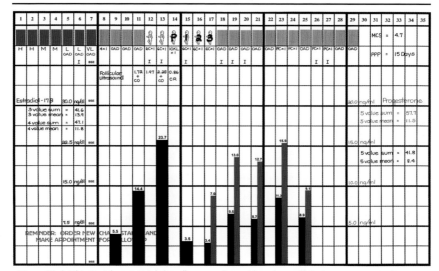

Figure 22-4: This Creighton Model chart from a patient with endometriosis shows a mucus cycle score of 4.7 and a post-Peak phase of 15 days. The follicle was mature, had a positive cumulus oophorus and ruptured completely. The periovulatory E_2, however, is somewhat decreased as is the postovulatory E_2 (From: Pope Paul VI Institute research, 2004).

In a group of patients who had endometriosis and were studied hormonally, the periovulatory E_2 peak was somewhat suppressed and the postovulatory progesterone profile was found to be markedly decreased. This suggests that there is a strong frequency of luteal phase progesterone deficiency (Type II) in patients who have endometriosis.

In a group of 228 patients, a luteal phase defect was observed in 54 percent of the patients studied. The most common type of defect was a Type II luteal phase deficiency. The progesterone profile during pregnancy also is decreased.

These patients with endometriosis also were studied from the point of view of the ultrasound characteristics of their ovulation patterns. In 331 patients who underwent serial ultrasound examination for identification of either an anatomically normal ovulation or a defective ovulation by ultrasound parameters, it was found that 60.3 percent of them had an abnormal ovulation pattern.

Finally, plasma β-endorphin levels also have been studied in patients with infertility who have endometriosis. The mid-luteal phase β-endorphin levels in those patients with infertility were significantly decreased from the normal fertility controls. This group of patients also has a high incidence of premenstrual symptoms, making the underlying hormonal abnormality similar to that observed in women with premenstrual syndrome.

Effects on Fertility

There is little question that endometriosis has an adverse effect on fertility by being strongly associated with infertility[32] and an association with a higher risk of spontaneous abortion.[33-36]

The peritoneal fluid in women with endometriosis increases in volume.[37] This is particularly true at and around the time of ovulation. In peritoneal fluid from infertile women who have endometriosis, it has been found that *it is toxic* to the growth and development of mouse embryos when compared to the fluid from normal women and infertile women without endometriosis.[38,39] Furthermore this fluid from infertile patients with endometriosis has been found to be detrimental to the mouse sperm-ova interaction.[40-42] It also has been suggested that the infertility may be due to poor quality embryos derived from impaired oocytes obtained from malfunctioning ovaries.[43]

Treatment

Ultimately, *endometriosis is a surgical disease.* Although medical therapy — such medications as danazol, leuprolide, oral contraceptives — may offer temporary pain relief, no medication can be used effectively for endometriosis-associated infertility. In addition, while pain relief may occur with medications, the medications are often given without a definitive diagnosis and they have a long list of side effects. In our studies the recurrence rate of the endometriosis is virtually 100 percent when treated with medications.

To improve fertility, endometriosis must be removed so that the inflammatory toxins can be removed, thereby improving fertility. An effective surgical treatment must consistently and reproducibly eradicate the disease. An extensive meta-analysis has shown convincingly the superiority of surgical treatment for the treatment of endometriosis-related infertility.[44]

Final Comment

Endometriosis is a condition that affects a large number of women and, in particular, adversely affects their quality of life and their fertility. It is a disease that should be aggressively identified and treated. In women of reproductive age, treatment should be aimed at preserving reproductive function if that is the patient's desire. By surgically excising the disease or vaporizing it, one can not only preserve fertility, but also enhance it. By treating the underlying hormonal and target organ dysfunction, fertility also is improved (Figure 22-5). The recurrence rate after the areas of endometriosis have been removed by laser at the time of laparoscopy in my practice is less than 20 percent. When the areas are surgically removed (which requires an abdominal incision), the recurrence rate is less than seven percent.

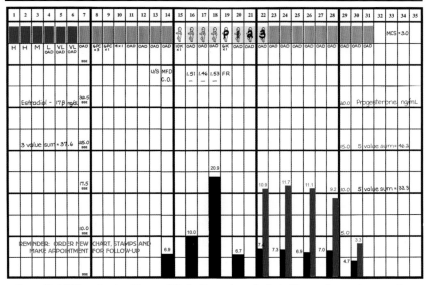

Figure 22-5: This patient is a 35-year-old infertility patient who had a history of severe dysmenorrhea, premenstrual syndrome and infertility. She had a diagnostic laparoscopy that revealed endometriosis, an immature follicle with complete rupture and a very suboptimal periovulatory E_2 profile and a suppressed postovulatory progesterone and E_2 profile. She was treated successfully for her endometriosis, limited mucus and ovarian dysfunction. She successfully achieved a pregnancy and delivered a normal full-term infant. Refer to page 83 for the Vaginal Discharge Recording System (VDRS).

Chapter 23

Polycystic Ovarian Disease

HE FOLLOWING CLINICAL rationale was presented to a patient of mine who had polycystic ovarian disease and had been scheduled for a bilateral ovarian wedge resection. It was written by a registered nurse, but it, in effect, quotes the Physician Review from the insurance company. It says:

> "Since fertility is not the reason for the evaluation, medical treatment should usually be used first to treat the abnormal uterine bleeding and dysmenorrhea/pelvic pain. This treatment would most commonly be oral contraceptives. The metabolic syndrome would most commonly be treated with metformin. Aldactone would most commonly be used for excess androgen problems (hirsutism). The laparoscopy two years ago did not show endometriosis, but this does not rule out endometriosis completely. Oral-contraceptive therapy is the most commonly used treatment for endometriosis, however. The laparoscopy did show pelvic adhesions, which may be the cause of the pain (but not the abnormal bleeding or metabolic problems). If medical therapy was not effective for the abnormal uterine bleeding and pain, then laparoscopy and possibly hysteroscopy might be indicated, but ovarian wedge resection and hysterosalpingogram would not be indicated."

The insurance industry has come to demand that a physician practice a certain way. They do this by withholding reimbursement if some other approach is used. The use of oral contraception for the treatment of polycystic ovaries *does not treat the disease.* The recurrence (persistence of the disease) is 100 percent. It is a cheap treatment that is not a treatment at all. The very best treatment is ovarian wedge resection.

In 1934, at the Central Association of Obstetricians and Gynecologists in New Orleans, Drs. Stein and Leventhal described a series of seven cases in which amenorrhea (the absence of menstruation) was associated with bilateral polycystic ovaries. They also reported surgical wedge resection as a treatment that "was successful in completely restoring physiologic function. Menstruation in every instance became normal and remained so during the period of observation."[1]

At that time, the condition was seen to be associated with hypertension (high blood pressure), hirsutism (increased hair growth), the absence or irregular nature of the menses, infertility and obesity, and became known as the *Stein-Leventhal syndrome*. For many years, polycystic ovarian disease (PCOD) was thought to be present only in those women who presented with all of the clinical aspects of this syndrome. We now know that this condition is more prevalent than previously thought and occurs in women who are not obese or hypertensive; although hirsutism, irregular cycles and some form of reproductive abnormality (usually infertility) are still quite common. We also know that it can occur in women who not only have long and irregular cycles, but in those women whose cycles are regular.

The hormone features of polycystic ovaries include elevated androgen and LH levels, an increased LH:FSH ratio, some increase in serum estrogens, increases in fasting or challenged insulin levels, and occasionally increased prolactin levels.

The incidence of polycystic ovaries (PCO) has been observed to be 14.2 percent in a group of otherwise healthy women. In symptomatic women, the incidence is higher. Using ultrasound, 87 percent of patients with irregular cycles and 92 percent with idiopathic (unknown cause) hirsutism had evidence of polycystic ovaries.[2,3] This is a condition that is more common than once thought and actually may exist in different stages of severity.

This is a condition that not only has fertility-related issues, but also has a significant impact on a woman's health. The incidence of adult-onset diabetes, elevated insulin levels for example, is estimated to be 11 percent. Cardiovascular disease, high LDL-C (bad cholesterol) and low HDL-C levels (good cholesterol) also are observed. There also is thought to be an increased risk in the long term of endometrial and breast cancer.

The prevalence of obesity in PCOD is rather high, ranging from 30 to 60 percent,[4] and insulin resistance is present in more than 50 percent of PCOD patients.[2] While 70 percent of obese PCOD patients exhibit exaggerated insulin secretion, it also is present in 20 to 40 percent of non-obese patients with PCOD.[5]

Diagnosis

Presumptive evidence of polycystic ovaries can be elicited when the following clinical manifestations are present:

- ◆ Clinical evidence of elevated male hormones (e.g., hirsutism, acne, male pattern hair loss) and/or elevated total or free testosterone levels.

- ◆ Irregular length menstrual cycle (i.e., cycle duration greater than 35 days in duration or less than eight cycles per year).

- ◆ Exclusion of other related disorders (e.g. elevated prolactin levels, thyroid dysfunction, androgen-secreting tumors).[6]

With advances in ultrasound technology, it is possible to visualize these ovaries very well. The volume often is exaggerated and the ovaries tend to be more spherical than ovoid.

More definitive evidence for the existence of polycystic ovaries can be obtained by measuring the ratio between pituitary hormones LH and FSH, a male hormone profile (including testosterone, free testosterone, androstenedione and DHEAs), performing a transvaginal ultrasound examination that looks for the classic appearance of the cystic arrangement within the ovaries, and a diagnostic laparoscopy that will reveal the classic pattern of this condition.

At the time of laparoscopy, the ovaries will be seen to be enlarged (Figures 23-1 and 23-2). These ovaries tend to be classic in appearance. They are enlarged, very smooth on their surface, usually quite white and have small gray areas seen through the surface of the ovary. These are the small cystic follicles present under the ovarian capsule. Ultrasound examination will reveal a classic "string of pearls" appearance of the immature follicles (Figures 23-4 and 23-5). Three dimensional ultrasound also is very dramatic (Figure 23-6).

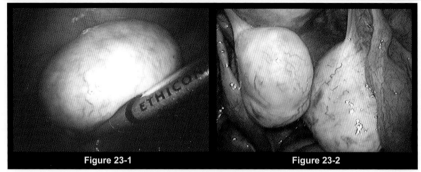

Figure 23-1 **Figure 23-2**

Figure 23-1 and 23-2: Laparoscopic photographs of polycystic ovaries. In Figure 23-2, the two large polycystic ovaries are seen "kissing" or touching each other in the pelvic cavity. These ovaries tend to be enlarged (from two to six times) and very smooth in appearance (From: Pope Paul VI Institute, 2004).

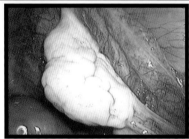

Figure 23-3: A normal-appearing ovary with the characteristic grooves that are seen on the surface. (From: Pope Paul VI Institute Division of Reproductive Ultrasound, 2004).

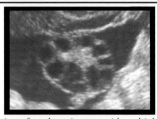

Figure 23-4: An ultrasound view of a polycystic ovary with multiple cysts located peripherally.

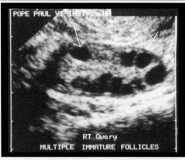

Figure 23-5: A standard two-dimensional ultrasound view of a polycystic ovary showing the peripheral "string of pearls" alignment of the small follicles. (From: Pope Paul VI Institute Division of Reproductive Ultrasound, 2004).

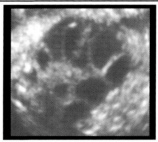

Figure 23-6: A three-dimensional (volumetric) ultrasound picture of a polycystic ovary (From: Pope Paul VI Institute Division of Reproductive Ultrasound, 2004).

The most striking feature of the hormone parameters are a reversal of the FSH-to-LH ratio. Normally FSH is produced in excess of LH, but in PCOD LH is produced in excess of FSH (a reversed FSH:LH ratio). Male hormone levels often are increased, but not always and need not be a part of the hormone parameters for making this diagnosis. The cycles are classically long and irregular.

PCOD is a condition in which the majority of women receive inadequate treatment in spite of the long-term risk factors.[7] Studies of electrologists suggest that education for them about the hirsutism associated with polycystic ovaries might be helpful. In these clients, a significant percentage are associated with polycystic ovaries and very few of them receive adequate medical care.[8]

Hormonal Correlates

Our studies, which agree with other published reports, show that total testosterone, free testosterone, androstenedione and DHEAs levels tend to be elevated in this condition. This is what leads to many of the symptoms associated with polycystic ovaries.

If one looks at the periovulatory estrogen (E_2) levels and the subsequent postovulatory progesterone and estrogen levels, one sees in patients with PCOD that E_2 levels in the periovulatory time period are significantly lower than in a normal ovulation pattern. The postovulatory progesterone levels also are significantly decreased although the E_2 levels are not. It also has been shown that LH receptors in the preovulatory follicles of patients with PCOD are decreased. Thus, the hypothalamic-pituitary dysfunction that exists in this condition exhibits abnormalities, which also affect the target organs.

These target organ effects also are reflected in a high frequency of ovulation-related defects. While most attention over the years has been placed on the obvious irregular nature of ovulation (oligo-ovulation) frequently seen in this group of patients, when the actual ovulation event is studied, it too, is frequently abnormal. While it is difficult to study these events by ultrasound because of the irregular nature of their occurrence, we have studied 18 cycles in patients with PCOD. In this population, 11 of the ovulations (61.1 percent) were defective.

The androgen levels can be treated medically, but the gonadotropin levels respond only to surgery. There is a significant decrease in testosterone, free testosterone, androstenedione and DHEAs following wedge resection. In addition, LH comes down significantly. FSH does not change, but the LH:FSH ratio is significantly reduced. This hormonal change is most likely what is responsible for the recurrence of regular menstrual cycles in a very high percentage of patients (over 90 percent) following ovarian wedge resection.

In 26 pregnant patients with previously documented PCOD, serum progesterone levels were found to be significantly lower during the course of their pregnancies. This suggests a degree of placental insufficiency that follows the luteal phase deficiency observed in these patients.

Endometriosis and PCOD

For many years it was the common belief that endometriosis was not associated with PCOD. This was thought to be the case because these women had very long and irregular cycles and their pelvic tissues were under-stimulated by the ovarian hormones. With this as a rationale, it was thought that endometriosis, which is a hormonally-dependent tissue, would not normally be observed.

It has now been shown, however, that endometriosis does co-exist at an increased incidence in patients with PCOD who also have infertility.[9] In our own population of patients, we have found an incidence of endometriosis in patients with PCOD of 50.9 percent.

Long-term Medical Impact

This condition has a number of implications for a woman's long-term health and quality of life. Not only is it associated with obesity, abnormal hair growth, skin problems and abnormal menstrual periods, but it also is associated with much more significant longer-term health consequences. Women who have PCOD have at least a seven times increased risk of heart attack and heart disease than other women.[10,11]

They are at risk for hypertension and, by the age of 40, 40 percent of them will develop Type II diabetes.[12] In addition, there is a long-term risk of endometrial cancer, which develops because of the unopposed low-dose estrogen stimulation and affects the endometrium.

While it is well established that PCOD constitutes a risk factor for endometrial (uterine) cancer due to the prolonged unopposed action of estrogens on the endometrium,[13,14] elevated insulin levels have been proposed as an independent risk factor for endometrial cancer.[13-16]

Insulin-like growth factors (IGFs) also seem to be implicated in the development of breast cancer,[17] another pathology that is more frequently observed in women with PCOD. A threefold increase in postmenopausal breast cancer has been observed in women with polycystic ovaries.[18] It also has been observed that breast cancer risk is increased in women with elevated male hormones.[19,20]

These women also have an increased risk of dysfunctional uterine bleeding (a form of estrogen breakthrough bleeding) because of the unopposed estrogen effect. In fact, this group of patients more frequently undergoes hysterectomy because of this type of problem.[21] Ovarian cancer also is increased.[22] HDL-Cholesterol is lower and triglycerides are elevated in this patient population. In addition, homocysteine levels are increased in this patient group, which may also increase their cardiovascular risk.[23] PCOD also is reported more often in women with chronic fatigue syndrome.[24]

Hirsutism

Hirsutism is characterized by the excess growth of hair in women and is largely defined by personal and social norms.[25] In women, the presence of terminal (coarse) hair in usually male hormone-dependent areas, such as the upper lip, chin, chest, areolas, abdomen and anterior thighs, denotes a hirsute state.[26]

In approaching the treatment of this condition, there are several different medical approaches. Quite often oral contraceptives are used to both regulate the menstrual cycle and suppress the androgens. The use of the combined oral contraceptives are associated with increased total cholesterol with a tendency towards increasing levels of triglycerides. Thus, it is not an ideal approach to treatment.[27] One of the more benign approaches is to use dexamethasone. This will decrease the adrenal production of male hormones and reduce the stimulation of the hair follicles; it will not eliminate, however, the hirsutism and it may aggravate the hyperinsulinism. If one uses dexamethasone on a long-term basis, then electrolysis also will be necessary. The major side effects to dexamethasone are weight gain and bloating.

Of the other approaches that have been used, spironolactone (Aldactone) seems to be one of the better approaches.[28-31] Spironolactone does affect the male hormone receptors and will, over a prolonged period of time, reduce the hirsutism on its own. Good results can be obtained from it as long as one is patient. The side effects are minimal. It is a category D drug, so it should not be taken in pregnancy.

Insulin Resistance

Polycystic ovary syndrome has major metabolic, as well as reproductive, morbidities. It is an important risk factor for those women who develop *Type II diabetes*. It is associated with insulin resistance, which will amplify reproductive abnormalities observed in PCOD. The insulin-sensitizing drugs may be helpful in the treatment of the insulin resistance related to PCOD.[32]

Insulin resistance is usually thought of as a condition in which the peripheral cells require more insulin to be able to maintain a normal blood sugar state. In such cases, the patients technically are not diabetic because their blood sugar levels are normal. In response to a sugar load, however, their insulin levels will be elevated because of the resistance that exists in the peripheral cells.

It is not necessarily easy to make this diagnosis correctly. In patients with documented PCOD, we have found that nearly all patients had normal blood sugars and slightly over 50 percent had elevated *fasting* insulin levels. When the insulin levels were evaluated further by the patient's weight, a significant association was observed between obesity and elevated fasting insulin levels.

A more specific way for identifying these patients is to use a standardized sugar load (75 grams of oral glucose) and to do a glucose tolerance test, measuring not only the glucose levels, but also the serum insulin levels over the period of a two-hour glucose tolerance procedure.[33] This has become our preferred way for evaluating patients who have polycystic ovaries and are suspected of being insulin resistant.

There is evidence to suggest that treating these patients with metformin (Glucophage) can be beneficial.[34] Metformin has been shown to directly inhibit androgen (male hormone) production. It also has an effect on lowering insulin levels. Along with this, metformin therapy has been shown to improve the menstrual pattern in patients with PCOD.[35-37]

It has been thought that increasing the regularity of the menstrual cycle with the use of metformin also will increase pregnancy rates, especially if used in cooperation with clomiphene citrate (Clomid).[38] The effectiveness and the role of metformin in the treatment of PCOD-related infertility, however, is difficult to assess from currently available research.[39] It does appear to improve ovulation rates, but its effect on pregnancy rates is not striking.[40]

PCOD, with its associated insulin resistance, does appear to be a risk factor for pregnancy-induced diabetes,[41,42] and the use of metformin therapy during the course of pregnancy will reduce the development of diabetes in these patients.[43]

Women who have recurrent pregnancy loss also have a significantly increased prevalence of insulin resistance.[44] Continuing metformin throughout the course of the pregnancy appears to reduce the incidence of spontaneous abortion. It does appear to be safe when given in pregnancy.[45]

CREIGHTON MODEL System in PCOD

The hallmark of a patient who is charting her menstrual and fertility cycles with the **CrMS** and who has PCOD will be long and irregular cycles usually greater than 38 days in duration. Cycles that are 32 to 38 days in duration often are associated with PCO as well, but more research is needed to clarify this. The average cycle length is 44.6 days, the average post-Peak phase is 15 days (but it can be highly variable) and the average mucus cycle score is 4.82. This is significantly decreased from normal.

If an ovarian wedge resection is performed, the effects of that also can be monitored and shown decisively when the woman is prospectively charting her biomarkers. Examples of charting associated with polycystic ovaries are shown in Figure 23-7.

If Clomid is used to stimulate ovulation, then the effects of Clomid can be followed and monitored with the use of the **CrMS**. In addition, post-peak progesterone levels can be used to monitor the biochemical effectiveness of the Clomid.

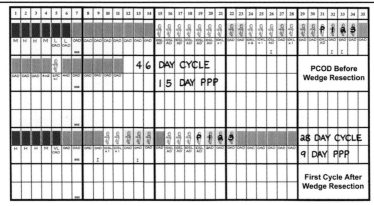

Figure 23-7: This CrMS chart shows a classic cycle that often is observed in women with PCOD. The cycle is 46 days in duration. In the second cycle, the first one following ovarian wedge resection, the cycle has shortened to 28 days. Refer to page 83 for the VDRS.

Progesterone Prophylaxis

Because women with polycystic ovaries have long and irregular cycles and do not ovulate regularly, the endometrium is exposed to low thresholds of estrogen stimulation without opposition from progesterone, which usually comes with the formation of the corpus luteum. This unopposed estrogen stimulation is what is thought to be associated with the formation of adenomatous hyperplasia and subsequently, adenocarcinoma of the endometrium (cancer of the uterus). As a result, women with long and irregular cycles should be regulated with IMH progesterone in a regular fashion so that a regular opposition to the estrogen stimulation is provided. This will give some degree of protection to the formation of adenomatous hyperplasia and endometrial cancer.

Infertility and PCOD

It is common for women with polycystic ovarian disease to have problems with infertility. There are several reasons why this might occur:

1. Because of the long and irregular cycles, ovulation is occurring irregularly and not as frequently as usual, thus decreasing fertility.

2. When ovulation does occur, it often is abnormal. Ovulation defects are common in women with PCOD.

3. Endometriosis is common in women with PCOD.

4. Women with PCOD have limited mucus cycles suggesting target organ dysfunction (the cervix is not functioning normally).

5. Hormone profiles show abnormal function of the developing follicle and subsequent corpus luteum.

In addition to the above, there are undoubtedly other factors that may contribute to the infertility. Among these would be the insulin resistance that often is associated with this condition.

Evaluation of these patients begins by seeing them in the doctor's office and taking a pertinent history. At that time, they should begin tracking their fertility cycles using the **CrMS**. After two months of charting, they can return for evaluation of their charting and a complete physical examination. At that time, the following tests should be performed:

- Seminal fluid analysis (which also can be performed prior to this time)
- An amenorrhea profile
- A pelvic ultrasound examination
- A diagnostic laparoscopy, hysteroscopy and selective hysterosalpingogram

The amenorrhea profile includes a complete evaluation of those hormones that might be involved in creating the hypothalamic dysfunction that results in long and irregular cycles. This would include a FSH and LH level, prolactin, β-endorphin, an androgen profile and complete thyroid profile.

With the FSH and LH profile, one is looking for a reversal of the FSH:LH ratio. Usually FSH is produced in excess of LH, but in PCOD, LH is produced in excess of FSH. Prolactin levels usually are normal, but β-endorphin levels often are quite low. Androgen levels may or may not be elevated and thyroid disturbances may or may not be detected.

On ultrasound examination, one looks for the type of changes described previously in this chapter. In ordering such a pelvic ultrasound examination, it is good for the ordering physician to discuss with the radiologist or the ultrasonographer the type of evaluation you are requesting and the type of clinical findings you are working with. By describing PCOD to the radiologist and the type of ultrasound findings characteristic of this condition, the examination will turn out to be much more productive.

A diagnostic laparoscopy is performed for several reasons. First of all, this provides the definitive diagnosis of polycystic ovaries. In addition, with 50 percent of women with PCOD also having endometriosis, this usually can be identified and treated at the time of the laparoscopy with laser. Hysteroscopy and selective hysterosalpingography also is helpful in further evaluating the inside of the uterus and the patency of the fallopian tubes.

When this evaluation is completed, the patient returns for a comprehensive management review, which reviews the findings of the laparoscopy and all of the other tests including the **CrMS** charting. A treatment plan then is outlined.

In treating these patients, ovulation induction with clomiphene is the first line of treatment if it has not been used yet. This treatment program should continue for approximately six cycles. An approximate 30 percent pregnancy rate can be expected. There are many women with PCOD, however, who are resistant to clomiphene. In those cases, the only treatment that really is effective is ovarian wedge resection. In the case of clomiphene resistance, ovarian wedge resection should be the treatment of choice. In fact, because of the many positive and long lasting effects of ovarian wedge resection, it can be considered the first line of treatment in many patients.

When using ovulation-inducing medications, especially clomiphene, it almost always requires some type of mucus-enhancing medication because of the anti-estrogen effect of the clomiphene.

An example of a woman who has achieved a pregnancy without medication following ovarian wedge resection is shown in Figure 23-8.

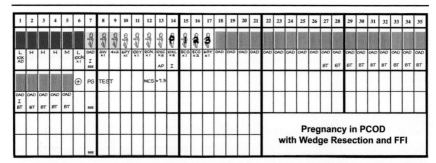

Figure 23-8: This chart shows a pregnancy occurring in the second cycle following ovarian wedge resection for PCOD. No medications were used in the cycle of conception. Cycles prior to the wedge resection were consistently 50-60 days in duration (From: Pope Paul VI Institute, 2004). Refer to page 83 for the VDRS.

For the Doctor

1. The mucus cycle score can be calculated from the types of mucus observations recorded by the vaginal discharge recording system. The highest score is 16.0 and the lowest score is 0.0 (a dry cycle). A regular mucus cycle scores 9.1 or greater, a limited mucus cycle 7.5 or less and a dry cycle 0.0.

2. There are two main ways a period can be induced with progesterone in women with PCOD and long cycles. The preferred method is to give IMH progesterone in a dosage of 100 mg on day 18, 21 and 24 of the cycle. In this way, at about the 28th or 30th day of the cycle, another menstrual period will occur. This intramuscular progesterone will regulate the menstrual cycle and provide protection to the endometrium. It is given long-term, so long as the menstrual cycles remain long and irregular.

3. An alternate approach to this is to use vaginal IMH progesterone in a dosage of 300 mg capsules every day at bedtime from day 18 through 27 of the cycle. Usually one or two days after the last progesterone dose, the menstrual period will begin. If ovulation begins to occur on this dosage, then the dosage should be changed to Peak +3 through 12.

Absence of Menstrual Periods

AN UNCOMMON CAUSE of infertility is the *absence of ovulation* (anovulation) associated with the *absence of menstruation* (amenorrhea). If the underlying cause can be identified, however, it represents one of the most successful groups of patients to be treated.

There are a variety of different causes associated with this, but four will be considered here:

- polycystic ovary syndrome
- hypothalamic amenorrhea
- hyperprolactinemia
- premature onset of menopause

In *polycystic ovary syndrome,* the most common cyclic pattern observed is one of long and irregular cycles. The actual occurrence of amenorrhea is not common, but it can, on occasion, occur. Thus, an evaluation for polycystic ovaries is important in the overall evaluation for this condition (see chapter 23).

In *hypothalamic amenorrhea,* the standard amenorrhea (hormone) profile (Table 24-1) will be normal. This type of amenorrhea is caused by a dysfunction between the hypothalamus and the pituitary gland secondary to chronic stress. One of the more common associated stressors is the college student who is under stress in taking examinations. Prolonged absence of ovulation in these patients, however, can be a

Table 24-1: Amenorrhea Hormone Profile		
FSH	Testosterone	Total T_4
LH	Free testosterone	Free T_4
Prolactin	Androstenedione	TSH
β-endorphin	DHEAs	Total T_3 Reverse T_3 T_3:rT_3 ratio

cause of infertility. It also can be a pre-condition towards the development of osteoporosis because of the low estrogen state.

In patients who have *hyperprolactinemia,* their prolactin level will be highly elevated in the face of what otherwise are normal hormone levels. Usually this is caused by a prolactin-secreting microadenoma (a generally benign tumor) of the pituitary gland. Evaluation includes not only prolactin levels, but also a MRI of the pituitary gland, which will reveal the presence of the tumor.

Another condition to be discussed in the conditions of amenorrhea is Kallmann syndrome. This is a condition of amenorrhea and anovulation associated with anosmia (the inability to smell). These patients have primary amenorrhea, which means they never develop menstrual periods. They need supplemental estrogen to develop secondary sexual characteristics when they are teenagers.

A final consideration in the diagnosis of amenorrhea is the question of the *premature onset of menopause.* This actually is one of the more common associated causes of amenorrhea although by itself it is quite rare. The difficulty with the premature onset of menopause is that it almost always comes unexpectedly. The periods stop, the woman begins to have hot flashes and upon evaluation her FSH and LH levels are highly elevated. On occasion, these hormonal characteristics will disappear on their own and normal function will resume, but most often it is permanent. In addition, it is resistant to treatment. These patients need to be treated with hormone replacement therapy so as to prevent bone loss since this occurs so early in their life.

The **CREIGHTON MODEL** charting patterns that are seen in this population of patients are shown in Figure 24-1 A and B. In Figure 24-1A, the pattern is one of predominant dryness in the absence of menstruation. In Figure 24-1B, a pattern more consistent with the variable return of Peak-type mucus is illustrated. This latter pattern is

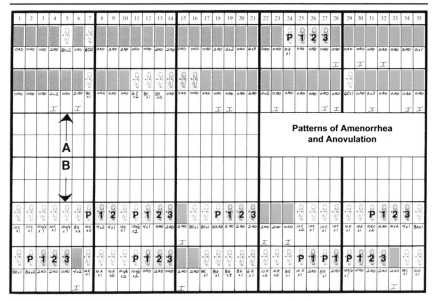

Figure 24-1 A and B: Two different CrMS patterns observed with amenorrhea/anovulation. The upper pattern (A) is dry in the absence of menstruation. The lower pattern (B) shows a variable return of Peak-type mucus in the absence of ovulation and menstruation (From: Pope Paul VI Institute research, 2004). Refer to page 83 for the Vaginal Discharge Recording System (VDRS).

apparently due to a waxing and waning of low levels of estrogen, which are enough to stimulate the cervix and produce a mucus discharge.

There are, of course, other conditions that also might be associated with chronic anovulation. This might include conditions such as anorexia nervosa, malnutrition, Cushing syndrome, and the congenital absence of ovaries. In some rare cases, the anovulatory pattern may have an auto-immune cause.

Those patterns associated with polycystic ovaries, hypothalamic amenorrhea, hyperprolactinemia, and Kallmann syndrome all lend themselves nicely to **NaProTECHNOLOGY**-related treatment interventions for infertility.

For the Doctor

Treatment of hyperprolactinemia is either bromocriptine (Parlodel), which will suppress the production of prolactin and help shrink the tumor, or a newer medication called Dostinex. Almost always these tumors can be brought under control with these types of medications, although on occasion, they can cause fairly extensive damage. Once the cycle becomes regular, fertility is usually re-established.

Pregnancy can be achieved in patients with hypothalamic amenorrhea or Kallmann's syndrome with the use of pulsatile gonadotropin-releasing hormone to stimulate ovulation and the **CrMS** to identify fertility.

ERTILITY IS A biologic function of both a husband and wife who, through sexual intercourse, unite their gametes. When a woman has difficulty achieving a pregnancy, an evaluation for that problem must involve not only her, but also her husband. This evaluation can be helpful at giving important information to the couple so they may understand better the future capability of their procreative potential. At the same time, it can be a complex and difficult area to work with.

In 1677, Antoine van Leeuwenhoek, one of the inventors of the microscope, discovered the spermatozoa and described his findings in a letter to the Royal Society of London. He provided a detailed description of the living spermatozoon and their movement. He was the first to hypothesize that the sperm actually penetrate an egg at the moment of conception.[1]

Since that time, various attempts have been made to evaluate the male's fertility and also develop ways of treating it. Generally speaking, this has been left up to the urologist, but experience would suggest that most urologists have little interest in male infertility problems and are quick to refer patients to an artificial reproduction technologist. Thus, I usually recommend that patients see a urologist mostly for the purpose of a physical examination. Any further evaluation and medical treatment is something that I usually undertake myself. Family physicians are better qualified to undertake such examinations since this is a part of their scope of practice. For a gynecologist, however, while it is not a complex or difficult examination, it is out of their field of expertise. A urologist also is used for any surgical reconstruction that is necessary (for example, a varicocele repair or a reversal of a vasectomy).

The most common diagnostic categories observed in the evaluation of the male will be varicocele, idiopathic oligospermia, or obstruction of the vas deferens.[2]

There are a variety of different fertility-impairing medications that also need to be investigated. For example, anabolic steroids, cimetidine, steroidal antiandrogens (DES), cyclosporine, and phenothiazine will suppress to some extent the hypothalamic-pituitary-gonadal axis. Such medications as ketoconazole, sulfasalazine, valproic acid, spironolactone and allopurinol are directly gonadal toxic. In addition, calcium-channel blockers, colchicine, nitrofurantoin and minocycline are known at least, on occasion, to impair fertilization.[3] Other factors such as marijuana use or the large ingestion of caffeine also can impair the formation of sperm.

It also is known that increased scrotal temperature can impair sperm development in men. It has been shown, for example, that the scrotal temperature of infertile men is significantly greater than that observed in men who are fertile. The higher the scrotal temperature, the more likely there will be alterations.[4] An exact cause of the hyperthemia is not known but may result in up to a 0.5°C elevation in temperature.

Varicocele (a vericose vein of the testicle), one of the more common findings in an infertile population, proves to be somewhat complex because it also may be observed in men who have normal fertility. In fact, studies on normally fertile men show that 61 percent may have some degree of a varicocele; although, most of these are subclinical. The subclinical varicoceles do not appear to have any impact on fertility.[5]

Seminal Fluid Analysis

To assess male fertility, short of a pregnancy, an analysis of the seminal fluid is helpful. This can be accomplished in a variety of ways, some of which are helpful and others that are not, while at the same time some are acceptable to patients while others are not.

The postcoital test (Sims-Huhner test) has been shown to have only a poor to fair reproducibility among trained observers using a standardized scoring system.[6] This particular test, which evaluates an interaction of the seminal fluid with the cervical mucus, is enticing because it involves the natural act of intercourse and does not involve masturbatory activity; the overall results, however, are not very useful. If it is to be done, it should be timed with the appearance of good mucus and not just the day of the cycle.

The American Society for Reproductive Medicine has the following recommendation: "At least two semen samples collected on separate days by masturbation are recommended."[7] Thus, encouraging men to masturbate becomes a part of the standard medical evaluation for infertility; this approach to semen collection, however, is dehumanizing and humiliating. Men are usually placed in a washroom with pornographic literature and asked to masturbate. Having spoken to many men about this over the years, it is not well received by most, though they often do not object because it is sort of the "macho" thing to do. It is not something that settles well with most of the male patients I have discussed this with. In fact, there are many men who refuse a seminal fluid analysis thinking that this is the only way that seminal fluid can be collected.

There is, however, an excellent alternative to collect seminal fluid that does not violate one's religious, moral or aesthetic beliefs and obtains reliable results. This technique is to use a perforated seminal collection device (SCD). This collection device can be purchased from: Apex Medical Technologies, Inc., 10064 Mesa Ridge Ct., Suite 202, San Diego, CA 92121. Phone: 1-800-345-3208. The perforations need to be placed by an assistant with a sterile needle because the SCD does not come pre-perforated. In this fashion, however, the seminal fluid can be collected with an act of intercourse, at home, in a way that is not contraceptive. When the seminal fluid is collected in this fashion, it needs to be brought to the hospital or to the laboratory within 30 to 45 minutes after collection and it should be kept warm during this time. It is preferable for the seminal fluid to be emptied from the collection device into a clean plastic container prior to being brought into the laboratory.

There have been a number of studies over the years that have shown this type of approach to the collection of the seminal fluid to be very reliable.[8-10] In fact, this technique has been found to be superior to masturbation or coitus interruptus for the collection of seminal fluid.[11,12]

Table 25-1: Semen Analysis Minimal Standards of Adequacy

Parameter	Adequate Values
On at least two occasions	
Ejaculate volume	1.5–5.0 mL
Sperm density	> 20 million/mL
Motility	> 60 percent
Forward progression	> 2 (scale 0-4)
and	
No significant sperm agglutination	
No significant pyospermia	
No hyperviscosity	

From: Sigman M, Lipshultz LI, Howard SS: Evaluation of the subfertile male. In: Lipshultz LI, Howard SS (Eds): Infertility in the Male, Ed3. St. Louis, Mosby-Yearbook, 1997, p 173-103.

The work done at our center, where the seminal fluid parameters using a perforated seminal collection device were compared with same patient results where the seminal fluid had been collected by masturbation and the analysis had been performed elsewhere, showed very interesting results. In this analysis, *no statistically-significant differences* were found in an evaluation of the following seminal fluid parameters: volume, viscosity, motility, percent of normal sperm (morphology), the total sperm count and the effective sperm count - ESC (the count/cc x percent motility x percent normals).

This brings us to a discussion of what should be considered a normal sperm count. The standard sperm count parameters are identified in Table 25-1. In these parameters, if the count is greater than 20 million, the motility is greater than 60 percent and the morphology reflects greater than 60 percent normal sperm, the seminal fluid analysis can be considered normal.

More recently, the World Health Organization has issued a different set of reference values. In this case, the sperm concentration of greater than 20 million is still present, but motility is considered normal if it is greater than 50 percent and the morphology is normal if greater than 15 percent. The World Health Organization criteria for normal semen reference ranges reflects an introduction of the *strict Kruger criteria* for sperm morphology. This development requires further comment (see Table 25-2).

In January 1988, Dr. T.F. Kruger introduced the concept that the sperm morphology of patients could only be considered normal if the morphology assessment was based on his "strict" criteria.[13]

Table 25-2: World Health Organization Reference Criteria for Semen Analysis[1]

Parameter	Reference Values
Volume	$\geq$ 2.0 mL or greater
pH	7.2–7.8
Sperm concentration	$\geq$ 20 million/mL
Total sperm count	$\geq$ 40 million
Motility	$\geq$ 50%
Morphology[2]	> 15% normal forms

1. From: WHO Laboratory Manual for the Examination of Human Semen and Sperm-Cervical Mucus Interaction. WHO. 4th Ed. Cambridge University Press. New York, 1999.
2. Adapted from Kruger.

Unfortunately, this approach to evaluating the seminal fluid now has been incorporated into most laboratories around the country. This produces seminal fluid testing results that, for example, may show a count of 98 million with a motility of 80 percent but a normal morphology of only 5 percent. Such an analysis is possible only with the utilization of the Kruger criteria. Most pathologists have fallen into the trap that has been set by these criteria. In fact, this criteria was *specifically established* to determine who would be a better candidate for *in vitro* fertilization, and the *criteria has little to do with the natural procreative act.* As a result, many patients now are getting very odd results from their pathologists or their laboratories and the results often do not legitimately make sense.

This idea of strict criteria has been further developed by the National Cooperative Reproductive Medicine Network.[14] *These strict criteria have had no evaluation in the group of infertility patients who are interested in achieving pregnancy with natural intercourse and thus have little or no application in that setting.* The move of many laboratories toward the adoption of these criteria is another example of the *insensitivity* that the medical community has shown to many patients who refuse to participate in any IVF or ART-type program. Furthermore, it is another example of how they have been *abandoned* by those in reproductive medicine. As an aside, the use of the Kruger criteria has led to a huge increase in the use of the ICSI form of IVF (see below).

Treatment: Intrauterine Insemination and ICSI

It has been suggested that if the individual male is identified as having male factor infertility (keep in mind that the *strict morphology tends to falsely encourage such a diagnosis*), treatment should include intrauterine insemination and, if this fails, *in vitro* fertilization with *intracytoplasmic sperm injection* (ICSI). Very little attempt is made at further identifying the underlying causes or treating men medically. Little attempt is made at trying to assist couples at achieving pregnancy naturally.

And yet, the success rates for intrauterine insemination for "male factor infertility" are very poor. When IUI is used in natural cycles, the pregnancy rate ranges from 0.0 to 9.0 percent. When IUI is used in clomiphene citrate-stimulated cycles for male factor infertility, the pregnancy rates range from 0.1 to 16.0 percent and with HMG-stimulated cycles, the pregnancy rate ranges from one to 15 percent. Thus, intrauterine insemination, with its very low success rate and patients with male factor-associated fertility problems (as determined by the Kruger criteria) are *primed to be directed into the artificial reproductive technologies.* A very high percentage of these patients eventually will have that recommendation presented to them.

ICSI also has been recommended for treatment of male factor infertility and the obstruction of the vas deferens (obstructive azoospermia). A recent cost-benefit analysis, however, demonstrated that microsurgical correction of this problem was more efficacious and cost-effective than ICSI for post-vasectomy infertility (a cost of $25,470 versus $72,521 per live birth). Furthermore, concerns have been raised about exposing women to the risks and complications that may be associated with ICSI. There is some concern about the transmission of abnormal genetic material in this procedure.[15] The overall completed pregnancy rate in patients being treated with ICSI ranges only from 15 to 19 percent.[16]

Medical Treatment

Azoospermia (the complete absence of sperm) has no known treatment unless this condition is secondary to obstruction. If it is obstructive in origin, then surgery can be helpful. For those people who are azoospermic (which is quite rare), counseling should be provided to encourage them to adopt. That is part of the approach in **NaProTECHNOLOGY**.

With those patients who have oligospermia (low sperm count), the most common medication used to help stimulate the sperm count is clomiphene citrate.[17,18] Approximately 55 percent of patients with oligospermia can expect an improvement in their sperm count with the use of clomiphene.

The most recommended dosage of clomiphene is 25 mg per day for 25 days followed by a rest period of five or six days; in our program, however, we have found that lower doses of clomiphene are, at least empirically, more successful. Our standard dose of clompihene in oligospermia is 5 mg by mouth two times a day. This can be prepared through a compounding pharmacy. Generally speaking, there are good data to support the effectiveness of clomiphene in improving the sperm count,[19] at least in some patients.

Human chorionic gonadotropin (HCG) has been shown to have a high grade of predictability concerning the restoration of fertility. While it is not nearly 100 percent effective, it does help the majority of men. When administered intramuscularly, HCG has a long circulating half-life (about 30 to 40 hours), significantly increasing plasma testosterone levels 24 hours after HCG application. Human chorionic gonadotropin has been used with success in patients with persistently low motility.[19] This also has improved pregnancy rates.[20] Attempts have been made to combine HCG treatment with various forms of FSH (either human menopausal gonadotropin or recombinant human FSH). Results from this, however, have not been encouraging.[21-23]

A variety of other approaches also have been utilized. For example, clonidine will improve spermatogenesis in patients who have maturation arrest. Clonidine is an alpha-adrenergic agent that stimulates growth hormone secretion.[24] Prostaglandin inhibitors have been used[25] and pentoxifylline has proved beneficial in oligospermia.[26,27]

Glutathione, in a dosage of 600 mg by intramuscular injection every other day over a period of two months, demonstrated a statistically-significant-positive effect on sperm motility. Glutathione has a number of physiologic and pharmacologic qualities. This recently has been found to be involved in sperm damage, resulting in a reduced fertilizing potential.[28]

Finally, vitamin E also has been used as an antioxidant to treat reactive oxygen species associated with male infertility.[29] An oral administration of vitamin E significantly improved the *in vitro* function of human spermatozoa.

Vaginal Lubricants

It has been shown in various studies that lubricants used to assist intercourse are, to varying degrees, spermatocidal.[30-34] Raw egg white is the only one that has been shown not to be deleterious to the sperm. The use of raw egg white, however, is *not* recommended because of the potential to have a foreign protein allergic reaction from placing this in the vagina.[32] In a study of 15 substances that have been used over the years as vaginal lubricants, petroleum jelly and glycerine have had the least detrimental affects on motility and were considered, at the time, to be the lubricants of choice.[31] It should be specifically noted that substances such as K-Y® Jelly or Surgilube® are especially spermicidal. A more recently developed lubricant, Pre-Seed, has been developed to be helpful to the sperm rather than being toxic (www.preseed.com).

CREIGHTON MODEL FertilityCare™ System and NaProTECHNOLOGY

The **CREIGHTON MODEL System** plays a specific role in patients who have difficulty achieving pregnancy when the seminal fluid parameters are abnormal. In such circumstances, identifying the time of fertility with accuracy will assist couples with severe oligospermia to achieve pregnancy. In Figures 25-1 and 25-2, four examples of successful pregnancies in these circumstances are shown. In Figure 25-1, the patient's husband had a sperm count done on day 10 of the pregnancy cycle. His effective sperm count (ESC) was 189,666/cc. This

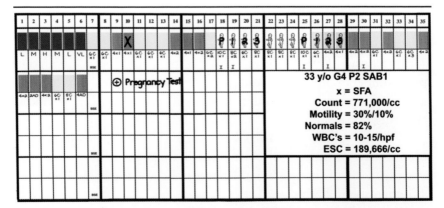

Figure 25-1: Patient whose husband has severe oligospermia. Effective sperm count (ESC) was 189,666/cc at time of pregnancy using natural insemination and properly-timed intercourse (From: Pope Paul VI Institute research, 2004). Refer to page 83 for the Vaginal Discharge Recording System.

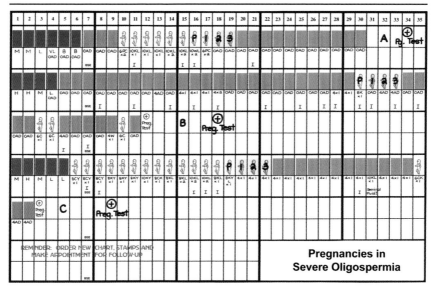

Figure 25-2: Patients with severe oligospermia and successful pregnancy using properly-timed intercourse and natural insemination: A) effective sperm count = 30,000/cc, B) effective sperm count = 116,850/cc, C) effective sperm count = 50,000/cc (From: Pope Paul VI Institute research, 2004). Refer to page 83 for the Vaginal Discharge Recording System (VDRS).

was not this patient's first pregnancy; it was her fourth. They had more difficulty achieving this pregnancy, however, than the others. Nonetheless, the only treatment eventually implemented after she had been evaluated and found to be within normal limits was *fertility-focused intercourse* through the **CrMS**.

In Figure 25-2, several similar examples are presented. In patient A, the effective sperm count was 30,000/cc, in patient B the ESC was 116,850/cc and in patient C, the ESC was 50,000/cc. These examples are presented to show that the **CrMS** and **NaProTECHNOLOGY** can be used to assist couples achieve pregnancy even when there is severe oligospermia.

In Figure 25-2, pregnancy cycle B, there are other findings. This patient's Peak Day occurred on day 30 of the cycle with an observation of "tacky clear" (8K x 1). This was the only peak mucus observation of the entire cycle. The couple used this day and successfully achieved a pregnancy. Later, with an ultrasound performed approximately four weeks following the estimated time of conception, verification of this conception date was achieved. The due date as estimated by ultrasound and the due date estimated by the Peak Day were identical within one day.

Over the years of our involvement in the treatment of infertility, we have consistently seen successes in patients who have severe oligospermia. These results equal or exceed the success rate of all of the artificial reproductive technologies.

Menstrual Cramps and Pelvic Pain

CHRONIC PELVIC PAIN is medically defined as pain in the pelvic region that is not menstrual in origin, but does have a duration of at least three months and/or menstrual pain that is at least six months in duration.[1] This chapter will focus on chronic pelvic pain that is predominantly menstrual in presentation, but often associated with pelvic pain throughout the course of the menstrual cycle as well. It will explain how surgical **NaProTECHNOLOGY** can help.

It is difficult to determine exactly how many women suffer from these types of problems or difficulties, but one estimate is that 9,200,000 women suffer from this each year in the United States and about one-third of them eventually will seek medical care.[1] In addition, there is a huge economic impact since this pain also can affect various components of a woman's life. If one puts the cost of medical care, the effect on a woman's life and her productivity at work, the economic impact would reach into the billions of dollars.[1]

In approaching this condition, one must obtain a good medical history. In the form used by the Pope Paul VI Institute, found in Figure 26-1, obtaining important information can be determined about the severity and location of the pelvic pain. Furthermore, one can determine if previous medications have been used, such as non-steroidal anti-inflammatory agents or oral contraceptives. Following this, a good physical examination also is important. This includes, of course, a pelvic examination, where masses in the pelvic area, such as ovarian cysts or other masses, might be identified. At the same time,

PELVIC PAIN SCALE
POPE PAUL VI INSTITUTE

Patient's Name:_____

Date:_____

Diagnosis:_____

Intervening Rx:_____

No Pain		Mild Pain		Moderate Pain			Severe Pain		Debilitating Pain

```
 |----+----+----+----+----+----+----+----+----+----|
 1    2    3    4    5    6    7    8    9   10
```

PAIN SCORE

1. Menstrual Cramps

2. Pelvic Pain (other than cramps) with menstruation

3. Low backache with menses

4. Are you genitally active? Yes_____ No_____
   If yes, pain with intercourse with deep penetration

5. Pain with bowel movements, especially during menstruation

6. Do you experience period pain or low backache during the week
   leading up to menstruation? Yes_____ No_____   If yes, how severe?

7. Do you have pelvic pain between menstrual periods? Yes_____ No_____
   If yes, how severe?

8. Do you have pelvic pain at the time of ovulation?   Yes_____ No_____
   If yes, how severe?

9. Do you have any of the following additional symptoms at the time of your period?

Constipation	Yes_____ No_____
Diarrhea	Yes_____ No_____
Intestinal Cramps	Yes_____ No_____
Pelvic Pain with Exercise	Yes_____ No_____

10. How many days each month do you experience some type of pelvic pain? _____

11. How many days each month do you feel good? _____

12. Which of the following medications have you taken for this pain and how effective have they been?

EFFECTIVENESS

MEDICATION	YES	NO	NO EFFECT	SOME EFFECT	GOOD EFFECT
Anaprox					
Motrin					
Aspirin					
Codeine					
Birth Control Pills					
Other _____					

THANK YOU FOR YOUR TIME!

Prepared by
Pope Paul VI Institute For the Study of Human Reproduction

Figure 26-1: The pelvic pain scale used at the Pope Paul VI Institute.

various types of tenderness within the pelvic area also can be ascertained, such as ovarian tenderness, tenderness or nodules behind the uterus, tenderness with manipulation of the uterus and tenderness over the bladder.

The first approach to most of these patients will be the use of non-steroidal anti-inflammatory agents (such as ibuprofen). Because of the increase in prostaglandins that are associated with menstrual cramps, these medications often will be helpful or effective because they inhibit the effect of the prostaglandins. Other approaches often promoted include the use of oral contraceptives or gonadotropin-releasing hormone agonists.[2] While both of those approaches can be temporarily helpful in pain relief, they offer no long-term effect. Furthermore, they only suppress the symptoms while ignoring the underlying disease.

In reviewing the patient's history, it also is important to inquire about premenstrual symptoms. It is quite common that women with severe dysmenorrhea (menstrual cramps) and pelvic pain also will have fairly significant premenstrual symptoms. In fact, it is not at all uncommon, when they begin to chart their cycles using the **CREIGHTON MODEL System**, to also have limited mucus cycles, variable length post-Peak phases and eventually, if measured, decreased progesterone production. It is thought that these symptoms occur as a result of the *chronic stress,* which occurs secondary to the presence of the chronic pain pattern. In addition to that, it also is important to investigate the possibility that there may be some past history of childhood sexual abuse or post-traumatic stress disorder.[3,4] Women with chronic pelvic pain can demonstrate alterations that parallel correlates of post-traumatic stress disorder.[4]

Abnormalities at the time of diagnostic laparoscopy have been reported in anywhere from 9 to 80 percent of the patients with chronic pelvic pain and menstrual cramps.[5,6] The *Association of Professors of Gynecology and Obstetrics* (APGO) have noted that such wide variability in the identification of intra-abdominal abnormalities suggests *a considerable variability in diagnostic skill, surgical skill and clinical expertise of the practitioners involved.*[1]

The need for laparoscopy for diagnosis and treatment of these women continues to be a subject that remains under considerable debate.[7] Nonetheless, a significant proportion of patients who undergo laparoscopy will be found to have endometriosis.[5,6] The inadequacies of the surgeon's experience and ability to identify endometriosis, however, must be taken into account and patients, specifically, should work toward seeing physicians who are specifically trained in the identification and treatment of endometriosis. Furthermore, it is suggested here that skills in "near contact" laparoscopy be available to the surgeon undertaking this care. I also think that laser skills are very important.

The causes of pelvic pain can be multiple. In my own experience, *the overwhelming majority of patients with these symptoms have endometriosis*. There may be other situations in which the cause is pelvic adhesive disease, perhaps secondary to either previous pelvic infection or a previous surgical procedure, such as the adhesions that form following cesarean section when the peritoneum is not closed.

We report here a series of 234 patients who have chronic and severe pelvic pain and dysmenorrhea (menstual cramps) secondary to endometriosis. These patients were treated either by laser laparoscopy (n=152) or by laser laparotomy (n=82). The age and gravidity of these two populations and the distribution of their symptom complexes were similar.

The decision to treat this either by laser laparoscopy or by laparotomy and excision of the endometrial implants is made based on the extent and location of the endometrial implants. If the endometriosis is fairly mild and does not involve the fallopian tube, ovary, anterior rectum (or any other part of the bowel), or is not overlying the ureter, then *laparoscopic laser vaporization* of the endometrial implants is used. When the endometriosis is more extensive involving endometriomas on the ovary (cysts of endometriosis), endometriosis on the rectum (which is particularly painful), fallopian tube endometriosis, or endometriosis on the bowel (the terminal ileum or cecum) or overlying the ureter, then laparotomy with *excision of endometrial implants* is used.

In both situations, a laser uterosacral nerve ablation (LUNA) also is performed. This procedure cuts a portion of the nerve supply to the pelvic area and assists in the reduction of pelvic pain.

A subgroup of the patients in this population were a group of women 20 years of age or younger (n=19). The average age of this group was 17.4 years and the breakdown of symptoms is somewhat different than in the older population. While menstrual cramps are still the prominent symptom, pain prior to the onset of menstruation was observed more commonly and low backache a little less common.

When considering such issues as absence from school or activity being clearly inhibited, there was a significant difference in those women who were 20 years of age or younger versus those who were over 20. In this case, the younger women missed school or work at a significantly higher rate than the older women did and indicated that their activity clearly had been inhibited at a much higher rate. It should be pointed out that this is, in some ways, not too unexpected in a younger population where the maturity level is lower and the coping skills are less refined.

Each of the women in the population previously had been treated with oral contraceptives and continued to have pain or did not wish to continue on oral contraceptives.

Results

The results of this approach have been outstanding. Of course, it is not just the result of a LUNA procedure, but rather the laser vaporization of all endometrial implants as identified by laparoscopy or the surgical excision and repair of the areas of endometriosis identified at the time of laparotomy along with the LUNA procedure that account for the success.

The average pain scores prior to laser laparoscopy averaged 2.71 (on a scale of 3 where 3=severe pain). Laser laparotomy was 2.74. But in the follow-up over the first year, the pain scores ranged from 0.84 to 1.4, which is in the mild range. In each case, the reduction in pain with this approach was statistically highly significant. For most patients, this results in long-term pain relief. In some cases, however, pain will return as the endometriosis returns and subsequent laparoscopy may be necessary. In our experience, however, the need for repeat laparoscopy has not been common (less than 12 percent come for repeat laparoscopy).

In the *19 teenagers* who were on birth control pills because of severe dysmenorhea (menstrual cramps) of unknown cause, *each of them (100 percent) had endometriosis* and were improved significantly after surgery.

There are some patients who do not get better following these treatments. The incidence of hysterectomy in the laser laparoscopy group was 12.2 percent, while in the laser laparotomy group was 10.2 percent (not significantly different). The incidence of hysterectomy is very low for this population of patients. Left untreated, the hysterectomy rate is generally considered to be 40 percent.

Final Comment

Many years ago, when I was in training as a young obstetrician-gynecologist, the thought of a woman with pelvic pain was, in some ways, quite disturbing. It was thought that no matter what anyone did, only 50 percent would get better, while 50 percent would continue to experience pain. This led to a generally defeatist attitude regarding surgical treatment. Over the years as more experience was obtained and the use of diagnostic laparoscopy was implemented to try to establish the underlying cause, the eventual outcome for these patients was *significantly better than previously thought.* In fact, with a good "near contact" laparoscopic procedure, one usually can identify the underlying causes of the pelvic pain. With treatment of those underlying causes, the patient can expect to become better. The most complex portion of this is the psychosomatic component of it. While I am hesitant to suggest that some of the pain factors may be psychosomatic, there clearly can be an overlying factor of a psychosomatic reaction to the pain in some patients. This often is difficult to pinpoint through the first several visits, and it only affects, in our experience, a small percentage of patients. It is good, however, if one can work closely with a clinical psychologist who might be able to be of assistance in cases such as this. With the appropriate psychological support and care, adopting certain coping strategies, these patients also can get better. It is important to keep in mind that whether or not the pain is organic or psychosomatic in origin, *it is still pain.* Thus, the pain and its underlying causes must be addressed. With a sound and organized approach to this and the use of good surgical technique, excellent results can be anticipated.

Commonly, women with severe pelvic pain and/or menstrual cramps can have significant associated hormone dysfunctions that cause *premenstrual syndrome,* which in time decreases their ability to cope. Having them chart their cycles and doing a targeted hormone assessment can be very helpful. Appropriate hormone support also can improve these symptoms and the ability to cope. An example is presented in Figure 26-2.

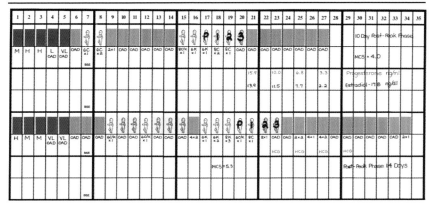

Figure 26-2: This 17-year-old woman has severe menstrual cramps and associated premenstrual syndrome. She had a laser laparoscopy and a LUNA procedure to treat her pain with excellent results. Her CrMS chart revealed a mucus cycle score of 4.0 and a post-Peak progesterone profile that also was decreased. In the second cycle of Figure 24-3, she was given HCG 2000 units IM on Peak +3, +5, +7, +9 with a prolongation of her post-Peak phase and an amelioration of her premenstrual symptoms.

Chronic Vaginal Discharges

THREE BASIC ABNORMAL discharge patterns seen in the **CrMS** charting can be correlated to various underlying problems. These patterns are a continuous cervical mucus discharge, the frequent appearance of wet without lubrication (2W) observations, and the presence of a green mucus discharge. Some women have a continuous mucus discharge in which there is no apparent correlation to abnormalities. A continuous pasty, cloudy discharge (PC) is most likely a normal variant. The presence of a continuous mucus-type discharge and the appearance of a normal cervix may, however, represent an abnormality.

Identification of Cervical Inflammation (Cervical Ectropion)

Women who have an *inflammatory condition of the cervix* may experience a characteristic discharge pattern. This inflammatory condition is commonly associated with a *cervical eversion* or *ectropion* or with a *cervical erosion*. These conditions may cause a discharge to occur at specific times during the course of the menstrual cycle. The Pap smear usually will be normal and cultures will be negative. The only indication of inflammation is the persistence of a discharge pattern, which is most likely the result of the constant exposure of the cervical cells to acidic vaginal fluids (these cells are used to an alkaline environment).

If the physician and the FCP know the specific *criteria* that have been developed to identify these cervical eversions, they can identify the presence of an eversion from the **CrMS** chart with a high degree of accuracy. In order to understand this capability, which is a constant companion of the **CrMS**, one must be familiar with the concept of criteria. *Criteria* are defined as *specific markers through which, by their presence or absence, a specific judgment can be made.*

The development of criteria is one of the fundamental principles of **NaProTECHNOLOGY**. Indeed, the **CrMS** chart must carefully be read looking specifically for the presence or absence of certain criteria. If the criteria are present, the potential increases that a particular gynecologic condition exists. Said in another way, the **CrMS** is a "criteria-driven" system.

Criteria for Identifying Cervical Inflammation (Cervical Eversion)

The following are the criteria for identifying a cervical eversion (inflammation) from the **CrMS** chart:

1.   A sticky (1/4 inch), tacky (1/2-3/4 inch) or gummy discharge present during the early pre-Peak phase of the cycle (those days prior to the sixth day before the Peak Day).

2.   Any sticky, tacky, stretchy (1 inch or more) or gummy discharge seen any time from the fourth day post-Peak.

3.   A pasty, cloudy discharge is *not* a criteria.

4.   Yellow discoloration of the mucus is *not* a criteria.

5.   Premenstrual mucus is *not* a criteria.

CERVIX GRADING

NORMAL	GRADE I up to 5 mm	GRADE II 5 mm to 1 cm	GRADE III 1 cm to 2 cm	GRADE IV over 2 cm

Figure 27-1: A simple grading system of the cervix that allows for a standardized assessment of the cervical eversion and the monitoring of its healing following treatment. The size represents the radius of the reddened area on the cervix.

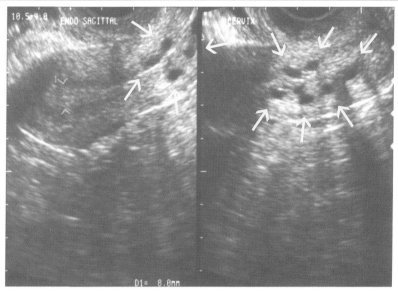

Figure 27-2: The uterus in a side view by ultrasound with several nabothian cysts located within the cervix (left, upper right) and a closer view of the same cervix showing the multiple appearance of these nabothian cysts (right) (From: Pope Paul VI Institute Reproductive Ultrasound Center).

If one or both of the first two criteria are present, then the criteria for a cervical eversion (inflammation) exists. During pelvic examinations for cervical assessment, a simple grading system can be used by your doctor to identify the grade (or the size) of the cervical eversion (Figure 27-1). One also can look for the presence of *nabothian cysts* on the cervix (these are cysts that are caused by a blockage of the duct that normally drains the mucus producing crypts) (see Figure 27-2). If the charting criteria for cervical inflammation are present, a grade II or larger inflammatory reaction in the cervix (cervical eversion or ectropion) will be present in over 75 percent of cases. Examples of cycles that do and do not meet these criteria and the grade of the cervix observed are shown in Figure 27-3.

I conducted a three-part study of the cervix to identify these correlations. First, a total of 381 patients participated where the presence of a cervical eversion (inflammation) was predicted from the **CrMS** chart. Second, another 103 patients participated where an absence of cervical eversion was predicted from the **CrMS** chart. Third, an additional 171 patients were evaluated for the condition of their cervix at the time of their postpartum examination (at four to six weeks postpartum).

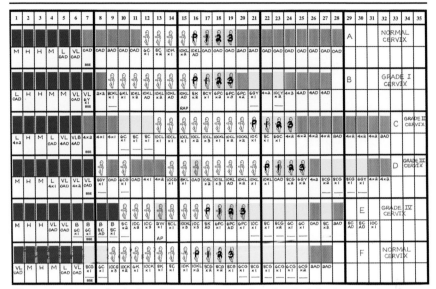

Figure 27-3: A series of cycles from different women who show the criteria for the presence or absence of cervical inflammation. Cycle A shows the absence of criteria and the cervix was normal. Cycles B - F show varying signs of both pre- and post-Peak criteria (From: Pope Paul VI Institute research, 2004).

The cervical inflammation criteria correctly predicted the *presence of a cervical ectropion* of grade II or larger in 292 of 381 cases for a positive predictive value (PPV) of 76.6 percent (292/381). The absence of the criteria correctly predicted *the absence of a cervical eversion* in 78 of 103 cases for a negative predictive value (NPV) of 75.7 percent (78/103). The difference between the two criteria was statistically significant.

In the third portion, 171 patients had their cervix evaluated at the time of their postpartum examination. These were performed following cesarean section and vaginal delivery. All of the 17 patients who had a cesarean section had a normal or grade I cervix. Of those who had a vaginal delivery in which minor cervical lacerations were not repaired (major cervical lacerations were repaired), 19.1 percent had a grade II through IV cervical eversion.

Management Concepts

When the women who appear to have a cervical inflammation as observed on their CrMS chart are seen by their physician, the physician does a pelvic examination and evaluates the presence or absence of a cervical eversion. If an eversion is present, it is then treated. The standard **NaProTECHNOLOGY** treatment *currently used* is to *hyfrecate* the cervix at monthly intervals until the cervix heals. Hyfrecation is a mild cauterization technique undertaken using local anesthesia. In some cases, cryosurgery (freezing of the cervix) may be used, but it is important that the cryosurgery unit be set on a superficial setting so that it does not deeply penetrate and destroy the cervical crypts. In the past, silver nitrate applications also have been used on the cervix. While this can be a very effective treatment, it does require multiple applications and can be cumbersome.

The end point of treatment is not necessarily to revert the chart completely to a "normal" appearance, where discharge is absent during the early pre-Peak and post-Peak phases of the cycle. With the treatment of a cervical eversion, a significant reduction in the amount of abnormal mucus discharge can result thus making the woman's ability to detect the points of change during both the pre-Peak and the immediate post-Peak phases of the cycle easier. This facilitates the woman's application of yellow stamps during the pre-Peak and post-Peak phases of the cycle, and it makes the system more applicable to the couple and significantly increases their confidence (Figure 27-4).

Side effects of the hyfrecating treatment include a watery discharge for seven to 10 days following the hyfrecation. Small amounts of bleeding (spotting) may be associated with the treatment for a few days. Over the years of experience, the treatment is avoided in women who are breast-feeding (and not ovulating or menstruating). In this case, the cervix seems to bleed more than usual and for a longer period of time—several weeks (thus, treatment is avoided). Once menses and

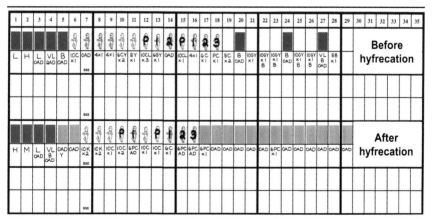

Figure 27-4: The CrMS chart in a patient prior to hyfrecation and following hyfrecation for a cervical eversion (From: Pope Paul VI Institute research, 2004). Refer to page 83 for the VDRS.

normal hormone function resumes in the breast-feeding woman, treatment can be used. The routine treatment of the cervix at the six-week postpartum checkup also may be considered.

About 25 percent of the patients who meet the criteria for cervical inflammation will have a normal-appearing cervix. In these circumstances or in circumstances where the cervix is treated followed by no significant change in the mucus pattern, post-Peak progesterone vaginal capsules can be used with some additional success.

When the physician has completed treatment for the patient, the patient should be referred back to the FCP because the basic pattern of discharges, which is important for her knowledge of fertility, will have changed. One or two follow-ups may be necessary to assist with this transition.

In a large number of cases with these criteria, the cervix has been cultured and found to be negative. A variety of different antibiotic approaches also have been used to treat this without success. Thus, the most likely explanation for this discharge pattern is the relationship of the glandular cells on the cervix and how they have been irritated by the acidic vaginal fluids. This creates a chronic irritation that results in a discharge from those cells at a time when a discharge would not normally be present.

Frequent 2W Observations

The frequent observation of *wet without lubrication* (2W) referred to as a "frequent 2W" pattern also has been studied. This pattern is one that may occur during the early pre-Peak phase of the cycle and during the post-Peak phase of the cycle from Peak +4 onward. When this pattern occurs, it usually is associated with a *low-grade infection of the cervix.*

In 18 consecutive patients where the cervix has been cultured for all bacteria (not simply a beta-strep culture), 15 of them had positive cultures (83.3 percent). In these cases, antibiotic-specific treatment can be helpful. An example of treatment is shown in Figure 27-5. With appropriate antibiotic treatment, the 2W discharge disappears.

Green Discharge

On occasion, the **CrMS** chart will reveal a persistent greenish discharge. Cases like this are rare, but we have had the opportunity to culture four of these patients. In three of them, positive cultures were

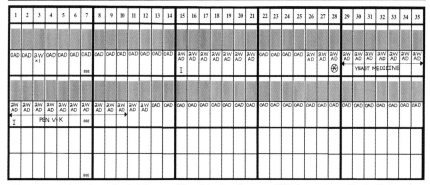

Figure 27-5: A patient who is 36 years old and having frequent 2W observations. She is 19.1 weeks pregnant and culture revealed yeast (Candida albicans) and Group B beta-strep. Treatment with yeast medication and penicillin reverted her observations back to dry (From: Pope Paul VI Institute research, 2004). Refer to page 83 for the Vaginal Discharge Recording System (VDRS).

obtained. An interesting feature of this particular circumstance is that in all three cases multiple organisms were observed. Again, antibiotic-specific treatment can be helpful in eliminating this pattern and the subsequent effects that result from chronic infection.

Implantation Mucus

There may be times when a chronic discharge pattern is completely normal although it might be interpreted as being related to a cervical inflammation. Such an example is present in Figure 27-6. In this case, the patient became pregnant during the course of the cycle, and *implantation bleeding* is identified in days 29, 30, and 31 of her cycle. On day 22 and 23 of her cycle, however, she had a Peak-type mucus discharge. This pattern, which has been observed in a number of patients in early pregnancy, is called *"implantation mucus."* The

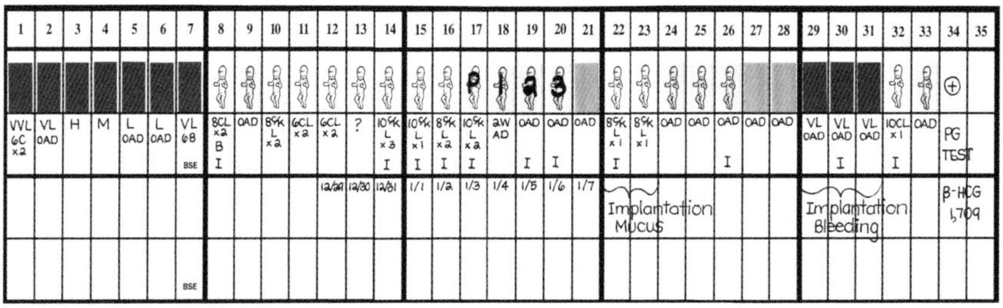

Figure 27-6: A conception cycle using the CrMS with Peak Day on day 17. Implantation mucus was present on days 22 and 23 and implantation bleeding on days 29, 30, and 31. A positive serum pregnancy test on day 34 (Peak +19) was identified. All of the dates were confirmed by ultrasound (From: Pope Paul VI Institute research, 2004). Refer to page 83 for the VDRS.

frequency of this has not been studied, but its existence has been clearly observed. In this case, the mucus discharge is a normal variant and most likely a discharge coming from the uterus. As a result, no treatment is necessary. Treatment of the cervix with any type of mechanical treatment would be contraindicated during pregnancy.

Chronic Discharges and Family Planning

For women who have chronic discharges, the **CREIGHTON MODEL System** (CrMS) can be used effectively as a family planning system. To do so requires the assistance of an adequately-trained **Fertility***Care*™ **Practitioner** (FCP) who understands the concepts used in implementing pre- and post-Peak yellow stamps for the identification of preovulatory and postovulatory infertility. These yellow stamps are used in the presence of a continuous mucus discharge that is considered infertile.

The use of *pre-Peak* yellow stamps in women who have a continuous discharge involves identifying a pattern of pre-Peak mucus that is *essentially the same from day to day* (what is referred to as an essential sameness pattern - ESP). These days are considered infertile because the ovary is quiet and ovulation has not begun yet. When the mucus pattern changes from this ESP a *point of change* (POC) is identified and marks the beginning of the time of fertility. The POC correlates with the rising levels of estrogen seen at the beginning of the ovulation phase.[1] Thus, a woman can be taught how to prospectively identify the days of *pre-ovulatory infertility* and the beginning of the days of fertility.

Post-Peak yellow stamps are implemented for those days during the *post-Peak* phase of the cycle that would be considered infertile. These are implemented once the woman has been properly taught and when she *confidently identifies her Peak Day*.

The proper use and implementation of yellow stamps can help the woman and the couple understand when their naturally-occurring phases of fertility and infertility exist. While the continuous discharge occasionally may lead to a decrease in overall confidence in the use of the system, because the system is standardized, it is possible to interpret the types of discharge and the patterns of those discharges. The types and patterns of discharge then can be correlated with normal or abnormal events that might be occurring. With this information, appropriate treatment modalities can help normalize the charting record and assist the couple in developing confidence in use of the system.

For the Doctor

Progesterone vaginal capsules (300 mg) can be administered during the post-Peak phase of the cycle from Peak +3 through Peak +12 every day at bed time (QD hs). The progesterone has a local drying effect on the cervix and often reduces the amount of mucus significantly or will completely dry up the pattern.

Special Acknowledgement

The author acknowledges the assistance of Joseph B. Stanford, M.D., MSPH, CFCMC, associate professor in the Department of Family and Preventive Medicine, University of Utah, Salt Lake City, Utah, in preparation of this chapter.

THE **CREIGHTON MODEL System** (CrMS), with its objective and standardized observational system, has opened up a whole new way of looking at various bleeding abnormalities that occur within the course of the menstrual cycle. In the **CrMS**, *the presence of bleeding that is different from a normal menstrual period* is called **unusual bleeding**. This term resonates with women because they have confidence in knowing their own menstrual periods (which is referred to as *usual bleeding*). Because the **CrMS** is objective and standardized, these bleeding episodes are revealed in an extremely accurate way and in a way that is very helpful for further evaluation.

Normal Menstruation

To understand unusual bleeding, one must recognize that *a normal menstruation is one that follows an "ovulatory event."* An *ovulatory event* is either ovulation itself or an event that mimics ovulation. For example, an unruptured follicle is an anovulatory situation, but it mimics ovulation from a physiologic point of view. In this case, an increase of progesterone and other signs follow the event and suggest that ovulation occurred even though it did not. Because the follicle did not rupture, the egg is trapped within it and not released.

Normal menstruation is a bleeding episode associated with all events where progesterone production follows the occurrence of the ovulation event (the development of a corpus luteum). This is a very characteristic-bleeding episode. Normal menstrual periods or bleeding episodes that follow the previous production of progesterone are *crescendo/decrescendo* or *decrescendo* in their patterns.

Crescendo/Decrescendo
L-H-M-L-VL

Decrescendo
H-H-M-M-L

The above bleeding patterns often are associated with other mild symptoms of menstruation such as premenstrual breast tenderness, mild low backache and mild menstrual cramps.

Characteristics of Unusual Bleeding

Bleeding that would be considered unusual often is light, very light or brown (black) in color. Usually, it is not crescendo/decrescendo or decrescendo in its characteristics. It tends to be similar from day to day. It is not necessarily associated with the menstrual period, although on rare occasions, it may have characteristics of a normal menstrual flow. Most unusual bleeding episodes have hormonal causes *(dysfunctional uterine bleeding),* but some may be organic.

The hormonal causes may include "ovulatory" bleeding. **Ovulatory bleeding** is a term given to a type of bleeding that is observed around the time of ovulation and is presumed to be associated with the various estrogen changes that occur at that time.

There are two basic types of ovulatory bleeding:

A. Estrogen-breakthrough bleeding:
This is unusual bleeding observed leading up to the time of the Peak Day.

B. Estrogen-withdrawal bleeding:
This is unusual bleeding that is observed immediately following the Peak Day in the count of three.

Another form of unusual bleeding that has a hormonal cause is that seen in women who are oligo-ovulatory or anovulatory. The most common situation is in women who have polycystic ovarian disease (PCOD) and long and irregular cycles. It is observed as periods of L, VL, or B bleeding unassociated with menses. It is a very characteristic type of bleeding pattern, which can be identified very quickly when looking at the **CrMS** chart.

Medical Definitions

To understand the various types of bleeding that occur during the course of the menstrual cycle, the following standard medical definitions are used:

Menorrhagia:
Heavier than normal bleeding.

Metrorrhagia:
Bleeding between menstrual periods.

Menometrorrhagia:
Heavier than normal menstrual periods and bleeding between menstrual periods.

Dysfunctional uterine bleeding (DUB):
Uterine bleeding associated with no identifiable organic condition; usually thought to be hormonal in nature.

To be certain about dysfunctional uterine bleeding, the woman must see her physician and have at least a pelvic examination that is negative. An ultrasound examination may be useful in further evaluating this condition.

CREIGHTON MODEL Definitions

In addition to the above, there are other definitions of bleeding that occur during the course of the menstrual cycle, which are referred to as **CREIGHTON MODEL** definitions:

Postmenstrual brown bleeding:
Two or more days of brown (black) bleeding appearing at the tail-end of the menstrual flow. Generally, the length of the menses in such cases is six days or longer, but this is not essential to the definition. Often this is referred to as *tail-end brown bleeding* (TEB).

Premenstrual bleeding:
> Three or more days of light or very light or brown
> (black) bleeding occurring prior to the beginning of the first
> moderate day of menstrual bleeding (PMB).

Excessively heavy menses:
> At least one 24- to 48-hour period where the woman must
> change pads, tampons or both more frequently than every
> two hours.

A typical pattern of unusual bleeding (dysfunctional uterine bleeding) is shown in Figure 28-1. In this case, a woman with polycystic ovarian disease and long, irregular cycles has multiple episodes of irregular bleeding. These bleeding episodes are characteristically different from her menstrual periods. Her true menstrual periods begin on day 1 of lines 1, 4 and 6. They are typical decrescendo bleeding episodes. In addition, the true menstruations, which are observed on line 4 and line 6 of Figure 28-1, also follow the occurrence of a Peak Day, which occurred repectively 14 and 13 days earlier. The

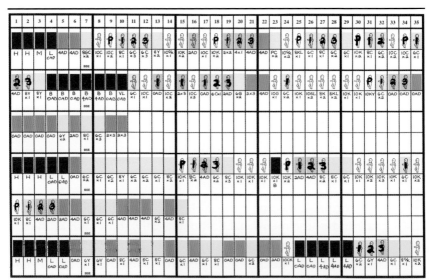

Figure 28-1: This series of cycles, from the same woman, is an example of a charting pattern observed in a patient who has polycystic ovarian disease. The cycles are very long and irregular. The first cycle is 80 days in duration. The second cycle is 50 days in duration and the third cycle is not yet complete. The bleeding patterns beginning on day 1 of lines 1, 4 and 6 are all classic usual menstrual periods. The bleeding from days 4 through 10 of line 2, day 23 of line 4 and days 25 through 29 of line 6, however, are all classic patterns of dysfunctional uterine bleeding (From: Pope Paul VI Institute research, 2004).

unusual bleeding episodes are light bleeding or brown bleeding episodes, which tend to be the same from day to day. These episodes usually are associated with the *unopposed* (by progesterone) *stimulation of the endometrium by estrogen*, which is being manufactured by the ovary during the course of these long preovulatory phases.

The causes of *premenstrual bleeding* are thought to result from the premature breakdown of endometrial capillaries secondary to an inadequate support by the corpus luteum during the luteal phase of the menstrual cycle. In addition, the *postmenstrual brown bleeding* (tail-end brown bleeding, TEB) may be due to an irregular sloughing of the endometrium with the retention of small fragments of endometrial tissue and associated necrosis and inflammation. This, too, may be associated with decreased progesterone production in the previous post-Peak phase of the cycle.

An example of this is shown in Figure 28-2. In this chart, the woman had three days of TEB at the end of her menstruation and her menstrual periods are somewhat longer than usual (eight days in duration).

The system for observing bleeding in the **CrMS** uses a recording of H = heavy; M = moderate; L = light; VL = very light; B = brown or black bleeding. This approach to the reporting of menstruation coincides with data that were generated on a subjective rating of the volume of menstrual discharge.[1]

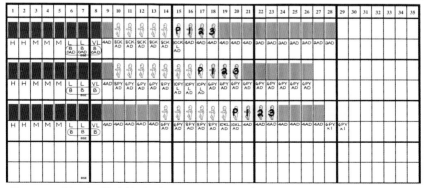

Figure 28-2: TEB (or black bleeding) in a woman with infertility and endometriosis. At D&C, the endometrium revealed retained fragments of necrotic endometrial tissue (From: Pope Paul VI Institute research, 2004). Refer to page 83 for the Vaginal Discharge Recording System (VDRS).

Organic Causes

A number of organic causes for various abnormal bleeding patterns may occur. We have developed a classification of unusual bleeding based upon the CrMS. The bleeding can be broken down into two categories: *perimenstrual bleeding (around the time of menstruation) and intermenstrual bleeding (between menstruations).* The premenstrual and postmenstrual brown bleeding and excessively heavy bleeding that have been mentioned previously falls into the category of the perimenstrual bleeding pattern. With intermenstrual bleeding, the bleeding episodes can occur in the following fashion: bleeding early in the mucus buildup, bleeding closer to the Peak Day, prolonged premenstrual bleeding, prolonged postmenstrual brown bleeding, and a variable return of unusual bleeding in long (anovulatory or infrequently ovulatory) cycles.

A review of the histologic tissue diagnoses in a group of 148 consecutive **CREIGHTON MODEL** users who exhibited various unusual bleeding episodes and had a dilatation and curettage (D&C) (and often a hysteroscopy) has been evaluated. No specific organic pathology was observed in 63 of the patients (42.6 percent), but evidence of organic pathology was identified in the other 85 patients (57.4 percent).

Chronic Cervicitis

An example of a chronic cervicitis causing abnormal bleeding and its subsequent treatment is shown in Figure 28-3. In this example, the patient had a large cervical eversion (ectropion) with a normal Pap smear, but the cervix was friable and bled easily. After the cervix was treated properly, the cervix returned to normal and the bleeding was brought under control.

Endometritis

Examples where endometritis caused unusual bleeding are shown in Figure 28-4 and Figure 28-5. In the first case, the bleeding was heavy and not typical of a standard unusual bleeding pattern. When the cervix and endometrium were evaluated, *Escherichia coli* was cultured and the patient was treated with cephalosporins (Keflex) and intramuscular progesterone. The outcome was excellent.

In Figure 28-5, the patient presented with prolonged post-Peak bleeding. A D&C was performed and chronic endometritis was identified. Culture at that time from the endometrium revealed *Enterococcus faecalis.* The patient improved dramatically following the D&C and treatment with Ampicillin.

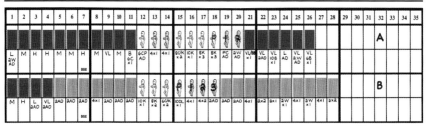

Figure 28-3 A and B: In cycle A, bleeding in this menstrual cycle is occurring in 21 of the 26 days of the cycle. This was observed in a woman who had a grade 4 cervical eversion with very friable tissue that bled easily. After having her cervix treated with hyfrecation and the cervix was healed, her cycle returned to the one shown as cycle B (From: Pope Paul VI Institute research, 2004).

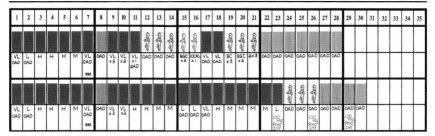

Figure 28-4: In these two consecutive cycles, the patient showed intermenstrual bleeding associated with her mucus cycle in the first cycle of this chart and in the second cycle, a nearly continuous 23-day pattern of bleeding. When she was evaluated, the endometrium was cultured and E. coli was found. This eventually was treated with cephalosporins and she also was given intramuscular progesterone on day 23, 26, and 29. This resulted in a normal pattern (From: Pope Paul VI Institute research, 2004).

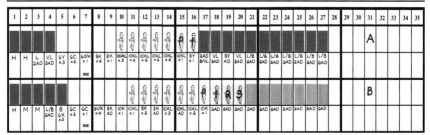

Figure 28-5 A and B: In cycle A, the cycle shows prolonged premenstrual spotting. The patient had a D&C and a positive endometrial culture for Enterococcus faecalis. After being treated with Ampicillin, her cycle became normal and is shown in cycle B (From: Pope Paul VI Institute research, 2004). Refer to page 83 for the Vaginal Discharge Recording System (VDRS).

Premenstrual Bleeding

A good example of *premenstrual bleeding* and its associated treatment are shown in Figure 28-6. In this case, suboptimal progesterone and estrogen levels were identified during the post-Peak phase of the cycle and the patient was treated with post-Peak HCG, 2000 IU, Peak +3, 5, 7, and 9. This eliminated her premenstrual bleeding and corrected the underlying hormone problem.

Endometrial Polyps

Figure 28-7 shows a patient who had *intermenstrual bleeding* that occurred immediately after the Peak Day and then again in the middle of the mucus cycle with the bleeding continuing despite post-Peak progesterone therapy. She had a D&C and a hysteroscopy. At the time of the surgical procedure, an *endometrial polyp* (a mass of endometrial tissue appended to the lining of the uterus by a pedicle) was identified. In the cycle following the surgery, the bleeding disappeared. The overwhelming majority of endometrial polyps are benign and often asymptomatic, but a small number can show malignant transformation. Thus, it is important to recognize them and treat them appropriately.

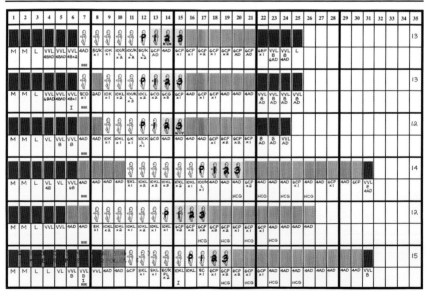

Figure 28-6: This patient had premenstrual spotting associated with decreased progesterone levels. Following that, she was treated with post-Peak HCG, 2000 units IM on Peak +3, 5, 7 and 9. This is shown in the last three cycles of this figure. This corrected her bleeding abnormality (From: Pope Paul VI Institute research, 2004). Refer to page 83 for the Vaginal Discharge Recording System (VDRS).

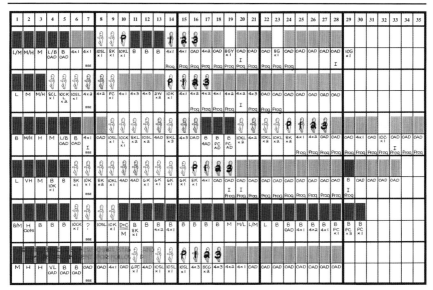

Figure 28-7: In this patient, the first five cycles revealed intermenstrual bleeding in a 48-year-old woman. She underwent a D&C in the fifth cycle and this corrected the bleeding as shown in the sixth cycle. On pathology examination, she had an endometrial polyp (From: Pope Paul VI Institute research, 2004).

Endometrial biopsy is not adequate for the treatment of endometrial polyps; the polyp itself must be removed.

Excessively Heavy Menses

Very heavy menstrual periods have many different causes. These can include uterine fibroids, adenomyosis, myometrial hyperplasia (hypertrophy of the uterus), or even coagulation disorders such as thrombocytopenia, systemic lupus, or von Willebrand disease.

There are three main types of uterine fibroids. These are *submucous, intramural and subserous.* The most complex, from a bleeding point of view, are the submucous fibroids. A small submucous fibroid can cause extremely heavy menstrual flow. Submucus fibroids are ones that are located immediately under the lining of the uterus.

The exact incidence of benign fibroid tumors within the general population is not exactly known. It has been estimated that 20 percent of all women over 30 have fibroid tumors. Some have estimated, however, that as high as 40 percent of women over the age of 35 have fibroids. Submucous fibroids are thought to compose about 5 to 10 percent of all fibroid tumors. With the advent of ultrasound, we now are able to see fibroid tumors better and it may change our views on this in time.

Figure 28-8 shows the **CrMS** chart of a patient with very large submucous fibroids. This particular patient was an intensive-care nurse and, on the day described as VH (very heavy), she actually measured the amount of blood discharged. In one cycle it totaled nearly 500 cc (over one unit of blood). She had a decrease in her hemoglobin with each of her menstrual periods and even myomectomy did not help. Submucous fibroids were identified and a hysterectomy was needed.

Treatment of uterine fibroids depends entirely on symptoms. Most women need no treatment at all if they are not symptomatic. Most often, fibroids do not interfere with fertility although submucous fibroids might lead to miscarriage. Fibroids have a very low malignant potential. Submucous fibroids are clearly the most problematic because of their ability to bleed heavily.

Treatment programs include everything from hysterectomy to myomectomy (removal of the fibroid while leaving the uterus). With regard to the latter procedure, many patients prefer a myomectomy over a hysterectomy. These women do not wish to have their uterus removed and want an alternative form of treatment. Most of the time,

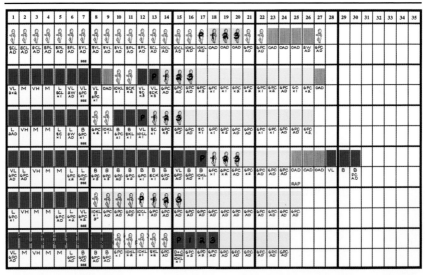

Figure 28-8: This patient had very heavy menstrual periods. The days labeled "VH" (very heavy) measured nearly 500 cc of blood flow. She also has prolonged tail-end brown bleeding. Diagnosis in this case revealed multiple submucous fibroids (From: Pope Paul VI Institute research, 2004).

a myomectomy will cause a reduction in the volume of menstrual blood loss. They may continue to have some increased bleeding, however, even with a myomectomy and may still require hysterectomy.

Endometrial Hyperplasia

Endometrial hyperplasia is a condition in which the endometrium exhibits excessive cellular proliferation. Pathologic interpretations of pre-invasive histologic changes or precursors to adenocarcinoma (cancer) of the uterus can be inconsistent.

Suspected endometrial hyperplasia must be thoroughly investigated. An ultrasound measurement of endometrial thickness that exceeds 8 mm or a morphologic irregularity in which one area is thicker than another indicates the need for further evaluation by biopsy or hysteroscopy. In fact, such evaluation is essential to a definitive diagnosis. [2-4]

Endometrial biopsies can be performed on an outpatient basis, but that procedure can be physically painful and psychologically stressful. In addition, diagnostic certainty is limited by the fact that it is a "blind" procedure and cannot sample all of the endometrium. Hysteroscopy is the optimal method of assessing endometrial hyperplasia because the entire surface of the endometrium can be visualized.[3] This then can be accompanied with D&C for endometrial sampling.

Figure 28-9 shows a **CrMS** chart in a woman diagnosed with endometrial hyperplasia.

Dysfunctional Uterine Bleeding
Secondary to Polycystic Ovaries

Figure 28-10 shows a dysfunctional uterine bleeding pattern seen in a woman who has polycystic ovarian disease. The endometrial biopsy was negative.

In this case, the treatment approach was to provide intramuscular, isomolecular progesterone 100 mg on days 18, 21 and 24. Repeating this from cycle to cycle allows for regularization of the cycle to occur and also provides the protection of progesterone to unopposed estrogen. It should reduce the likelihood of developing uterine cancer.

Thyroid

On occasion, treatment of thyroid dysfunction or supplementation with thyroid can be effective in reducing or eliminating unusual

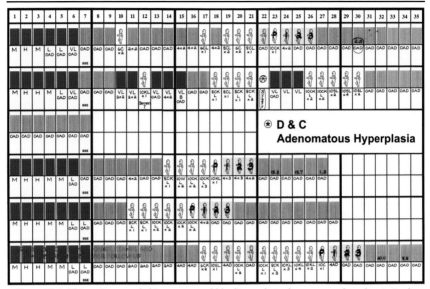

Figure 28-9: This patient revealed intermenstrual bleeding early in the mucus cycle and again in the middle of the mucus cycle. At the time of surgery (a D&C), pathology revealed endometrial hyperplasia without atypia. In the remaining three cycles, the bleeding corrected itself (From: Pope Paul VI Institute research, 2004). Refer to page 83 for the Vaginal Discharge Recording System (VDRS).

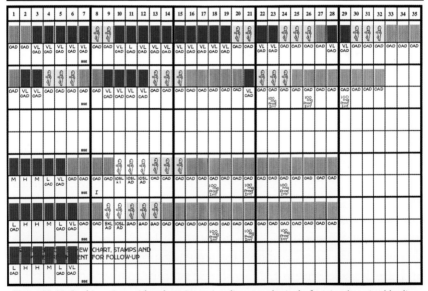

Figure 28-10: In this patient with polycystic ovarian disease, a classic dysfunctional uterine bleeding pattern is shown in the first two lines of charting. The type of bleeding seen is a continuous pattern of bleeding, which is the same from day to day. On days 23, 26 and 29 of the second line of charting, she was given isomolecular progesterone 100 mg IM. She then was managed on a cycle-by-cycle basis with isomolecular progesterone 100 mg IM on days 18, 21 and 24. This resulted in regular menstrual cycles and an elimination of the dysfunctional uterine bleeding (From: Pope Paul VI Institute research, 2004). Refer to page 83 for the Vaginal Discharge Recording System (VDRS).

bleeding observed with **CrMS**. In Figure 28-11, the patient has been supplemented with sustained-release triiodothyronine (T$_3$). With this supplementation, the bleeding improved significantly. One should always consider thyroid dysfunction as a possible underlying problem in situations of abnormal bleeding.

Adenomyosis

The patient shown in Figure 28-12 was followed for several years with very long menstrual periods. These periods were up to 13 days in duration and associated with prolonged postmenstrual brown bleeding. Over the years of observation, she was evaluated hormonally and found to have suboptimal progesterone production. Supplementation with both progesterone and HCG provided her with no benefit to her bleeding pattern. Eventually, the bleeding became heavier and the menstrual periods became more painful. This then necessitated a hysterectomy. At the time of hysterectomy, it was found that she had *adenomyosis*. Now in looking at similar charts, we have observed several patients with this type of bleeding pattern associated with adenomyosis. Adenomyosis is a condition related to endometriosis where the endometrial glands invade the muscle of the uterus.

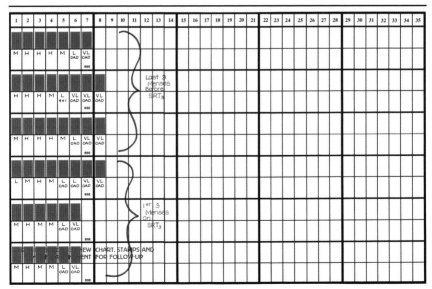

Figure 28-11: The menstrual periods of this woman before and after the implementation of T3 (sustained-release) therapy are shown. Her periods were very heavy in the first three cycles, but on SRT3 her menses decreased significantly in intensity (From: Pope Paul VI Institute research, 2004).

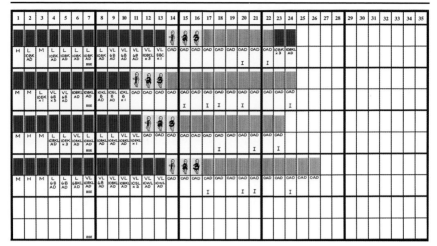

Figure 28-12: In this example, the patient's menstrual periods extended for 10 to 13 days. This ongoing pattern existed for many years and was resistant to treatment with luteal phase progesterone support. Eventually, it necessitated hysterectomy and, at the time of hysterectomy, she was diagnosed as having adenomyosis (From: Pope Paul VI Institute research, 2004). Refer to page 83 for the VDRS.

Truncated Menstrual Cycles

Sometimes a patient will say that she is having a menstrual period every two weeks. This is rarely an emergency. Having the patient chart her cycles is helpful for proper evaluation. In Figure 28-13, a woman who had been charting her cycles for some time began having very short cycles, 16 days in duration. We did a hormone evaluation on her and found, interestingly enough, that her post-Peak progesterone levels were in the preovulatory range, and yet, the bleeding pattern was characteristically similar to a true menstrual flow. This is one of the few situations that we have observed in which the bleeding is similar to a true menstruation. We have called this a "truncated" menstrual cycle. In these cases, the patients will respond favorably to three cycles of intramuscular isomolecular progesterone. Generally speaking, the progesterone should begin prior to the onset of her next anticipated menstrual flow. Thus, in a situation such as Figure 28-13, the progesterone should begin on day 12 or 14 in the first cycle of administration. The progesterone is then given on days 12, 15, and 18 in the first cycle. In the second cycle, it is given on days 15, 18, and 21 and in the third cycle on days 18, 21, and 24. After three cycles of intramuscular progesterone used in this fashion, the progesterone feeds

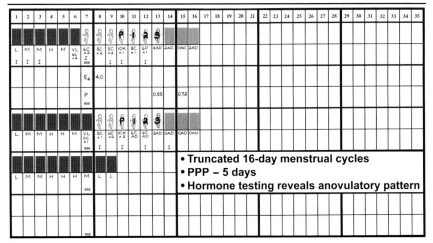

Figure 28-13: In this example of 16-day menstrual cycle, the patient had both estrogen and progesterone levels drawn. Her Peak +3 and Peak +5 progesterone levels in the first cycle were in the preovulatory range. These cycles, which can occur spontaneously, are referred to as "truncated" cycles. They can be treated by giving three cycles of intramuscular progesterone (see text) (From: Pope Paul VI Institute research, 2004).

back to the hypothalamus and restructures the hypothalamic pituitary ovarian axis, thus stimulating the return of a normal menstrual cycle.

Final Note

A good deal of gynecologic practice involves women who have abnormal bleeding episodes for a variety of reasons. Standard practice is to place them on oral contraceptives, which regulates their bleeding but neither pays attention to the underlying causes nor treats it. Some of these women end up with needless hysterectomies because of bleeding episodes that otherwise go undiagnosed and untreated.

When a woman begins charting her cycles with the CrMS, an objective and prospective pattern of bleeding can be observed and an eventual diagnosis can be made with the use of simple hormone studies or a diagnostic D&C and hysteroscopy. In addition, endometrial cultures can be helpful. Then appropriate management can be instituted and, most of the time without additional surgery, the problem can be solved.

Real Persons, Real Problems, Real Solutions

When I was in high school, my cycles were always regular, "like clockwork," I always said. When I started college, everything started to change and my cycles became more irregular. A doctor I went to in college attributed my irregular cycles to the stress of nursing school. Although I didn't feel particularly stressed, I believed him. After all, he was the doctor.

After college, my cycles became progressively more irregular. I went to an OB/GYN in my local area who promptly handed me birth control pills. He told me that not only would they regulate my cycle, but I would have birth control, too. I found that surprising since I had not said that I needed any birth control. I was already a little unsure of this doctor since he had laughed at me once because I was so nervous about my exam. After he would not return my call when I had questions about the birth control pills he had just given me, I decided it was time to find another doctor.

By this time, I was working as a nurse at our local hospital. I decided to go to one of the doctors who was on staff there. When she learned of my irregular cycles, she immediately put me on birth control pills. About a year after our wedding, my husband and I decided we would see if we could get pregnant, so I stopped taking the pill. I had been on it for about six years by that point. I immediately started having problems again, including some unusual bleeding. In less than a year I was in surgery having a D&C. My doctor told me that would "take care of me for a while." It didn't. I ran into her one day at the hospital when she was making rounds. When she found I was still having problems, she said she wanted to put me back on the pill "for three months." I told her I didn't want to do that (remember we wanted to get pregnant). She never asked me why I was opposed to taking the pill. She just told me to come into her office and we'd discuss my options. When I did, she sat me down at her big desk, handed me a three-month supply of birth control pills and walked out of the room. There was no discussion. I walked out of that office, too, and never went back.

My next doctor did listen to me to some extent. Rather than put me on birth control pills, he treated me with Provera, an artificial progesterone. We initially were able to get my unusual bleeding to stop. After that, my instructions became unclear. My doctor didn't want me to take the Provera every month because he wanted to see if I would cycle on my own. However, I was never told how long I should let things go before calling him. It wasn't long before I started bleeding again. Every time I thought I should call, the bleeding seemed as if it was going to stop. After four months of nonstop bleeding or spotting, I called the doctor. He stopped my bleeding by having me take four birth control pills a day for five days, which made me very nauseous. After seven years of being off the pill, I was put back on it.

At one point, I asked this last doctor if I could have polycystic ovarian disease (PCOD). His answer was that "it could be" and left the room. After 20 years and three doctors, I still didn't know what was wrong with me. None of them even tried to diagnose me.

In August 2001, my associate pastor gave a very pro-life, anti-contraception homily. That prompted me to make an appointment with him since I was being treated with the pill and had been told by another priest that it was okay. That appointment brought much emotional distress when I realized that I had acted against the teachings of my beloved Catholic faith by being treated with the pill. I believe it also saved my life, both physically and spiritually. I had already been treated for depression after restarting the pill and was being treated for high blood pressure. Both can be side effects. I've not had a problem with either after stopping the pill. At the end of the appointment, the priest handed me the phone number for the Pope Paul VI Institute.

My phone call to the Institute led me to charting my cycles with the **CREIGHTON MODEL Fertility*Care*™ System** and a referral to Dr. Hilgers. After reviewing my charting and medical records, Dr. Hilgers suspected PCOD. My blood work was so abnormal, it confirmed that diagnosis.

Dr. Hilgers immediately began treating me with compounded natural progesterone. Shortly after starting treatment with Dr. Hilgers, I expressed to one of the nurses my fear of having continuous bleeding again. She assured me that Dr. Hilgers wouldn't let that happen. She was correct. I've never had better care.

About two years after being under Dr. Hilgers' care, I began experiencing unusual bleeding again. After a few short phone calls and a check about our insurance, I was planning a visit to Omaha and Dr. Hilgers for a D&C and hysteroscopy (a procedure where he would look at the inside of my uterus through a scope). I felt the doctors in my local area had had their chance and I didn't want to have this surgery with them. During my surgery, Dr. Hilgers found polyps, which he removed. Not only did he go to the waiting room to tell my husband this, but he also gave him pictures of my polyps!

We also decided that it would be beneficial for me to have an ovarian wedge resection, a surgery where a wedge of the oversized polycystic ovary is removed to make it a more normal size. We returned to Omaha three months later for that. After that surgery, I began cycling on my own! A recheck of my blood work showed a dramatic improvement. For the first time since high school, I finally felt normal again!

During the continuing course of my care through the Pope Paul VI Institute, Dr. Hilgers has evaluated me and is treating me for thyroid system dysfunction. This has dramatically increased my energy. He also is treating me for insulin resistance, which can be found in women with PCOD.

I can't put into words the emotional well-being and gratitude that come from having a diagnosis and the proper medical care to fit that diagnosis. I only wish I had found Dr. Hilgers and the Pope Paul VI Institute 20 years earlier. Hopefully, as a **FertilityCare™ Practitioner** and **Educator**, I can help other women find the proper diagnosis and care sooner.

Kathy Hirkala, RN, BSN, CFCP, FCE
Weirton, West Virginia

For the Doctor

1.　In our research, the average duration of tail-end brown bleeding in those cycles that are considered to be abnormal is 2.2 days. In those women who said they had "heavy menstrual periods," the average length of time in which they had to change pads, tampons or both was every 77 minutes. It ranged from every half hour to every four hours in 23 patients studied. Of those 23 patients, however, 20 of them changed every two hours or less.

2.　The menstrual discharge itself is made up of both blood and endometrial fluids as the major contributors. The hemoglobin (Hb) level of a menstrual discharge ranges from 4 to 5. The hemoglobin level in the bloodstream normally runs between 12 and 16 in healthy woman. Minor contributions to the menstrual discharge also may come from cervical fluid, vaginal secretions, endometrial fluids, and perhaps even fluid from the fallopian tube.

3.　The most common finding was an endometrial polyp (n=31). Hormonal imbalance (mostly disordered proliferative endometrium) (n=18), endometrial hyperplasia without atypia (n=14), and chronic endometritis (inflammation of the lining of the uterus)(n=10) also were seen frequently. Other changes that were observed but were not as common included cystic hyperplasia (n=4), endometrial hyperplasia with atypia (n=2), adenocarcinoma (n=1), and carcinosarcoma (n=1). The latter two are cancers of the uterus.

4.　Some prostaglandin inhibitors also have been used to reduce the amount of blood loss. These would include drugs such as mefenamic acid (MFA) (Ponstel) and meclofenamate sodium (Meclomen). Studies conducted on the use of these medications in women with excessively heavy menses have been done. In all categories of very heavy bleeding, mefenamic acid decreased the amount of menstrual flow. This also has been observed with meclofenamate sodium (Figure 28-14).

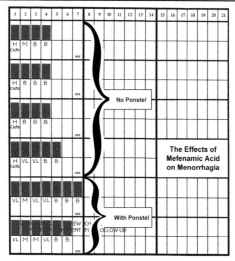

Figure 28-14: The effects of medication (mefenamic acid—Ponstel) in a patient with severe menorrhagia. In the first four cycles without Ponstel, the periods were very heavy. With the addition of medication in the last two cycles, her periods decreased their intensity significantly (From: Pope Paul VI Institute research, 2004).

THE PREMATURITY RATE *in the United States is a national tragedy* (Figure 29-1)! While the American College of Obstetricians and Gynecologists said in 2003 that the incidence of preterm birth has "changed little over the last 40 years,"[1] it actually increased from 6.7 percent in 1967 to 12.7 percent in 2005.[2-6] It represents the *leading cause of neonatal mortality*[7] and the *second leading cause of infant mortality* (death during the first year of life) and, for the first time since 1958 there has been an increase in the infant mortality rate between 2001 and 2002.[6]

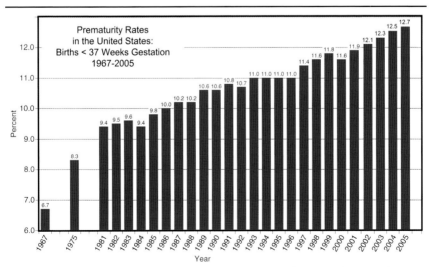

Figure 29-1: The prematurity rate in the United States (birth less than 37 weeks gestation) 1967-2005.[1-4]

351

While modern obstetrics has been interested mostly in the severely premature infant born at less than 32 weeks gestation, even those infants born from 32 through 36 weeks gestation are at increased risk. The relative risk for infant death from all causes among singletons born between 32 and 33 gestational weeks in the United States is 6.6 and among those born from 34 through 36 weeks, the relative risk is 2.9.[8]

It is estimated that the national hospital bill for prematurity totalled *$13.6 billion* in 2001.[6] In addition to increased mortality, there are many medical and developmental problems that are associated with premature birth.[9-16] There is an increased rate of *intraventricular hemorrhage, respiratory distress, cerebral palsy and visual and hearing impairment.* In fact, the rate of cerebral palsy in neonatal survivors who weigh between 500 and 1500 grams at the time of birth is *10 to 50 times higher* than for full-term infants.[17,18] Developmentally, *abnormal cognitive function, academic skills, poor visual motor, gross motor and adaptive function* also are associated with preterm birth. In addition, *mental retardation* and *developmental delay* are more frequent in infants born prior to 37-weeks gestation.

All in all, *prematurity carries with it enormous risks* along with the extraordinary utilization of health care resources. And yet, its causes have been complex and difficult to pinpoint. Clearly, the increased rate of multiple pregnancies secondary to the use of the artificial reproductive technologies has added to the prematurity rate. It is quite possible that the epidemic of sexually-transmitted diseases and induced abortion also has had an impact on this situation.

The current approach to preterm birth appears to be more of an acceptance of its inevitability and then preparation for early delivery.[19] While various risk factors are recognized, programs are recommended to anticipate the delivery of the premature infant. The recommendations often made are the timely administration of corticosteroids, heightened surveillance with monitoring of maternal and fetal well-being, referral to a perinatologist or neonatologist on a non-emergent basis, preparing the patient and her family, arranging for delivery at a tertiary care center (if necessary) and in some cases undertaking interventions that may delay or prevent preterm delivery.[19]

Many attempts have been made to implement programs for the prevention of preterm birth. Often, these either have not been successful[20] or have been only minimally successful.[21] While prenatal care has been shown to improve infant mortality rates,[22] more and more there is a recognition that neither preterm birth nor intrauterine growth restriction can be prevented effectively by prenatal care in its present form. A recent call has been made for the reconceptualization of prenatal care as part of a strategy to promote optimal development of women's reproductive health in order to prevent preterm birth and low birth weight delivery.[23]

In our program, a comprehensive and integrated strategy for the prevention of preterm birth has been developed, implemented and tested. It has resulted in a 71.4 percent decrease in the overall prematurity rate with deliveries at ≤ 36.9 weeks and a 142.1 percent decrease in the delivery of infants at ≤ 34.9 weeks gestation and a 200 percent decrease in delivery at ≤ 33.9 weeks. This chapter will present this approach to the prevention of preterm birth along with the overall context within which such a program exists locally, as well as its potential application on a wider level.

Our Prematurity Prevention Program

For more than 25 years, I have been interested in the question of preventing preterm labor and delivery. For the last 23 years, a specific protocol for the prevention of preterm labor and delivery has been instituted. This protocol is outlined in Table 29-1.

The program begins by identifying those patients who are at *high risk* for going into preterm labor. These patients then are taught how to *self-monitor their uterine contractions*. When indicated, *supplemental intramuscular progesterone* is provided while monitoring serum progesterone levels and *tocolytic therapy* (usually with the drug terbutaline) is used for symptoms of uterine irritability (contractions).

**Table 29-1: Prematurity Prevention
Program of the Pope Paul VI Institute**

---

1. Identify patients who are at high risk

2. Uterine contraction self-monitoring (patient education)

3. Supplement with IM progesterone while monitoring serum levels

4. Tocolytic therapy (usually terbutaline) for symptoms of uterine irritability (contractions)

5. Antibiotic therapy when patient breaks through tocolytic therapy

6. Ultrasound assessment of cervix when dictated by risk criterion, symptoms or pregnancy condition

7. Cerclage when indicated by ultrasound assessment

In addition to the above, *antibiotic therapy* is provided to those patients who break through their tocolytic therapy. Ultrasound assessment of the cervix also is used according to risk criterion, symptoms or pregnancy condition. If ultrasound assessment of the cervix indicates, a *cervical cerclage* is placed. Each of these will be taken individually.

Identifying Patients at Risk

Many risk factors may precede the onset of premature labor and delivery. The NICHD maternal fetal medicine network has carried out a preterm prediction study, which found that *fetal fibronectin* and a *short cervix* documented by ultrasound examination were strong predictors of preterm labor. Other predictors included *previous spontaneous preterm birth, uterine contractions, vaginal bleeding, pelvic infection* and *bacterial vaginosis.*[24]

Additional risk factors include such conditions as *infertility, abortion, adolescence, multiple pregnancy, premature cervical dilatation, history of previous stillbirth, malpresentation, maternal age of greater than 35 years,* and a *gestational age at which the mother was born of at less than 37 weeks.*[25-38] When one of these risk factors are identified at the initial intake of the new obstetrical visit or during the course of the pregnancy, the patient is entered into the next phase of the program.

Uterine Contraction Self-Monitoring

It seems quite clear that women who are destined for preterm delivery have more uterine activity on average than do other women of comparable gestational age. Although there may be a considerable amount of overlap,[39,40] various approaches to monitoring this increased uterine activity have been used.

Using external electronic monitors, even by long distance and at home, suggested that this could be a reasonable means for monitoring this activity.[41-44] There appeared to be some early enthusiasm for this approach and it appeared to be somewhat effective in identifying early the woman who might go into preterm labor.[45-47] Reports then were published that showed that this measurement clinically was not useful for the prediction or prevention of preterm delivery.[48,49] This approach also began to utilize nursing intervention. The initial reports were hopeful,[50] but it was shown to result in no better outcome than those who have less frequent nursing contact.[51-54].

The bulk of this work brought to the surface a series of symptoms that were associated with uterine contractions and the possibility that they may herald the onset, some time in the future, of preterm labor.[55,56] While there was continued controversy with regard to these signs and symptoms, because of their low positive predictive value, their use for the purposes of screening for the possibility of preterm labor was defended.[57] This all presented certain challenges. As obstetricians, it has been thought that *"Braxton Hicks contractions"* were normal, but there was a call for the discontinuance of the term "Braxton Hicks contractions."[58]

In our program, patients are instructed on the symptoms of uterine contractions during pregnancy (Table 29-2). These include *pelvic pressure, low backache, the uterus knotting up like a ball, uterine contractions (or cramps), a vaginal discharge (especially the "2W" discharge) and vaginal bleeding,* which is otherwise unexplained. They are instructed in the following fashion:

Pelvic pressure:

Sometimes uterine contractions are felt simply as a significant pressure in the pelvis that tends to come and go. Sometimes women will describe this feeling as "something falling out." Sometimes they are rhythmic, occurring two to three times an hour, or perhaps only two to three times a day.

Low backache:

Low backache is another sign of uterine contractions, especially if it is periodic. Sometimes uterine contractions are best felt in the back and are not felt in the front. Again, one's awareness that this may occur and is associated with contractions can be very helpful.

Table 29-2: Symptoms of Uterine Contractions during Pregnancy[55,56]

- Pelvic pressure
- Low backache
- Uterus knots up into a ball
- Uterine contractions (or cramps)
- Vaginal discharge (2W)
- Vaginal bleeding otherwise unexplained

Uterus knots up like a ball:

Sometimes the only symptom of contractions is the tightening of the uterus in which the uterus seems to "knot up like a ball." In a situation like this, it is easy for the woman to touch the uterus through the abdominal wall and to determine its firmness. Again, if these are rhythmic, they are important.

Uterine contractions (cramps):

The uterus is a muscle and when it contracts, there may or may not be a feeling that the woman will perceive as a contraction. When the woman is in labor, the contractions are easily identified, but in the earlier stages of pregnancy, they may easily go unnoticed unless she develops an awareness of these contractions and a realization of their importance. Uterine contractions cause the uterus to tighten and release in a periodic fashion. Uterine contractions are not constant (generally speaking) and occasional and irregular contractions are of less significance.

The woman can appreciate the presence of uterine contractions by simply realizing the importance of this kind of tightening that occurs in her abdomen that comes and goes over a period of time. This also can be identified by lying on one's left side with fingertips pressing against the uterus. If the uterus indents softly and easily, then there are no contractions. Once the uterus tightens, it will feel more firm and that firmness is a contraction whether or not the woman interprets it as a contraction or not. One can time these contractions with this type of monitoring.

In some women, the uterine contractions feel close to intermittent menstrual-like cramping. When cramps occur during the course of the pregnancy, they should *not* be ignored.

Vaginal discharge (2W):

Generally, there is no discharge during the course of pregnancy, although on occasion a mucus discharge might occur. When a *watery discharge (wet without lubrication)* begins to occur, it is important to be notified. It may be a sign of a low-grade infection and these infections can be the early stimulus to the development of premature labor.

Vaginal bleeding otherwise unexplained:

There should be no vaginal bleeding during the course of pregnancy until a woman goes into labor. On occasion, however, bleeding may occur sometime during the second or third trimester of pregnancy. It may be the only sign of the uterus contracting and often is a sign of low-grade infection. If a woman observes this, it should be reported to her physician.

The patient is educated in monitoring these symptoms of uterine contractions during pregnancy. Most importantly, *she is encouraged to notify our office when they occur.* A uterine contraction self-monitoring form is provided to the patient so she can maintain this monitoring during the course of the second and third trimesters of her pregnancy. This form is shown in Figure 29-2. If the symptoms are essentially the same from one day to the next, they are most likely not important. Once they change or become more severe, however, it is *extremely important* that the physician's office be notified.

If these symptoms are the same from one day to the next, they are most likely not very relevant. But *once the pattern changes,* it is important to pay attention to it. It also is important to *allow the woman* not only *to decide these issues,* but also provide her the freedom to call the office and have the office nurses, who should be properly trained in eliciting and interpreting these symptoms, assess them and report to the physician.

A Prematurity Prevention Office Visit Assessment Form also is utilized. This makes it easy at the time of the prenatal visit to review the patient's self-monitoring (Figure 29-3). *No prenatal visit should be complete without reviewing these symptoms with the patient.* Furthermore, the patient should be told that prenatal visits can only occur on an every-other-week to four-week basis, and yet these symptoms may occur at other times. Thus, when they do occur and when they worsen, it is important for the patient to call the office because intervention is based on this interaction.

The Use of Progesterone

The assessment and utilization of progesterone in pregnancy has been reviewed already. It will not be reviewed again at this time. But it should be reinforced that the ability of progesterone to effectively treat threatened premature labor has been in the medical literature since at least 1956.[59] It was reinforced in 1979 when decreased progesterone and 17-hydroxyprogesterone levels were observed in those patients who delivered prematurely.[60] Subsequently, a number of additional studies have reinforced these findings.[61-63]

Obstetrical Health Maintenance

Uterine Contractions Self-Monitoring System

Name: _____

Due date: _____

Month: _____

Sign	Date of Month																														
	1	2	3	4	5	6	7	8	9	10	11	12	13	14	15	16	17	18	19	20	21	22	23	24	25	26	27	28	29	30	31
1. Pelvic pressure																															
2. Low backache																															
3. Abdomen knots up like a ball																															
4. Cramps or contractions																															
5. Vaginal bleeding																															
6. Vaginal discharge (2W)*																															
7. Generally not feeling right (+ or −)																															
Is today the same as yesterday? (Y or N)																															
Total score																															

0	=	not present (absent)
+1	=	occasional or irregular
+2	=	more regular, more intense
+3	=	rhythmic (come and go), stronger

* Use Vaginal Discharge Recording System from your CREIGHTON MODEL FertilityCare™ System

Prepared by
Pope Paul VI Institute
for the Study of Human Reproduction
2004

Figure 29-2: Uterine Contractions Self-Monitoring System

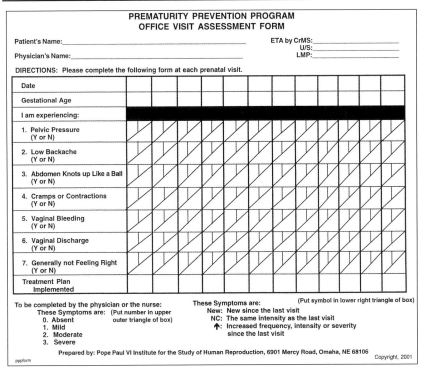

Figure 29-3: A prematurity prevention program office visit assessment form used at the Pope Paul VI Institute.

More recently, in 2003, the use of either progesterone[64] or 17 α-hydroxyprogesterone caproate[65] were shown to be effective in decreasing the incidence of preterm labor. And yet, even before the second of these two latter studies was published, it was declared that it was "too soon to adopt progesterone for the prevention of preterm delivery."[66] The American College of Obstetricians and Gynecologists (ACOG), in their May 2003 Practice Bulletin on the prevention of preterm labor, did not even mention progesterone.[1] In November 2003, the use of progesterone to reduce preterm birth finally was assessed by the ACOG, but then only with a caution that it should be restricted in its use only for women with a *documented history of a previous birth* at less than 37 weeks of gestation. The ACOG Committee on Obstetric Practice cites "unresolved issues" and these include "optimal route of drug delivery and long-term safety of the drug."[67]

And yet, *progesterone has been used in pregnancy for over 60 years with no known short- or long-term safety issues.* The ACOG approach to preterm birth appears to be without urgency. To them, a patient first needs to suffer through a preterm birth and its known neonatal and long-term problems before she can be considered a candidate for supplementation with a hormone that is normally produced in large quantities in pregnancy and where it has been shown that patients who go into preterm labor have decreased progesterone levels. *Not only does progesterone quiet the uterus,* but *it also may cause the narrowing and lengthening of the cervix* in a somewhat similar fashion to its effects in the postovulatory phase of the normal menstrual cycle.[68] It is troubling that a hormone that is produced in as large a quantity as progesterone is in normal pregnancy and carries with it virtually no known maternal or fetal side effects is so roundly ignored or de-emphasized.

Further study of the integrity of the corpus luteum in the cycle in which pregnancy was achieved also has shown the importance of progesterone. Dr. Jerome Check has shown that patients with *luteal phase deficiency* who did not receive progesterone in the pregnancy that occurred had a significantly higher prematurity rate including severe prematurity at less than 32-weeks gestation.[69] This has been reproduced by others[70] who also have shown that premature labor occurred in patients who had significantly lower progesterone levels during the luteal phase of their menstrual cycle in which pregnancy was achieved than those who delivered at full term. Taking this information and combining it with the knowledge of serum progesterone levels during the course of the pregnancy in certain types of luteal phase deficiency and in those patients with known types of infertility due to endometriosis, for example, shows the importance of progesterone in these situations.

More recently, HCG also has been shown to have very potent tocolytic effects.[71] In a placebo-controlled trial, the use of HCG (one single dose of HCG 5,000 units IV and 10,000 units of HCG in 500 cc of dextrose as a drip of 20 drops/minute) resulted in a delay in delivery of 28.8 days versus only 15 days for the placebo-treated group. This suggested that human chorionic gonadotropin also exhibits potent tocolysis with no fetal side effects.[72]

Tocolytic Therapy

Over the last 40 years, there has been an effort made to identify a pharmacologic agent that would stop uterine contractions and prevent preterm birth. The litany of pharmacologic agents includes the following: isoxsuprine, ethanol, morphine sulfate, terbutaline, ritodrine, indomethacin, magnesium sulfate and atosiban.[73,74] Extensive evaluation of these agents, alone or in combination, has been conducted over this period of time.[75-86] By 1993, the three most commonly used drugs were ritodrine, terbutaline and magnesium sulfate.[87]

In a critical and comprehensive review of the efficacy and safety of these agents in 1993,[88] it was concluded that "The only tocolytic drugs that might be effective are the prostaglandin inhibitors. Tocolytic agents should only be used between 24- and 32-completed weeks of gestation. Magnesium sulfate should not be used to treat premature labor. Oxytocin antagonists should be used only in experimental clinical trials. Calcium channel blockers and beta adrenergic receptor agonists inhibit uterine contractions, but do not prolong gestation for longer than 48 hours." Although tocolytic agents were shown to prolong pregnancy, their biggest criticism has been their inability to improve perinatal or neonatal outcomes and potentially the adverse affects on women in preterm labor.

In our program, a slightly different approach has been taken. The drug chosen for use is the β-mimetic agent terbutaline. This drug is provided to patients who have positive signs or symptoms of uterine contractions (uterine irritability) because it will quiet uterine activity. It is used in a dosage of 2.5 mg every four hours around the clock. Rarely is a higher dose *ever* used and then only on a very short-term basis. This drug in higher doses can be associated with significant side effects. At this lower dose, however, the only side effects observed usually are edginess or jitteriness, which usually dissipates within seven days. Thus it has been, in our experience, a safe drug to use!

Terbutaline is provided as a means of both *quieting the uterus* while, at the same time, *testing it*. In many cases, the treatment of the uterine irritability stops with the use of progesterone and terbutaline. *But if the patient's contractions or irritability begin to "break through" the terbutaline and progesterone, then a move toward the use of antibiotics is initiated.*

The Use Of Antibiotics

Up to 80 percent of early preterm births are associated with an intrauterine infection that *precedes* the rupture of membranes.[89,90] While there have been many trials of antibiotic therapy in women with preterm labor, most have found that such therapy does not prevent premature birth.[90] Some have questioned whether this failure is due to the selection of inappropriate antibiotics, the initiation of treatment too late in the cascade of events leading to spontaneous preterm labor or other factors that are unknown.[91]

A clue to possible identification of those women who have "silent chorioamnionitis" as a cause of preterm labor was published and virtually ignored in 1984.[92] This study showed that those women who were *refractory to tocolysis* with ritodrine had indicators present that suggested a *silent chorioamnionitis* (an infection of the membranes or fluid surrounding the baby). These included an elevated maternal C-reactive protein, positive amniotic fluid gram stain, greater than 100 mm^3 white blood cells in the amniotic fluid, positive bacterial growth and histopathologic evidence of chorioamnionitis at the time of delivery. This study and others that pointed to similar findings[93-95] provoked me to begin to use the clinical sign of *a breakthrough in uterine activity while on tocolytic agents (specifically terbutaline) as a clinical indication of silent chorioamnionitis.*

When one reviews the types of microorganisms that have been identified in chorioamnionitis, one sees a great variety. While antibiotics have not usually been successful, it is likely that they have either been started too late or the choice of antibiotic has not had a broad enough spectrum.

Prior to initiating any antibiotic therapy, urine cultures and sensitivities need to be done because of the possibility that an asymptomatic urinary tract infection may be present. These asymptomatic infections have been shown to be associated with both preterm delivery and low birth weight infants. Antibiotic therapy in those situations directed specifically at the causative organism is effective in reducing the occurrence of low birth weight.[96]

While many antibiotic trials have not shown satisfactory results, the use of a combination of ampicillin-sulbactam has been shown to be effective in prolonging pregnancy in the presence of premature rupture of membranes.[97] This combination antibiotic has a broader spectrum than many used in the past.

The antibiotic program I have used began in December 1985. At that time, the third generation cephalosporins were just becoming available. Because of a long half-life, broad spectrum and high intra-amniotic fluid levels, cefoperazone sodium (Cefobid) was chosen for use.[98] At the time this antibiotic was initiated, the concept of "pulsed antibiotic therapy" was initiated. Once the patient had breakthrough contractions on terbutaline, she was considered a candidate for the initiation of pulsed cefoperazone therapy. The therapy began as an outpatient intravenous application giving two grams IV every other day for three doses over a course of two to three weeks (usually Monday, Wednesday and Friday). Once there was symptomatic improvement, the antibiotic therapy was decreased to two grams IV twice a week. If uterine contractile activity increased symptomatically again, the antibiotic therapy was increased again to three times a week. This continued until 37 weeks when it was discontinued.

Cefoperazone has a very broad spectrum of activity, one that will cover most of the aerobic and anaerobic bacteria often found in these situations. A comparison could be made between the early delivery rate prior to the introduction of cefoperazone into the regimen and again afterwards. The incidence of premature delivery at ≤ 35.9-weeks gestational age after initiation of cefoperazone therapy was 2.8 percent. Prior to that time, it had been 6.6 percent.

A similar analysis was done for patients who delivered at ≤ 34.9-weeks gestation. Here the difference was even more striking as the incidence prior to cefoperazone therapy was 4.9 percent and afterwards, 1.7 percent.

The patients also exhibited superb symptomatic improvement in the presentation of their symptoms of uterine contraction irritability. In a study of 82 consecutive patients receiving cefoperazone therapy, 69 of them had good to excellent symptomatic improvement (84.1 percent). In those who had improvement, the average number of days required until improvement was attained was 10.3.

In addition, the incidence of the premature rupture of membranes *prior to 37 weeks gestation* significantly decreased from 4.9 percent prior to the introduction of cefoperazone therapy to 2.3 percent afterwards.

Another experience also was obtained with eight patients who had prolongation of their pregnancy for greater than seven days after spontaneous rupture of membranes prior to 37-weeks gestation. With the use of cefoperazone, the pregnancy was prolonged on an average of 11.8 weeks. Without cefoperazone, the prolongation was only 5.9 weeks. In one case, the patient's membranes ruptured at 16-weeks gestation and with pulsed cefoperazone, she delivered a full-term, healthy male infant. In another case, with ruptured membranes at 26-weeks gestation and failure of Augmentin therapy by the perinatologist, pulsed cefoperazone therapy was given and within four weeks she sealed her membranes and eventually delivered at 38 weeks.

Unfortunately, cefoperazone was removed from the market approximately six years ago. Since that time, our protocol has used ceftriaxone (Rocephin) as its main antibiotic treatment. This antibiotic is similar to cefoperazone in that it has a long half-life (24 hours) and a similar spectrum of activity. Because the half-life is so long, the regimen also was changed. It is given intravenously for 10 to 14 days at two grams per day. This all can be done on an outpatient basis. In a few cases, we have used intravenous metronidazole or ampicillin-sulbactam with similar effectiveness but not as the first-line approach.

To our knowledge, there have been no neonatal side effects from the use of this therapy. Some have cautioned that drug resistance could develop when maternal antibiotics are utilized.[99-100] While this is a legitimate concern, no drug resistance has been observed in the 23 years of application of this protocol. Furthermore, the overall neonatal morbidity and mortality is *significantly reduced* because of the advanced gestational age at the time of delivery. In addition, the use of outpatient antibiotic therapy has been found to be safe and economical.[101-103]

Use of Cervical Cerclage

In 1986, the use of ultrasound to evaluate the length of the cervix was reported[104] and found that preterm delivery was significantly higher in those patients who had a *shortened cervix*. Early in the study, they realized that ultrasound-observable changes of cervical incompetency, when left untreated, could result in second trimester losses. The study design, therefore, could not incorporate a randomized treatment and non-treatment group. Nonetheless, this study began our interest in the evaluation of the cervix by ultrasound associated with the use of cervical cerclage (a surgical procedure where a suture is placed around the cervix to give it greater strength).

In 1996, a report for the Maternal Fetal Medicine Unit Network showed that the risk of spontaneous preterm delivery is increased in women who are found to have a short cervix by vaginal ultrasound during pregnancy.[105] In the meantime, indications for a cervical cerclage were being expanded beyond the traditionally-accepted diagnosis of classic cervical incontinence (documented by a previous pregnancy loss during the middle trimester). Its use has been recommended in placenta previa,[106] uterine malformations,[107,108] previous DES exposure or cervical cone biopsy with cervical changes in pregnancy.[109] In spite of these expansions, concern continued to exist with regard to the overall safety of cervical cerclage and whether or not it might be associated with chorioamnionitis, premature rupture of membranes, premature labor or other concerns that might be avoidable.

There was, in fact, the classic randomized control trial of cervical cerclage that suggested that there is no evidence that cerclage either prolonged gestation or improved survival.[110] A *major methodological flaw* in the study, however, included the *ineligibility* of most of the high-risk groups including recurrent spontaneous abortion, multiple pregnancy, congenital anomalies, uterine fibroids, previous surgery on the cervix, or a short or dilated cervix. This trial, in effect, showed that the use of cervical cerclage for the prevention of preterm labor in individuals who *were not at high risk and did not need a cerclage* resulted in a higher incidence of problems in the study group. It did not address the actual population of patients who might be in need of cervical cerclage. A similar study from France had similar results and similar flaws.[111] The final report of the Medical Research Council/Royal College of Obstetricians and Gynecologists Multicenter Randomized Trial of Cervical Cerclage[112] showed that it had a beneficial effect in a small number of cases, but was associated with puerperal fever. In none of these three studies was ultrasound used to assess the cervix or were prophylactic antibiotics used. Furthermore, in the Royal College's Multicenter Trial, no special tests or special followup visits were required.

When comparing the use of cervical cerclage with and without prophylactic antibiotics (cefoperazone), I found a much higher risk of premature birth in patients who did *not* receive prophylactic antibiotics. When evaluated further, the average gestational age at delivery with cerclage and prophylactic cefoperazone was 38.5 weeks. The average gestational age at delivery of those patients who received cervical cerclage without the use of prophylactic antibiotics (cefoperazone) was 34.7 weeks.

It also was identified that patients had difficulty adjusting to the cerclage if they were mobilized too quickly following the surgery. Thus, **a protocol was developed for all patients who receive cervical cerclage**. This involves the following:

1. The cervix must measure less than 3 cm or exhibit greater than 6 mm of endocervical funneling (nippling) on ultrasound examination.

2. These changes must be present prior to the 28th week of pregnancy.

3. Prophylactic antibiotics are given prior to the time of surgery in preop holding [currently two grams ceftriaxone (Rocephin) IV].

4. The cerclage is performed.

5. The patient is kept at *total bedrest* except for bathroom privileges for the first 36 hours following the placement of the cerclage.

6. Ceftriaxone (Rocephin) is continued at two grams, intravenously, every 24 hours for three doses.

7. After the 36-hour quiet period, the patient is allowed to be up and around, but not at complete activity for another seven days.

The type of cerclage we use is referred to as a "modified McDonald" cerclage. A 5mm mersilene band (looks a bit like a shoelace) is placed in a purse string-like fashion around the cervix to give it added strength. It is done in the operating room under anesthesia and it takes only five to 10 minutes to place.

The cerclage is removed by placing a ring forceps on the knot and pulling gently so that the loop of the cerclage can be identified. Using a long, sterile scissors that loop is cut and the cerclage is removed. This can be done, usually without difficulty, in the office and is performed at 36 weeks if there is no previous history of cervical incompetence and at 37 weeks if there is a previous history of pregnancy loss.

The length of the cervix as measured by ultrasound in patients whose cervix was initially less than or equal to 3 cm, both before and after cervical cerclage. The average length of the cervix was 2.27 cm prior to the cerclage and 3.32 cm after the cerclage. This is a statistically significant improvement in the length of the cervix.

The nippling of the membranes down the cervical canal, as measured by ultrasound, was 14.2 mm prior to the cerclage and 7 mm after the cerclage. It has been reported that the increase in the length of the cervix correlated with improved pregnancy outcome.[113] This is definitely what we have observed.

Our program considers the proper placement of a cervical cerclage to provide *excellent reinforcement* to the cervix in an appropriately identified population using ultrasound parameters with the *use of prophylactic antibiotics* and *short-term bedrest* following the procedure. In most cases, the patient eventually will resume normal or near normal activity.

Twin Pregnancies

In twin pregnancies, it has been found that supplementation with progesterone is helpful in prolonging the length of the gestation. In those patients who had progesterone during the course of their pregnancy, the average gestational age at the time of delivery was 36.5 weeks. In those patients who did not have progesterone, the average gestational age at the time of delivery was 34.6 weeks. This is a statistically significant lengthening of the pregnancy. So it is now routine with our Prematurity Prevention Program to supplement all twin pregnancies with intramuscular progesterone throughout the course of the pregnancy. If indicated by ultrasound or other parameters, the use of cerclage or intravenous antibiotics, as previously described, also would be utilized, but often is not necessary.

Results of the Program

The results of the Prematurity Prevention Protocol outlined in this chapter are presented in Table 29-4. The overall prematurity rate (delivery at $\leq$ 36.9 weeks) using the Pope Paul VI Institute Protocol was 7 percent (n=775). In a comparison group of patients who also received their prenatal care at our center, but where the protocol was not utilized, the corresponding prematurity rate was 12 percent (similar to the national average). Overall, this represents a 71.4 percent decline

Table 29-4: Summary of Delivery Rates Pope Paul VI Institute Prematurity Prevention Protocol vs. Comparsion Group

Delivery at (weeks gestation)	Comparison Group[1] %	PPVI Protocol[2] %	p-value[3]
$\leq$36.9 weeks	12.0	7.0	.0032
$\leq$35.9 weeks	6.4	3.6	.025
$\leq$34.9 weeks	4.6	1.9	.008
$\leq$33.9 weeks	3.9	1.3	.0031

1. Total N=435 deliveries
2. Total N=775 deliveries
3. Chi-square analysis

in the prematurity rate using this protocol. A similar analysis also was conducted with regard to delivery rates at ≤ 35.9 weeks, ≤ 34.9 weeks, or ≤ 33.9 weeks.

The most significant reduction in prematurity rates occurred at the lower gestational ages; 96.4 percent of babies were born at 36 weeks or greater. At ≤ 34.9 weeks, there was a 142.1-percent decrease and at ≤ 33.9 weeks, a 200-percent decrease in delivery rates.

Special Case Examples

The work presented in this chapter is summarized with the following case presentations:

Case 1

This is a 26-year-old woman who exhibited in her first pregnancy preterm labor, uterine irritability and premature changes in her cervix. She was at bedrest for the last 2-1/2 months of her pregnancy and delivered at 36-weeks gestation, while being cared for elsewhere. In her second pregnancy, her cervix measured 2.89 cm at 14.1 weeks without endocervical nippling. A cervical cerclage was placed, she was managed with oral Terbutaline, progesterone and eventually pulsed cefoperazone. Her hsCRP (high sensitivity c-reactive protein–a test for inflamation) decreased from 9.1 mg/L to 4.1 mg/L. She continued to work full time throughout the course of that pregnancy and delivered at 41 weeks. A similar management scheme was used for her third pregnancy. She delivered at term after working up to the time of delivery.

Case 2

This is a 36-year-old woman who had three previous spontaneous abortions. She was given progesterone and HCG support during the course of her pregnancy. At 12-weeks gestation she began having severe menstrual-like cramps and vaginal bleeding. Her hsCRP was 8.5 mg/L. She was given 10 days of Rocephin two grams IV. Her symptoms disappeared; her hsCRP decreased to 5.1 and she delivered at full term with a repeat cesarean section.

Case 3

This is a 26-year-old woman who began having significant uterine irritability at about 14-weeks gestation. At 16 weeks, a large retroplacental hematoma was identified on ultrasound. She was managed with intramuscular progesterone and complete bedrest for six weeks and the hematoma resolved. She went on to deliver a full-term, healthy baby. In a series of 23 such patients, the full-term delivery rate in our program is 82.6 percent. This compares to a term delivery rate of 44.4 percent as presented in the medical literature.

Case 4

This is a 44-year-old woman who had had six previous spontaneous abortions. Her one and only child was delivered by emergency cesarean section at 36-weeks gestation because of a pronounced decrease in fetal heart tones. She was evaluated and found to have suboptimal progesterone production during the luteal phase of her menstrual cycle and also endometriosis. The endometriosis was laser vaporized and her luteal phase deficiency was treated with HCG.

During the course of her pregnancy, she was managed with progesterone and HCG supplementation. An ultrasound at 22.4 weeks, after several episodes of symptoms of uterine irritability, showed a cervix that measured 2.45 cm with 12.5 mm of endocervical nippling and dilatation of the internal cervical os of 16.9 mm. A cervical cerclage was placed and at 27.6 weeks, her cervix was now 3.63 cm with no endocervical nippling. She also was treated with terbutaline and pulsed cefoperazone. She delivered at 38 weeks a healthy female infant by repeat cesarean section. For much of the pregnancy (especially the second and third trimester), her progesterone levels were in low zone 2 or high zone 1.

Case 5

This is a 24-year-old woman who had one previously-induced abortion, one ectopic pregnancy, a stillborn at 19 weeks and a delivery at 24 weeks with spontaneous rupture of membranes at labor. With the last delivery, at 24 weeks, she was sent home by the perinatologist until she went into labor.

With her fifth pregnancy, she was followed carefully by us and by 10.2 weeks, already had evidence of endocervical nippling. Because of her extremely poor obstetrical history, she was given three days of ceftriaxone prior to placement of the cervical cerclage. This was followed by an additional 10 days of treatment. The cerclage, in her case, was placed at 10.2 weeks. While this is unusual, because of her poor obstetrical history, it was thought to be justified.

In this pregnancy, she had spontaneous rupture of the membranes at 38.1 weeks, and eventually had a cesarean section for failure to progress. She had a 6-pound, 7-ounce baby boy with Apgar scores of 7 and 9.

Case 6

The final case presentation is a 41-year-old woman who had one previous spontaneous abortion along with a long history of infertility. At the time of evaluation, she had endometriosis, severe bilateral salpingitis isthmica nodosa with occlusion of both fallopian tubes, decreased pre-Peak and post-Peak estradiol levels and a normal progesterone profile. Her T_3:rT_3 ratio was 3.7 and her β-endorphin level was less than 8.8 pg/mL. She was treated with post-Peak HCG, amoxicillin and guaifenesin for mucus enhancement, T_3, naltrexone 16 mg by mouth two times a day and estradiol-17β, 1 mg by mouth every day at bedtime Peak +3 through 12. She also had been tried for many months on low-dose Clomid, but its effect on the mucus was so poor it had to be stopped.

With this treatment program, she did achieve a pregnancy, but at 16.7-weeks gestation, she began having symptoms and her cervix measured 2.65 cm with 19.1 mm of nippling and dilatation of the internal cervical opening at 15.7 mm. She underwent a cervical cerclage and four weeks later, her cervix was 3.13 cm with no endocervical nippling and the internal opening was closed. She also had, at 22 weeks, a recurring problem with uterine contractions and was treated with ceftriaxone two grams IV x 14 days. Many of her symptoms disappeared. She went full term without additional symptoms and delivered a healthy baby girl. Her progesterone levels in this pregnancy were consistently suboptimal.

One of the important features of this case is her **CrMS** chart, which prior to her pregnancy, is shown in Figure 29-4. This chart shows multiple signs of infection present in advance of her pregnancy. The prolonged episodes of premenstrual brown bleeding, the "frequent 2W" observations and the tail-end brown bleeding all can be signs of low-grade infection that are otherwise asymptomatic. A focus of research in the future will be the evaluation of the **CrMS** and its standardized vulvar observations with the subsequent outcome of pregnancies. If, in fact, much of prematurity is caused by low-grade infection, which is, of and by itself, very difficult to diagnose, the best of all worlds would be to identify this in advance of pregnancy, treat it effectively and prevent the entire spectrum of uterine irritability, uterine contractions, premature labor and premature birth.

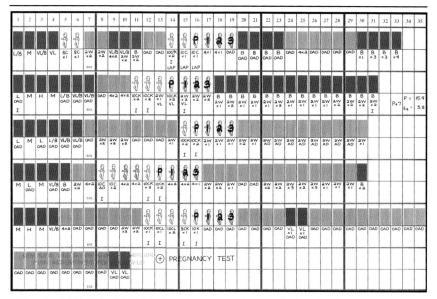

Figure 29-4: This is the CrMS chart from the patient in Case No. 6. This is her chart leading up to the time of her pregnancy. Noteworthy is the presence of prolonged premenstrual spotting, tail-end brown bleeding and "frequent 2W" observations. All of these observations are consistent with a low-grade infection being present prior to the onset of her pregnancy. Further research is necessary to determine the ability of this type of prospective tracking of vulvar observations to be helpful in the identification of low-grade infection prior to the onset of pregnancy and, hopefully, subsequently treated (From: Pope Paul VI Institute research, 2004). Refer to page 83 for the Vaginal Discharge Recording System.

Conclusions

This work has shown that it is possible to make a significant impact in reducing the escalating incidence of preterm births. It does require, however, a specific commitment to see that it is accomplished. This particular program has worked because it uses a *comprehensive and integrated approach.* It also is made possible by incorporating the pregnant woman, through pregnancy-related education, into the role of a meaningful partner in her own health care and that of her new baby. Patients will respond when given this opportunity and without them, it is not possible. It should be pointed out that others have used successfully a somewhat similar approach.[114]

In addition, the physician and others in the prematurity-prevention program cannot accept preterm labor and birth as a *fait accompli.* It *must* be viewed as an intensive care situation and *must* be correspondingly addressed. Most of this effort can be accomplished through an outpatient effort. It is not common for one of our patients to be managed in the hospital and when it does occur, it is usually only for one or two days, enough time to give a dose of subcutaneous Terbutaline (0.25 mg SQ), hydrate the patient and give her one dose of ceftriaxone.

This chapter began by pointing out that *the prematurity rate in the United States is a national tragedy.* Unfortunately, it does not get enough publicity to arouse the public to greater action. Some of the increase is iatrogenic (caused by physician-instituted "therapies," especially with the increase in multiple pregnancies from ART) and some is self-imposed by what appears to be pregnancy-associated infection, some of which is most certainly secondary to sexually-transmitted diseases. Some of it, too, is undoubtedly related to the widespread use of first trimester-induced abortion by the medical profession to solve what ultimately is a social problem (as opposed to a medical problem). But most of it appears to result because of a *lack of will* on the part of the medical profession and the community to make a defined impact. It is hoped that our work will stimulate others to develop meaningful programs for the prevention of preterm birth.

Real People, Real Problems, Real Solutions

Around 25 weeks, I started having contractions. All day, I had flu-like symptoms and mild cramping. By evening, the contractions were two to three minutes apart. I called my local doctor who said that I was probably having Braxton Hicks [contractions]. I told him that they were very regular and I could time them. He said that if I wanted to, I could go to the hospital. I could tell from the tone of his voice that he thought I was overreacting. At the hospital, the nurses saw that I was in labor. My contractions were two to three minutes apart and my cervix was softening. They gave me shots of terbutaline to stop my contractions. After a few hours, the medications stopped my contractions. When the doctor came in to discharge me, he never checked my cervix, he sent me home with no medications and he told me to ignore the contractions. He told me to relax and the contractions would go away.

I called Dr. Hilgers' office and talked to Cheryl. She could not believe that the local doctor did not treat my preterm labor. Immediately, Cheryl phoned a prescription of terbutaline to my local pharmacy. I started taking it every four hours around the clock. Dr. Hilgers also recommended an IV treatment that would calm my uterus in case I had an infection. Cheryl set up everything for me and kept me in her prayers. The next day, I had a nurse in my home administering my IV treatment. My local doctor was upset that I went over him. He said that he had never heard of such a treatment, but when I asked him if this treatment was harming my baby, he had no comment. He said that if it eased my mind, I should continue treatment. I knew that his feathers were ruffled so I did not comment on his sarcastic remark. Unfortunately, he was like so many of my previous doctors who misdiagnosed me or thought I was overly anxious about my health. He called this a 'paranoid pregnancy.' He did not even know about the shots of hCG and progesterone.

Thanks to Dr. Hilgers, I delivered at 37 weeks. As soon as I stopped the terbutaline, I went into labor. Robbie was born by emergency C-section due to very strong and irregular contractions that made his heart rate drop. He is a healthy, beautiful baby.

I cannot thank Dr. Hilgers enough for everything that he has done for me. He had answers to what was causing my infertility and treated me. I guess I was not paranoid after all! His treatment helped my body become healthy so that I could become pregnant. His preterm labor treatment made sure I was able to maintain my pregnancy. I have a wonderful son to show for all of Dr. Hilgers' care, hard work and dedication to women's health. I prayed to God to show me the way, and he led me straight to Dr. Hilgers.

Jeanine Jahaske
Roselle, Illinois

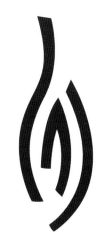

The Future

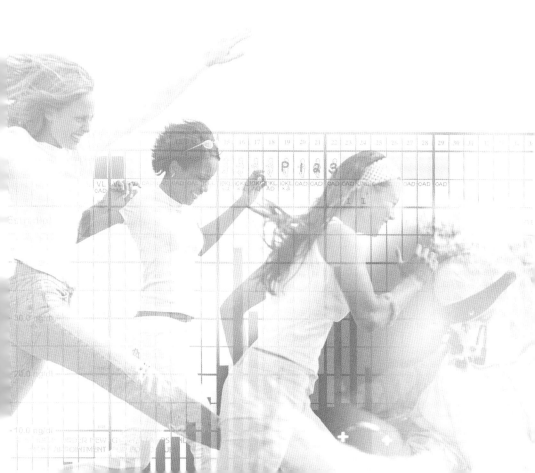

BASIC PRINCIPLE FOR the analysis of the economic aspects of medical care includes choices that involve alternative uses of resources and decisions that must consider both cost and outcome.[1] In addition, there is a move towards creating a health care system based on treatments that work, whether they are conventional, complimentary, alternative or integrated medicine.[2] In **NaProTECHNOLOGY**, we have a new women's health science that works. The question now is, "Is it affordable?"

It is impossible to review the cost effectiveness status of the entire spectrum of **NaProTECHNOLOGY** as it relates to conventional forms of evaluation and treatment because it has such a very broad scope of application. A sampling of several of the major areas of involvement of **NaProTECHNOLOGY**, however, can be calculated. In this chapter, we will calculate the use of the **CREIGHTON MODEL System** (CrMS) for family planning purposes and **NaProTECHNOLOGY** for the treatment of premenstrual syndrome, prematurity prevention and infertility.

Family Planning

The **CrMS** is an educational form of family planning that provides information in a standardized fashion to the patient and to her husband. It does this in such as way as to provide services that, for the purposes of avoiding pregnancy, can be compared economically to the use of artificial contraceptive methods. The main cost involved in providing the **CrMS** is in the provision of the educational services. In comparing the cost of tubal sterilization, a progesterone-releasing intrauterine device, and an oral contraceptive over a five-year period of use, the **CrMS** compares very favorably. The five-year cost for tubal sterilization is $2,835; the progesterone IUD $2,300; and the oral contraceptive $1,890. The **CrMS**, based upon an introductory session and eight individual follow-ups during the first year of use and an individual follow-up each of the four succeeding years, totals $494 (with an estimated cost of $37 per follow-up and $50 for the Introductory Session). This is a cost factor that is considerably less than that of the artificial methods.[3]

Premenstrual Syndrome

In reviewing the costs of premenstrual syndrome, it is important to take into consideration a variety of different components of this condition. This includes the current use of family planning, the supportive use of over-the-counter medications, the use of antidepressants or antianxiety medications, the number of work days that may be missed per month or work days that have reduced productivity. This all has been evaluated by others.[4,5] In **NaProTECHNOLOGY**, additional factors have to be taken into consideration that include the cost of hormone evaluation and the cost of treatment. Benefits come with an estimated decrease in the number of work days missed and the increased productivity that goes with it. The *cost savings* per woman using **NaProTECHNOLOGY** approaches has been calculated at $1,886.01 per year.[3]

Prematurity

The cost of premature birth in the United States is extremely high. The March of Dimes clearly has identified these factors. In an average week, there are more than 9,000 babies born prematurely in the United States. The total yearly number of preterm births exceeds 470,000.

The cost of medical care for these premature babies has been estimated at $13.6 billion. If the March of Dimes 2010 United States objective of a prematurity rate of 7.6 percent were reached, this cost could be reduced to $8,684,960,000. The projected cost using the Pope Paul VI Institute Prematurity Prevention Program, which has already established a prematurity rate of 7 percent, would reduce the costs even further to $7,999,520,000. The *savings* to the national health expenditure with the March of Dimes projection (a projection that has not been achieved) would be $4,915,040,000. The *savings* with the projection of the Prematurity Prevention Program operative at the Pope Paul VI Institute (a projection that already has been achieved) in its **NaProTECHNOLOGY** program would be $5,600,480,000.[3]

These savings do not take into account the extraordinary cost of long-term debility that occurs as a result of premature birth and the health of the infant. The estimated cost for the care of infants with cerebral palsy in the United States (for the year 1992) has been calculated at $2,426,000,000. This also does not take into consideration other problems that might be associated with premature birth, such as the development of learning disorders, abnormal motor function and mental retardation.[3]

It should be pointed out that the financial ramifications of prematurity are well documented. Gestational age at delivery, survival, length of nursery stay, the presence of Respiratory Distress Syndrome (RDS) and pneumonia are strong predictors of hospital charges. *Of the five most expensive hospital diagnoses in the United States, RDS and low birth weight (both associated with prematurity) are number 2 and 3 respectively.*[6]

Furthermore, the actual costs of premature birth, which take into account the cost of care for newborn infants, does not take into account the expenditures for hospitalizations related to preterm labor. The estimated costs for hospitalizations relative to preterm labor in the United States, on a yearly basis, is $820,000,000.[7] As has been pointed out, hospitalizations with the Institute's Prematurity Prevention Program are extremely rare and, when they do occur, are usually only 24 to 48 hours in duration. Almost all of the management of a Prematurity Prevention Program, modeled after the one at the Pope Paul VI Institute, can be undertaken as an outpatient.

Infertility

There are three major costs incurred in the evaluation and treatment of infertility:

1. The cost of the evaluation of the various aspects of the infertility problem and the treatment of the anatomic, organic, and functional abnormalities associated with it.

2. The per-cycle cost for the treatment of the infertility.

3. The estimated additional cost for treatment of multiple pregnancies.

A comparison of the costs for the evaluation and treatment of the various abnormalities in an IVF program vs. a **NaProTECHNOLOGY** program have been identified and enumerated. In comparing the two groups, including diagnostic laparoscopy and surgical intervention, if needed, the cost is $1,561,352 for an IVF program in comparison to $2,640,402 in a **NaProTECHNOLOGY** program (this is based per 100 patients in each group). The costs are higher in the **NaProTECHNOLOGY** program because the evaluation is more thorough and the treatment approach for the underlying disease is much more aggressive. On the other hand, many women who undergo IVF also are subjected to a variety of different evaluation protocols and subsequently to various surgical procedures.

The per-cycle cost of IVF has been identified as $9,226. The average per-cycle cost of **NaProTECHNOLOGY** will depend somewhat on the type of medical treatment utilized. If a progression in the use of the drug clomiphene is used, the average cost per cycle (including hormone monitoring and physician/nurse interaction) is $322.38. If an FSH/LH progression is used, the average cost per cycle is $992, including ultrasound, hormone testing and medication.

The estimated additional cost for treatment of multiple pregnancies in IVF and **NaProTECHNOLOGY** per 100 patients who become pregnant also has been calculated. The cost in an IVF program is $1,443,429.63. In the **NaProTECHNOLOGY** program, because the multiple pregnancy rate is so low (3.2 percent and the average gestational age at the time of delivery of twins in our program is 36.5 weeks), the cost is much lower at $33,680.00 per 100 pregnant patients.

The costs can be estimated for every 100 patients who achieve pregnancy and deliver a baby in comparing IVF and **NaProTECHNOLOGY**.[3] Taking into account the estimated costs for the medical evaluation and treatment, the various cycles of treatment and the multiple pregnancy care, the overall costs per 100 patients of IVF is $4,757,721. In **NaProTECHNOLOGY**, the cost in the clomiphene progression group is $3,060,938 per 100 pregnant women and in the FSH/LH progression it $3,864,482.3

The average per-patient cost per successful pregnancy with IVF using the previous calculations is $47,577.21. The cost of a clomiphene progression is $30,609.38 and for a FSH/LH progression is $38,644.82. It should be pointed out that *in the IVF group, that cost does not include the identification of the problem or its treatment, which usually goes unresolved.* With **NaProTECHNOLOGY**, however, the cost does include identification of the underlying problem and its treatment along with the pregnancy.[3]

In considering costs of the infertility program overall, it also is important to consider the cost to those patients who do not achieve a pregnancy with the type of infertility care provided. For purposes of calculation, it is presumed that 70 percent of the women who enter an IVF program do not achieve a pregnancy while only 40 percent of those entering a **NaProTECHNOLOGY** program do not achieve a pregnancy. The average per-patient cost for IVF for those patients who do not achieve a pregnancy is $33,143. In **NaProTECHNOLOGY**, with a clomiphene progression (which is by far the most common utilized at the present time), the cost is $30,348 and with an FSH/LH progression, it is $37,468. The clomiphene progression is less expensive than the IVF approach, while the FSH/LH progression is more expensive. *There is one major difference between these approaches.* In the IVF approach, once again, it is unlikely that *the patient will find out what the underlying cause is and thus, it will not be treated. For about the same number of dollars, in* **NaProTECHNOLOGY** *the patient will have a good understanding of the underlying causes, those causes will be treated and her health will be improved.* It is difficult to put a price on one's improved health. It is, as the ad says: "Priceless!"

Summary of Costs

A summary of costs comparing these different approaches results in a cost savings for **NaProTECHNOLOGY** for the items analyzed at $31,774.36 per person. This analysis does not include an anticipated reduction in the surgical rate for ovarian cysts and a reduced rate for hysterectomies. It does not include a reduced need for obstetrical intervention because of more accurate obstetrical dates. It does not include an analysis of costs for postpartum depression with progesterone being relatively inexpensive. It is important to keep this in mind as one considers these comparisons.

It also should be pointed out that while the insurance industry loves to exclude "fertility-related issues" from coverage, including anything related to the treatment of infertility, as soon as a multiple pregnancy is delivered prematurely through *in vitro* fertilization and the babies go to the neonatal intensive care unit, the insurance industry is quick to provide insurance coverage. I am not arguing here that such coverage should not be given, but as with most of these issues, it is important to keep everything in perspective. The care of these infants is one of the major expenditures of the current health care system in the United States and thus, this places an enormous amount of stress on third-party payers and the overall cost of health care. This is a stress which, quite frankly, does not have to be there. A significant reduction in these costs could be anticipated if **NaProTECHNOLOGY** programs were introduced.

Insurance Reform

A number of studies have been conducted that have tried to identify the average cost on a per-member basis to a health care plan if infertility coverage was provided.[8-12]   The estimated cost ranges from $0.10 to $1.71 per-member month or an average per-member month charge of $0.71.

This is an extremely important finding because infertility is the result of underlying disease and it's a very common abnormality experienced by women of reproductive age. The current health insurance climate that predominantly discriminates against women with fertility-related abnormalities withholds the availability of health care to this large class of women with real diseases. In fact, it is the largest single class of women with health care problems in our society. For this form of discrimination – which is gender specific – to be corrected, an investment needs to be made in the health care of women. These studies suggest that the cost of doing so actually is very low and most likely would be even lower if a **NaProTECHNOLOGY** approach were taken.

One of the major obstacles confronting contemporary medicine is the introduction of managed care programs that are fundamentally based in "cookbook medicine." If the doctor does not manage patients within the context of the computerized protocols that are housed within the insurance industry (to which physicians have no access), the patient or the doctor is penalized. *Unfortunately, protocols such as this are often years behind the progress that is made on a daily basis in medicine.* Thus, we now have developed a third-party reimbursement program within the United States which, by its very nature, establishes medical service that is generally out of date or significantly behind advances that are being made within the field.

The original design of managed care programs was to reduce the cost of health care. There is good evidence to suggest that this has not happened. While early development suggested that costs were being kept under control, it seems quite clear that the current rising costs of health care, once again, are out of control.

The exact direction to which insurance reform should go is not entirely known. Many are in favor of a nationalized health service. I do not believe that this is the answer to the problem, and this debate is raging as this book goes to press and as the Obama health care plan takes shape. In fact, it is strongly suggested that a nationalized health care program would only institutionalize on a more wide-ranging scale, this type of protocol-driven, cookbook medicine approach that the current managed care programs have developed. In addition, this medical care would be delivered by forcing a medical ethic on patients who often reject such an ethic. This would institutionalize, in a way which is even worse than exists currently, a group of patients that *medicine has abandoned.*

What needs to be developed is some type of hybrid structure where private insurance and government work hand-in-hand. One of the most important ingredients of this, however, should be the development of *"Centers of Excellence."* It is clear from my 38 years of medical practice that many physicians feel very comfortable delivering medical services that are basic. There is, on the other hand, another group of physicians who are clearly capable of managing more complex and advanced problems. These physicians and their programs need to be recognized as "Centers of Excellence," which would allow for the further establishment and expansion of third-party reimbursement policies for those centers.

To develop such a program would allow some inroads to be made in some of these more complex and difficult areas without physicians fearing inadequate reimbursement for their services. These are real issues that cannot be denied. Some would say that such should not be mentioned in a book of this type, and yet, there is a reality that needs to be addressed in this regard. One of the strong negative motivations in the lack of physician effort for treating the underlying causes of infertility in patients has been the constant hassle and antagonism that develops as the result of the physician's and the patient's interaction with the health insurance industry. *These conflicts must be resolved and they must be resolved in favor of the patient!* In fact, an underlying principle of a *good* health care system is its willingness *to advocate for the patient.*

It has been interesting to me to observe over the years the women's movement and how inoperative it has been when it comes to gender-specific discrimination in women within the health care reimbursement system. For example, it is not at all unusual for health care reimbursement to be given to men who suffer from erectile dysfunction and require medication, men who have chronic prostatitis who require long-term use of antibiotics, or men who have a varicocele that requires surgery. All of these treatments enhance the man's fertility, but almost universally, the health care reimbursement industry does not reject claims for evaluation and treatment of such conditions.

If you are a woman, however, who suffers from endometriosis or polycystic ovarian disease or you are a woman who has severe hormonal dysfunctions, or a woman who suffers from pelvic pain due to the presence of pelvic adhesive disease or endometriosis, it is likely that your claim for reimbursement will either be rejected or it will require a very confrontational approach with your health insurance program. Ultimately, these issues need to be resolved in favor of women because these are significant medical conditions that should require evaluation and treatment regardless of their association with fertility. There should be no double standard when it comes to the reimbursement of health care expenses for women. Ultimately, it will be up to women to lead the fight on this. *It is extremely important that women understand this!* Furthermore, the women's movement has let women down in this regard. In fact, they are a "no show" when it comes to this particular area – this widespread area – of gender discrimination.

Other Issues

There are many other issues that can be taken into consideration when looking at a cost-effectiveness equation. For example, cost-utility analysis looking at the *quality of life outcomes* generally has not been applied to reproductive medicine and infertility treatments specifically.[1] With the focus on women's health, identifying the underlying problems, providing appropriate medical remedies and improving one's quality of life, however, one would think that there would be an improved Quality-Adjusted Life Year (QALY) with a **NaProTECHNOLOGY** approach.

In addition, $8.4 billion is spent annually in the United States on the treatment of sexually-transmitted diseases. If one could produce a 25-percent decrease in the incidence of sexually-transmitted diseases because of a more responsible approach to the selection of sexual activity, one could anticipate a cost savings of $2.1 billion yearly. In **NaProTECHNOLOGY**, with its emphasis on responsible sexual interaction and responsible choices through the use of a natural means of avoiding pregnancy, such is potentially possible.

Finally, how can one put a price tag on a decrease in the divorce rate or the number of children affected by divorce; on an increase in the percentage of children living with both biologic parents; on a decrease in the number of abortions performed each year in the United States; on a decrease in the number of births to unmarried women; on a decrease in child abuse and neglect; on a decrease in the violent crime rate and the rate of drug use; on a decrease in the suicide rate amongst our teenagers; on a decrease in breast cancer and cervical cancer; and on a decrease in the number of individuals acquiring the AIDS virus? The *seismic shift* that has occurred in the past 40 years towards the endangerment of women, children and families all comes with a price tag. In many cases, it has a dollar value. In other cases, it has a relationship value or a quality of life value or a health value. *How does one put a price tag on this?* The answer is that it is difficult to do so; in fact, next to impossible. But each of these areas would be generally recognized as positive outcomes and it is up to all of us to work more vigorously and diligently because the overall cost benefits are truly enormous.

New Insights from Current Research

THE RESEARCH THAT IS stimulated by a **NaProTECHNOLOGY** approach to women's health care continues forward. In fact, it will continue forward for many, many years to come because the challenges that it presents are really significant. In this final chapter, I want to address some of the current research that is ongoing that will help us better identify, evaluate and treat women who have uterine cancer, breast cancer and osteoporosis. And then, as a close to this book, I would like to make a few comments related to the "protection of conscience" and the current move toward "evidence-based reproductive medicine."

Uterine Cancer

Cancer of the uterus is a disease of mostly postmenopausal women, but can occur during the years prior to menopause. Obesity, diabetes, and polycystic ovaries are all risk factors to the development of this cancer. The chronic absence of ovulation with its chronically unopposed (by progesterone) estrogen effect appears to be one of the major underlying factors.

Early detection is the best prevention for developing invasive uterine cancer. As the disease progresses, the chance of survival decreases significantly. Average five-year survival rates for endometrial cancer are 90 percent if it is caught in Stage I (an early stage), but only 5 percent if it's Stage IV (an advanced stage).

Abnormal vaginal bleeding is one of the major symptoms. Because the **CREIGHTON MODEL System** teaches women how to observe vaginal discharges, which includes the observation of bleeding, it is easy to detect bleeding when it first begins and when the symptom is in its very earliest stages. The CrMS is able to identify those women who have long and irregular cycles, irregular breakthrough bleeding and other types of abnormal bleeding (unusual bleeding). When that is observed, appropriate testing can be done and long-term progesterone treatment can be implemented or, if indicated, definitive surgery can be performed. We have been able to document several instances where women identified the symptoms related to a uterine cancer when it was very early in its development, and, because of that, all of these women are long-term survivors.

Breast Cancer

Breast cancer is the second most common cancer in women and the second leading cause of cancer-related death. One in eight women in the United States will develop breast cancer during their lifetime. The diagnosis of Stage I breast cancer increased 113 percent from 1983 to 1997. The number of new cases in 2002 was 205,000 and the women dying from breast cancer during that year numbered 40,000. Breast cancer is second only to lung cancer as a cause of cancer death.[1]

Risk factors for the development of breast cancer include a family history of the disease, a history of moderate use of alcohol (two to five drinks daily), obesity, a personal history of the disease (women with a history of breast cancer are three to four times more likely to have a recurrence), race (slightly more common in Caucasians), and sedentary lifestyle. Also, benign proliferative breast disease and mutations of the breast cancer gene also are thought to be risk factors.

Often not mentioned in discussions of breast cancer are its known associations with the use of oral contraceptives[2] and with induced abortion (a decision to abort and delay pregnancy). These can result also in an increased risk of breast cancer.[3,4] Irregular menstrual cycle patterns also are associated with increased risk but rarely studied.[5]

The diagnosis of breast cancer is made in a variety of different ways. Breast self-examination, physician breast examination, mammography, breast ultrasound, MRI and biopsy are used. While various studies have suggested that breast self-examination is not very helpful, it is still the recommended exercise. Mammography, too, often is criticized and yet it is one of the few techniques that allow for the early detection of breast cancer. A definitive diagnosis is made by breast biopsy. This is where a piece of the abnormal tissue is removed and examined under the microscope. But, of course, the area to be studied first must be identified in order to biopsy it. The key to long-term survival with breast cancer is the same as for uterine cancer: its early detection and treatment. The ability to accurately identify those individual women who are at risk for developing breast cancer and to treat them before they get the disease is very important.

Progesterone deficiency may be a prerequisite to the development of some forms of breast cancer. In comparing two groups of infertile women, one whose infertility was associated with progesterone deficiency and the other whose infertility was related to non-hormonal causes, women with progesterone deficiencies had a 5.4 times increased incidence of premenopausal breast cancer.[6]

This finding led us to evaluate the **CrMS** charting and hormone production of women who subsequently developed breast cancer. This pilot study took approximately 15 years. During this period of time, we collected 28 patients who were charting their cycles and who eventually developed breast cancer. Thus, we collected objective parameters of the menstrual and fertility cycles during the pre-breast cancer phase and compared it to women who did not develop breast cancer.

In this group of 28 patients, 27 of them had regular cycles. Only one had irregular cycles and that patient did have PCOD. In addition, 18 patients had charting information, 10 patients had targeted post-Peak progesterone profiles and seven patients had targeted post-Peak estrogen profiles prior to their development of the breast cancer.

From this information, we were able to evaluate the length of the post-Peak phase, the mucus cycle score, and a comparison of the post-Peak progesterone and estrogen profiles. The profiles of the breast cancer patients were compared to a normal control population. The post-Peak estrogen profiles were within the normal range, but the progesterone levels obtained on Peak+5, 7 and 9 were significantly lower than the control group. In fact, the Peak+11 progesterone level also was decreased, but numbers were insufficient to determine statistical significance.

When looking at the **CrMS**, a major identifiable biomarker was the variation in the length of the post-Peak phase of the cycle. In 16 patients with breast cancer, 13 of them had a post-Peak phase that varied four or more days in duration. When compared to a control group, only two of 20 patients had this type of variability. This variation in the length of the post-Peak phase (which is usually a sign of significantly-decreased progesterone production) was statistically highly significant.

When we looked at the mucus cycle scores, the score in the breast cancer patients was lower than that in the control group. This also was statistically significant.

If an increased variability in the length of the post-Peak phase and the presence of other biomarkers (such as premenstrual spotting, limited mucus or tail-end brown bleeding) could be shown to be associated with women who develop breast cancer, then one could have the opportunity to intervene and eventually prevent it. If these women are taught to chart their cycles and observe these markers, a Peak+7 progesterone level could possibly screen their luteal phase. If a woman has a decreased progesterone production, then post-Peak progesterone support could stabilize that phase of the cycle and *possibly* prevent breast cancer. More research is clearly needed in this area. *Nonetheless, this preliminary data strongly suggests that such research should be done.*

Osteoporosis

Osteoporosis is a skeletal disease characterized by low bone density and a deterioration in the micro-architecture of the bone leading to bones that are fragile and at an increased risk of fracture.[7] It is estimated that 10 million individuals have the disease and nearly 34 million (or 55 percent of those 50 years of age and older) have a low bone mass, which puts them at an increased risk of developing osteoporosis and related fractures. Of the 10 million Americans estimated to have osteoporosis, 80 percent are women and 20 percent are men.[8]

For women, the risk of hip fracture is equal to her combined risk of breast, uterine and ovarian cancer.[2] One might wonder how the topic of osteoporosis could fit into a discussion of the biomarkers of the menstrual and fertility cycle. Well, it is really very fascinating. We began an interesting bone-density evaluation of our patients who were undergoing hormonal evaluation. The most significant hormone finding was a decrease of the post-Peak estrogen levels along with a decrease in androstenedione and DHEA levels. Patients with a decreased post-Peak estrogen profile had significantly lower bone densities in the spine and the femoral neck (of the hip). Lower levels of androstenedione on Peak+7 were associated with significantly lower bone mineral density of the spine and lower levels of DHEAs were associated with statistically lower bone mineral densities in the femoral neck and the total hip. The decrease in estrogen in this situation is consistent with what we now classify as a Type V luteal phase defect: that is, a specific *estrogen* deficiency during the postovulatory phase of the cycle.

Because these findings are preliminary in nature, more research clearly needs to be done in this area. If it could be identified that women in the premenopausal years could be screened for being high risk for the subsequent development of a decreased bone mineral density and the early development of osteoporosis, then the possibility exists for implementing early therapy during the premenopausal years when women are still in the reproductive age group. It has been shown that a low bone mass prior to the menopause is associated with early postmenopausal fractures;[9] thus long-term analysis of hormone function in the reproductive-aged woman needs adequate evaluation because of the potential for implementing treatment strategies during the reproductive years to reduce significantly the impact of osteoporosis in the postmenopausal woman.

With these findings, the **CrMS** may become an important tool for the further evaluation of women with this difficulty or problem. Because the luteal phase can be targeted selectively with the **CrMS** for hormone evaluation, it is possible that screening programs could be established to identify the women at risk. *Supplementation with cooperative estrogen replacement therapy* in this patient group might be beneficial and could possibly reverse this effect, but more research is definitely needed.

Protection of Conscience

When Roe v. Wade was made the law of the land by the United States Supreme Court on January 22, 1973, there was a move among most states to develop what are referred to now as "conscience clauses." These conscience clauses tend to protect physicians and other allied health professionals from working in or being involved in abortion procedures, but the conscience clauses generally do not go far enough.

It is clear, as time has progressed since the ill-fated abortion decision of January 22, 1973, that physicians, nurses, hospitals and other institutions of health care provision, including residency education programs, feel threatened by the physician who might be opposed to the use of contraceptive agents. As a result, for example, there is not one Catholic medical school in the United States that approaches reproductive health care from the singular perspective of Catholic teaching. Many of the physicians in control of these programs would say that the Church is erroneous in their position. They certainly do have a right to that opinion. At the same time, however, even if they were in support they would be afraid of not being recognized by the accrediting bodies of the American Board of Obstetrics and Gynecology or other accrediting agencies. This obstacle needs to be overcome.

Contemporary reproductive medicine accepts abortion, contraception, sterilization, artificial reproductive technologies, embryonic stem cell research, embryo and fetal experimentation and artificial insemination as universal values. But they are not universal and they never will be!

Physicians must not be forced to abandon their ethical and moral principles. When I graduated from medical school at the University of Minnesota, we took a pledge called the *Declaration of Geneva*. This declaration was developed as a direct outcome of the Nuremberg trials that occurred after World War II. In this pledge it said: *"I will have the utmost respect for human life from the moment of conception."* Ultimately, it is my view that the right of physicians to practice medicine within the context of their moral and ethical beliefs is a basic human right, especially if founded in a strong and defined concept of medical ethics that should be protected by the First Amendment to the U.S. Constitution.[10] In addition, physicians should not be forced to violate their most solemnly taken vow.

In addition to the above, it is important that *patients be protected.* They have a right to receive medical evaluation and treatment that also are within the context of their own moral and religious beliefs. This is especially true for Catholic patients where their religion has a long-held and well-developed approach to medical-ethical and moral problems. The reason people believe in what the Church has said is because it makes sense to them. Its long-held and well-developed concepts of medical ethics are somewhat unique to the Catholic Church. Not all religions have such a foundation. The patients need to be protected in their right to go to the physician of their choice (a right that managed care often denies). Because there are two obstetrician-gynecologists within the managed care program, the insurance industry can say there is equal care available to the patient if physician A is included in the program and physician B is excluded. Physician B, however, is most likely going to be a Catholic physician who is being discriminated against and whose approach to medical evaluation and treatment is clearly different from other physicians. These sensitivities and approaches are not well provided by those physicians who do not believe in them. These physicians can, on the one hand, seem to support the patient, while on the other hand, be very antagonistic to the patient's beliefs. Another portion of insurance reform that will be necessary is allowing those physicians who represent certain medical/moral traditions to be represented within their programs.

Evidence-Based Reproductive Medicine: A Note of Caution

There has been a definite move over the last five to 10 years in the direction of "evidence-based medicine" and it has been applied to the field of reproductive medicine.[11] I would like to offer a statement of caution with regard to this trend. There has been a strong tendency in reproductive medicine over the last 40 years to accept certain types of research while not paying attention to other types. I often have stated that I do not know a physician who does not have an opinion on the natural means to regulate fertility. At the same time, I rarely have found a physician who knew very much about them. Physicians have a greater responsibility than to react in this way.

In fact, there has been a considerable amount of research over the last 25 years that has been published in peer-reviewed medical journals on the various natural means to regulate fertility (see Interent Appendix). These studies include the correlation of the mucus observations with the events occurring in endocervical mucus production,[12] the correlation of the Peak Day to the timing of ovulation,[13] the measurement of fecundability rates, and the measurement of use effectiveness.[14] Yet, most of this work has been ignored.

At the same time, in the first 39 years of the availability of oral contraceptives with well over 100,000 studies published there were *only* two double-blind, placebo-controlled studies on the effectiveness of the oral contraceptive in the treatment of any medical illness.[15] And so, the various medical indications for the use of the oral contraceptive that are applied to its "non-contraceptive health benefits" has remained "off-label" except for the treatment of acne.[15,16] It could be claimed legitimately that the oral contraceptive has an adequate amount of funding to be able to do trials such as this (whereas **NaProTECHNOLOGY** is only in its beginning stages and one of its major weaknesses is the general lack of funding).

Another flaw to the promotion of the oral contraceptive for the treatment of what are referred to as "non-contraceptive health benefits" has been the absence of its comparison to other approaches to treatment in which no contraceptives are being used at all. In this latter case, it would be an approach where the underlying condition is investigated and the underlying problem is treated. The promotion of oral contraceptives in the absence of such studies gives the false impression that this is the only effective treatment approach, and it is often quoted as "evidence-based medicine."

While randomized control trials (RCT) have been promoted in evidence-based medicine as being the best in study design, such RCTs are not always perfect, and in fact, can lead to false conclusions. An example of this would be the RCT that involved cervical cerclage and was published in 1984. This study made patients who were most in need of a cerclage ineligible for the trial. While the study showed that those patients who received a cerclage had more problems than those who did not, the study only showed that those people who really did not need a cerclage (but one was placed) had more difficulty than those people who did not receive a cerclage (and did not need it).[17] Nonetheless, this one study, along with its counterpart published in the same journal at the same time[18] and having some of the same limitations, suggested that cerclage was not a helpful tool for a technique in reducing the prematurity rate. This, in effect, removed cervical cerclage as a medical treatment for those patients who might risk premature delivery.

The study of the Medical Research Council/Royal College of Obstetricians and Gynecologists published a few years later showed some value to cerclage, but in general found the support to be weak. The eligibility criteria for entering into this study were extremely vague: "A woman was eligible for entry to the trial if her obstetrician was uncertain whether to advise her to have cervical cerclage."[19]

In all three of these trials, ultrasound was *not* used to assess the cervix, prophylactic antibiotics were *not* used at the time the cerclage was placed, and tocolytics (medications that help quiet uterine contractions) and progesterone support were *not* used. These types of trials, basically because of their study design (even though they were legitimately randomized controlled trials), produced what I believe to be flawed results. And yet their influence was striking when it came to the profession's view of the use of cervical cerclage in pregnant patients and the prevention of preterm birth.

A final example of how the profession has looked with a strong sense of bias against a particular approach to treatment is the proclamation made by the Association of Professors of Gynecology and Obstetrics (APGO) in their statements on the use of progesterone in women who have premenstrual syndrome[20] and the "British Medical Journal's" meta-analysis on the use of progesterone for the treatment of premenstrual syndrome. In the first case, APGO relied on a study that suggested that "normal ovarian function" was the cause of premenstrual syndrome. But that very study did not represent normality at all as all patients in the study were on leuprolide acetate to suppress ovulation at the time they took the progesterone. In the case of the "British Medical Journal,"[21] the timing on the use of progesterone was completely ignored in the meta-analysis and yet the only double-blind, placebo-controlled trial that ever showed progesterone was significantly successful, was one in which the timing was impeccable.

These issues are important as one looks at evidence-based medicine. It would be hoped, for example, that **NaProTECHNOLOGY** would be given the same 39-year reprieve that the oral contraceptive received (and still receives). At the same time, I completely recognize the need for research to advance in this area. Such research will require funding and an attention to the interests of the patients and their health.

It has been said that lack of funding can be an important barrier to the conduct of randomized controlled trials.[22] In fact, that is another major reason why trials of this nature cannot be the only means on which ultimate clinical decision making is made. While there is definitely a need for good and advancing research, and this book is a testimonial to a commitment to such, at the same time, medicine advances with evidence that, at times, is short of the ideal.

It is important that the *whole body of clinical evidence* be taken into consideration. Far too often fields of interest or studies that never have been adequately funded are ignored, even though good science may support their use. What has become quite commonplace in this day and age is the publication of "committee opinions" by various professional organizations. This is particularly true when it comes to The American College of Obstetricians and Gynecologists, which strongly supports contraception, sterilization, abortion and the artificial reproductive technologies, and, in fact, often is financially supported by these modalities. Thus, their "committee opinions" often ignore the "whole body of clinical evidence" and present an opinion that is *biased* in support of their own world view and the world view of their financial supporters.

One of the major tasks of this book and its allied medical textbook has been an attempt to integrate the findings of **NaProTECHNOLOGY** with the existing medical literature. There is a great deal of support for an approach such as **NaProTECHNOLOGY**, which is already within that medical literature, but one must become familiar with it and not ignore it. Sometimes our biases keep us from seeing all that is there.

Final Note

In **NaProTECHNOLOGY**, we have introduced a new women's health science that *thinks* from a different point of view. It *thinks* about *fertility* as something that is normal and not a disease. It *thinks* about the menstrual cycle as a normal physiologic occurrence as opposed to a "curse." It is not afraid of discussing the discharge of cervical mucus while others may call this an "unmentionable." And in reality, patients are not afraid to discuss these things either. We now have more than 30 years of experience in this regard. Our patients, in fact, have been our most valuable allies as we have worked at discovering this and understanding it better. They have been more than interested in helping us with this research.

There are many physicians who simply do not believe what we tell them about this. They do not believe the statistics that we have available to show them. The success we can achieve with **NaProTECHNOLOGY** goes beyond what is currently available. Those who have never experienced a natural method to regulate fertility, have never had a patient who has used the **CREIGHTON MODEL System**, or who has never been involved in a **NaProTECHNOLOGY**-oriented medical practice, or has not been trained in the science of this new approach will have difficulty understanding and seeing this. *In fact, it is more than believable! It is common-sense science!* And for those who are interested, they can read the stories of those who have benefited from this in a book titled **"In Their Own Words: Women Healed"** (Packard, J: *In Their Own Words: Women Healed*. Pope Paul VI Institute Press, Omaha, Nebraska, 2004).

Eventually, it will be up to the **women of the world** to take a look at the type of reproductive health care they are currently receiving and see whether or not they are satisfied with it. If they are unsatisfied, they need to look in a different direction and **NaProTECHNOLOGY** is an approach that can be extremely helpful. If **NaProTECHNOLOGY** is not available, and you would like to find it, you need to insist on its availability. *The women are the ones who will eventually see to it that this will become more and more available.* We cannot leave it directly to the physicians because they have never been able to show this type of leadership in the past. We cannot leave it to the insurance industry because they really do not care, as a primary issue, about your health. The leadership must come from outside the medical profession and the insurance industry and it must be based on the ethical principles and medical success principles that **NaProTECHNOLOGY** involves.

So, one last thought. The **CREIGHTON MODEL System** with its standardized and objective monitoring of various vaginal discharge patterns has allowed us to *unravel the mysteries of the woman's cycle.* With a sense of awe, we have had the opportunity to investigate these and work with patients who have, themselves, been deeply grateful for the added knowledge and the application of good medical principles. **NaProTECHNOLOGY**, as a new women's health science that involves state-of-the-art surgical techniques, hormone strategies, and ultrasound procedures, along with patient education about the biomarkers of her menstrual and fertility cycle, has truly *unleashed this power (knowledge, understanding, and medical application) that exists in a woman's cycle. It produces revolutionary answers to a woman's reproductive health and we will never be the same again.*

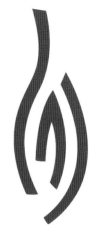

Internet Appendix
(www.unleashingthepower.info)

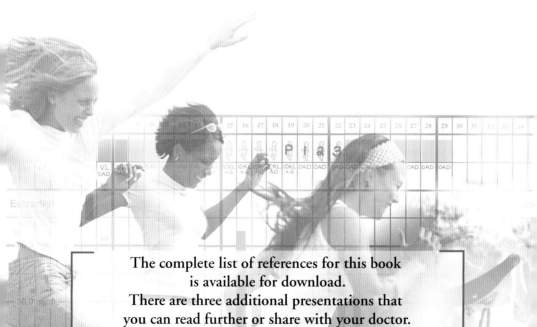

The complete list of references for this book
is available for download.
There are three additional presentations that
you can read further or share with your doctor.
These can be downloaded at no charge from our internet site:
www.unleashingthepower.info.
The presentations are called: "Introduction to the CrMS,"
"Scientific Foundations of the Creighton Model System,"
and "Medical Risks of Infertility."

Glossary of Terms

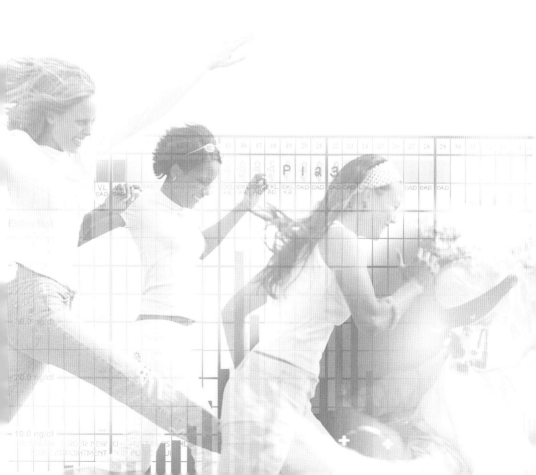

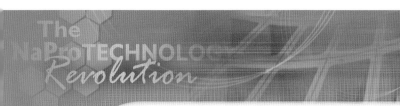

17-OHP-C: This abbreviation stands for 17-hydroxyprogesterone caproate. This is an artimone which is used in progestational support of pregnancy.

17-OHP-H: This abbreviation stands for 17-hydroxyprogesterone hexonate. This is an artimone which is rarely used in clinical medicine.

A

Abortifacient: An agent that produces abortion.

Acquired Immune Deficiency Syndrome (AIDS): This is a clinical syndrome which has immunologic and respiratory components and is caused by the HIV virus.

Adenocarcinoma: This term refers to a glandular-type cancer.

Adenomatous hyperplasia: This is an overgrowth of the glandular components in the lining of the uterus. It can be premalignant.

Adenomyosis: A condition in which the lining tissue inside the uterus (endometrial cell glands) penetrate into the uterine muscle. When this happens, it usually results in painful and very heavy menstrual periods. It is difficult to diagnosis because these glands in the muscle of the uterus are not visible by looking at the uterus from the outside.

Adherent placenta: This is a placenta that does not deliver itself spontaneously following delivery of the baby. Generally speaking, it is called adherent if it does not deliver on its own within 30 minutes following delivery.

Adhesions: This is scar tissue that connects one organ to another.

Adnexa: This includes the structures that are in the position to the right or the left of the uterus. This usually includes the tube and ovary.

Alprazolam: This is an antianxiety medication that comes under the commercial name of Xanax.

Amenorrhea: This is the absence of menstrual periods for at least one full year.

Ampicillin: This is a penicillin-related broad-spectrum antibiotic and it is used to treat any number of pelvic and urinary tract infections.

Androgenic: This refers to hormones that have a masculinizing effect.

Androstenedione: This is a male hormone (androgenic hormone) that is produced both in the ovary, as well as the adrenal gland. It tends to be elevated in women who have polycystic ovaries.

Anovulation: The absence of ovulation. This may occur within a given menstrual cycle or in prolonged periods of amenorrhea.

Apgar score: This is a score given to newborn babies generally at 1 and 5 minutes after birth. The perfect score is 10. It is based on various parameters of color, respirations, and the baby's activity. It is named after Dr. Virginia Apgar who first described it.

Artificial insemination: This is the placement of the sperm directly into the uterus (intrauterine insemination – IUI). Inseminations are performed by the physician and carry with them relatively low pregnancy rates. The physician may use the sperm from the husband (AIH) or from a donor (AID).

Azoospermia: A condition in which the sperm count is zero.

B

Bacterial vaginosis: This is a bacterial infection of the vagina which can be caused by several different organisms and gives some symptoms such as itching, discharge, etc.

Basal body temperature (BBT): This is a body temperature taken usually upon awakening in the morning. The BBT increases following ovulation because of progesterone that can increase body temperature.

Biological valve: The cervical mucus changes its physical characteristics around the time of ovulation allowing sperm to penetrate the cervix. At other times in the cycle, the cervical mucus will not allow the sperm to penetrate. Thus, this activity of the cervical mucus is called the biological valve.

Biomarker: This is a physical sign that shows up on the **CREIGHTON MODEL** charts and has a specific set of medical reasons for being there. For example, a limited mucus cycle, premenstrual spotting, tail-end brown bleeding, the post-Peak phase, etc., are all biomarkers.

Biophysical profile: This is an ultrasound examination done in pregnancy, usually after the 32nd week of pregnancy and it is a test for fetal distress. It is somewhat similar to an Apgar score but performed while the baby is in the uterus.

Breast-feeding: The woman is feeding her newborn baby with the milk from her own breasts. This either can be total breast-feeding or partial breast-feeding.

C

Cecum: This is the portion of the large intestine which is on the right side of the body and ascends upward to the transverse colon. The appendix is at the tip of the cecum.

Ceftriaxone: This is a cephalosporin antibiotic which has a very broad range of activity and can be given once daily. The trade name is Rocephin.

Cephalosporins: This refers to a group of antibiotics which obtain their activity by interfering with the synthesis of the cell wall of the bacteria.

Cerclage: This refers to a shoestring-like stitch that is placed around the cervix to help reinforce the cervix and prevent premature birth.

Cerebrocentric sexuality: This is a total person view of human sexuality taking into account the spiritual, physical, intellectual, communicative and emotional aspects of the individual man or woman.

Cervical canal: This is the channel that traverses the cervix and enters into uterine cavity.

Cervical crypts: These are outpouchings that line the cervical canal and they contain mucus-producing cells. These cells differ depending on what type of mucus is being produced.

Cervical mucus: This is a mucus that is produced in the cervical crypts and is discharged to the opening of the vagina.

Chlamydia: This is an obligatory intracellular bacteria which comes in different forms. *Chlamydia trachomatis* is a bacteria that infects the genital organs and is considered to be a sexually-transmitted disease.

CHO: This is an abbreviation for carbohydrates.

Clomiphene: This is a drug that stimulates the production of FSH and is used to stimulate ovulation. It is a medication that has been around for 40 years and has been used extensively in the treatment of infertility. One of the drawbacks of clomiphene is its negative effect on the production of cervical mucus. This is also known as clomiphene citrate with the trade name being Clomid or Serophene.

Conception: This refers to the union of the sperm with the ovum and marks the beginning of human life. In recent years, there has been an attempt to redefine conception to mean the implantation of the early blastocyst (about 6-9 days after conception). The reason for this was to avoid the label "abortifacient" which could be given to various contraceptive agents such as the intrauterine device or the oral contraceptive. However, the beginning of life is at the time when the egg and sperm unite.

Conization: This refers to the removal of an ice cream-shaped cone of tissue from the cervix. It is used for establishing a better diagnosis of precancerous or cancerous conditions of the cervix. In some of the early cases, it can also be therapeutic.

Corpus luteum: These are Latin words which mean "yellow body." This is the structure formed in the ovary following ovulation that produces both progesterone and estrogen.

CREIGHTON MODEL Fertility*Care*™ System (CrMS): This is a standardized modification of the Billings Ovulation Method and, because of its standardization, has multiple medical aspects to its use.

Cumulus oophorus: This is an accumulation of cells which surrounds the ovum and is present within the developing follicle.

Cystic hyperplasia: This is an overgrowth of cells in the lining of the uterus which is characterized by the formation of cystic structures.

D

D&C: This refers to the dilatation and curettage of the lining of the uterus. D&Cs are performed for diagnostic purposes, as well as for completing a miscarriage.

Decidual changes: This refers to the changes in the lining of the uterus (the endometrium) in a pregnant woman.

DHEAs: This is a hormone usually produced in the adrenal gland. It is thought of as a male hormone (androgenic), but both men and women have this hormone. It is sometimes referred to as a "mother hormone" because it helps in the production of other hormones.

Dilatation: This means to dilate. In the case of a D&C (dilatation and curettage), it means to dilate the cervix (dilatation) and scrape the lining of the uterus (curettage).

Double ovulation: This is a condition in which ovulation occurs twice in a given cycle. When that occurs, the two ovulations occur within the same 24-hour time period.

DPC-Immulite: This is a machine manufactured by Diagnostic Products Corporation (DPC) that uses a technology referred to as chem-immunoflorescence.

DSM-IV: This is an abbreviation which refers to the 4th Edition of the Diagnostic and Statistical Manual of Mental Disorders.

Dysfunctional uterine bleeding: This is a type of bleeding that usually occurs in women with long and irregular cycles (although it can be seen in regular cycles as well) and is usually hormonal in origin, as opposed to being due to some organic cause.

Dysmenorrhea: Severe menstrual cramps.

E

Ectopic pregnancy: This is a pregnancy located outside of the uterine cavity. The most common location is in the fallopian tube. However, it can also be in the cervix or the abdominal cavity.

Ectropion: An eversion of the cells that line the cervical canal out onto the surface of the cervix; most often seen following childbirth or following the use of birth control pills.

Electrologist: This is an individual who practices electrology. This is a technique which is used to remove excessive hair growth.

Encyclical letter: This is an official letter written by the Pope of the Catholic Church which conveys a particular teaching of the Church.

Endocervical: This refers to the cervical canal which leads up to the cavity within the uterus.

Endocrinology: This is a science which involves the study of the action and reaction of different hormones.

Endogenous: This refers to substances that are produced within the organism.

Endometrial hyperplasia: This is an overgrowth of the cells that are involved in the lining of the uterus. This type of overgrowth can be a premalignant condition.

Endometrial polyp: This is a tongue-like piece of tissue that originates from the lining of the uterus and projects itself into the uterine cavity. It is a common cause of abnormal bleeding during the course of the menstrual cycle. There also are micro-polyps that are much smaller versions and are associated with chronic endometritis (inflammation or infection of the endometrial tissue).

Endometrial stroma: The framework, usually of connective tissue of the endometrium.

Endometriosis: This is a condition in which the cells that are normally inside the uterus and slough with the menstrual period get onto the outside of the uterus where they do not belong.

Endometritis: This is an infection or an inflammation of the lining cells in the uterus.

Enterococcus faecalis: This is a bacteria often found in the gastrointestinal tract, but can contaminate the vagina, cervix or endometrium and cause infection.

Escherichia coli: This is a bacteria that is a frequent cause of infections in the urinary tract and the pelvis.

Esophageal atresia: This is a blockage of the esophagus which runs from the oral cavity to the stomach. It is a congenital anomaly.

Estimated time of arrival (ETA): This is the due date for the delivery of an individual baby. In medical terms it also is called the estimated date of confinement (EDC).

Estimated time of conception (ETC): This is a calculated time of conception that can be generated from the **CREIGHTON MODEL** charts. It generally is considered to be a highly accurate means of dating the beginning of pregnancy.

Estrogen: This is a female hormone that is produced mostly in the ovary during the course of the menstrual cycle.

Eversion: This is a condition in which the cells inside the cervical canal migrate out onto the surface of the cervix. Sometimes this is referred to as an ectropion.

Evidence-based medicine: This refers to a particular form of medical evaluation or treatment that has been subjected to scientific verification through different means of study.

Exogenous: This pertains to different substances that are produced outside of the organism.

F

Familiaris Consortio: This is a document written by Pope John Paul II that talks about marriage and family.

Fertility cycle: This refers to the cycle from one month to the next in which a woman (and thus the couple) is fertile.

Fertility*Care*™ **Educator**: This is a **Fertility***Care*™ **Practitioner** who has received one additional year of advanced education and is able to implement the **CREIGHTON MODEL** Core Curriculum in other parts of the country or the world.

Fertility*Care*™ **Medical Consultant:** This is a medical professional who has completed a six-month training program in the **CREIGHTON MODEL System** and the medical aspects of **NaProTECHNOLOGY**. In addition, they are certified through the American Academy of Fertility*Care* Professionals.

Fertility*Care*™ **Practitioner**: This refers to an individual who has been through a 13-month training program as an Allied Health Professional to teach the **CREIGHTON MODEL Fertility***Care*™ **System**.

Fetal fibronectin: Fibronectin is the high molecular weight multifunctional glycoprotein which is found on cell surface membranes and other body fluids. In the case of fetal fibronectin, it can be found in the cervix and can be somewhat helpful in predicting when a pregnant woman will go into premature labor.

Fibroids: These are fibrous, benign tumors usually in the uterus. Their medical name is leiomyoma. They can grow to be very large and can be located at different positions within the uterus, sometimes causing very heavy bleeding.

Fluoxetine: This is an antidepressant medication whose trade name is Prozac. It also has been released for use under the name Sarafem.

Follicle: This is a cystic structure on the ovary that develops every month and contains the egg. With the rupture of the follicle, the egg is released (ovulation).

Follicle-stimulating hormone (FSH): This is a hormone produced in the pituitary gland that stimulates the ovary to develop a mature follicle in a given cycle.

 Follicular phase: This is the phase of the menstrual cycle where there is the development in the ovary of the follicle which contains the egg.

Follicular Phase Deficiency: This is a condition in which the growth, development and function of the follicle is deficient. This can be determined either by hormonal analysis or by daily ultrasound exams around the time of ovulation.

Follow-up Form: This is a form developed for use in the **CREIGHTON MODEL System** that documents the teaching that is given to a client.

Follow-up: In the **CREIGHTON MODEL System**, the learning is done on a one-on-one basis and it is conducted at sessions that are referred to as follow-up sessions.

G

Genitocentric sexuality: This is a form of sexuality that revolves mostly around the physical aspects of sexuality. It is short on the view of the whole person.

Gestational diabetes: A form of diabetes that develops during the course of pregnancy. It usually goes away following pregnancy, but women who develop gestational diabetes are prone to become diabetic later in life.

Gonadotropin-releasing hormone (GnRH): This is a hormone produced in the hypothalamus. It is produced in pulses from one week to the next during the course of the menstrual and fertility cycle and is responsible for the stimulation of the production of both FSH and LH by the pituitary gland.

Gravida: This refers to a woman who either is or has been pregnant.

Gynecology: The medical science which devotes its efforts to the evaluation and treatment of the female reproductive system.

H

Hormone: A chemical produced in one part of the body but effects its action in another part.

Human chorionic gonadotropin (hCG or HCG): A hormone produced in large amounts during pregnancy. Pregnancy tests measure this hormone. It is a hormone that is very similar in its chemical structure to the luteinizing hormone (LH) and thus can be used as an LH substitute in the treatment of various conditions. Giving hCG during the post-Peak phase of the cycle will stimulate the ovary to produce both progesterone and estrogen.

HDL-C: Refers to high-density lipoprotein-cholesterol. This is a form of "good" cholesterol.

Hematoma: This is a collection of blood at some location in the body. In reference to a retroplacental hematoma, this is a collection of blood behind the placenta.

Hirsutism: Refers to excessive hair growth and is particularly significant when it occurs in women.

Histologic tissue diagnosis: This is a diagnosis which is made by reviewing tissue preparations under the microscope by the pathologist. Histology is the study of tissues under the microscope.

Humanae Vitae: The papal encyclical letter of Pope Paul VI published July 25, 1968. It outlined the Catholic Church's opposition to contraception and abortion while also giving the theological foundations to that decision.

Human papilloma virus (HPV): A sexually-transmitted virus which is thought to be the cause of cervical dysplasia and cervical cancer.

Hydrocephalus: A condition, usually seen in a newborn, in which fluid accumulates in the brain and can actually increase the size of the head.

Hyfrecation: A cautery-like technique which does not need a grounding pad.

Hyperprolactinemia: This is a condition where the prolactin level (the milk-producing hormone) is increased above normal.

Hypoglycemic: This refers to a condition where the blood sugar is very low.

Hypothalamus: This is a small gland just behind the pituitary gland that manufactures and releases gonadotropin-releasing hormone (GnRH). At times, because of a dysfunction of the hypothalamus, a woman may stop menstruating. This can be referred to as hypothalamic amenorrhea.

Hypospadias: A developmental anomaly where the opening of the urethra in the male is underneath the penis.

Hysterosalpingogram: An x-ray technique where dye is injected into the uterus and out the fallopian tubes. The dye injection on a hysterosalpingogram is done at the level of the cervix. In selective hysterosalpingography, the dye is injected directly into each fallopian tube selectively.

Hysteroscopy: This is a surgical procedure in which a small scope is inserted into the uterine cavity and the cavity can be observed for various changes that might be diagnostic.

I

Ibuprofen: This is a commonly recommended pain-relief medication (Advil, Motrin, etc.)

Idiopathic: This refers to a disease of unknown origin.

Induced abortion (IAB): An abortion that is consciously undertaken by the physician and patient for the sole purposes of ending the pregnancy.

Insomnia: This refers to the inability to sleep.

Intermenstrual: Refers to the time between the menstrual periods.

Intramuscular: This refers to the use of a hypodermic needle when an injection is given deep into the muscle. This is referred to as an intramuscular injection.

Introductory Session: This is a one-hour slide presentation in which couples are introduced to the **CREIGHTON MODEL FertilityCare™ System**.

In-vitro **fertilization (IVF):** This refers to test-tube babies. The ovum is taken from the mother's ovary and the sperm from the father and the two are united in a test tube; then after undergoing some development, are reinserted into the uterus. This falls under the generic classification of an artificial reproductive technology (ART).

K

Kallmann syndrome: This is a condition in which the woman never menstruates on her own and has difficulty differentiating odors.

Keflex: This is the trade name of one of the cephalosporin antibiotics.

L

Laparoscopy: A surgical procedure in which a small incision is made under the belly button and a scope is inserted so that the pelvic organs can be evaluated. Sometimes referred to as "same-day" surgery or "Band-Aid" surgery.

Laparotomy: A surgical procedure in which the abdomen is entered through an incision.

Laser: A form of light which can incise tissues with very little collateral damage or can vaporize tissues. The term laser stands for: Light Amplification With Stimulated Emission Radiation.

Last menstrual period (LMP): This is the last menstrual period that is recalled by a woman who is currently pregnant. It is a retrospective piece of information (and it relies on the woman's memory). It is often used to date the beginning of pregnancy.

LDL-C: Low-density lipoprotein cholesterol. This is the form of "bad" cholesterol.

Libido: This refers to the sexual energy and interest of an individual (man or woman).

Limb reduction: This means that one or more of the limbs is missing in a fetus. It is often thought of as being a congenital abnormality related to the use of various medications. It is very rare.

Lipoprotein-A: A specific form of compound which contains both a lipid and a protein. Elevated lipoprotein-A levels is a strong, independent risk factor for coronary artery disease and possibly stroke.

Lumen: Refers to the internal space of a tubal-like structure. An example would be the lumen of the bowel or the lumen of the fallopian tube.

Luteal phase: This refers to the phase in the ovary in which the corpus luteum is formed following ovulation.

Luteal Phase Deficiency: This refers to a dysfunction in the production of the hormones by the corpus luteum following ovulation. There are at least five different forms of Luteal Phase Deficiency.

Luteinized: The area in the ovary in which luteal tissue has been formed.

Luteinizing hormone (LH): This is a hormone produced in the pituitary gland and has several responsibilities during the course of the cycle. One of these is the LH "surge" that stimulates the mature follicle to rupture and release the ovum (ovulation).

M

Meconium: The first intestinal discharges of the newborn infant. It is usually greenish in color and consists of cells, mucus and bile.

Medroxyprogesterone acetate (MPA): This is a C-21 progestational agent and is an artimone. It is commonly used as a substitute for progesterone but it is 50 times stronger than progesterone.

Menometrorrhagia: This is a condition in a woman who is experiencing both heavy periods, in addition to bleeding between her periods.

Menorrhagia: Heavy menstrual periods.

Menstrual cycle: This is the period of time from the first day of menstrual bleeding up to and including the last day before the beginning of the next menstrual period.

Menstruation: This is the sloughing of the lining cells inside the uterus and results in external bleeding. Typically, it lasts from three to seven days in duration.

Mesentery: A double layer of tissue (peritoneum) which is attached to the abdominal wall and encloses in its fold a portion or all of one of the abdominal viscera (organs) and conveys its vessels and nerves. Commonly used in relationship to the bowel or the fallopian tube.

Metrorrhagia: This is a condition in a woman who is experiencing bleeding between menstrual periods.

Micronized: This is a pharmacologic technique in which a medication is pulverized into very, very small particles. The particle size is so small that it assists in the absorption of the medication from the stomach.

Morphology: This refers to the shape of a particular entity. It often refers to the shape of the spermatozoa observed at the time of a seminal fluid analysis.

Mucinous cystadenoma: This refers to a histologically-benign tumor derived from glandular elements in which cystic accumulations of retained secretions are formed. When it is a mucinous cystadenoma, it usually collects a mucinous-like material within the cyst. This is a tumor which contains mucin (a secretion containing carbohydrate-rich glycoproteins).

Mucus: A biophysical fluid which is produced in many types of organs such as the lung, the bowel, and of course, the cervix. Cervical mucus is important to the facilitation of sperm migration.

Mucus cycle: This is the period of time measured from the beginning of the mucus build-up to and including the Peak Day.

Mucus cycle score: This is a score that is obtained directly from the **CREIGHTON MODEL** charts that allows for an objective reading of the mucus cycle.

Myomectomy: This refers to a surgical procedure in which a fibroid tumor is removed.

N

Nabothian cysts: These are cysts that form in the cervix as the result of the closure of a cervical crypt and the backup of cervical mucus. This usually is due to a chronic inflammation.

Naltrexone: A drug which attaches itself to the opiate receptors in the brain. Its originally use was in helping heroin addicts stop their heroin addiction. However, it has also been used to treat premenstrual syndrome because of the role of beta endorphins (which is a naturally-occurring opiate).

NaProEducation TECHNOLOGY: This is the advanced form of educational technology used in the **CREIGHTON MODEL FertilityCare™ System**. It utilizes such tools as the

Picture Dictionary, the Vaginal Discharge Recording System, the Follow-up Form, Pregnancy Evaluation Form, etc.

Necrosis: Pathologic death of one or more cells or a portion of tissue or organ, resulting from irreversible damage.

Neural tube: The structure in the embryo which becomes the spinal cord.

Non-Peak-type mucus: This is mucus that is not stretchy, not clear and not lubricative.

O

Obstetrics: This is the medical field that specializes in the care of pregnant women.

Oligohydramnios: Refers to a pregnancy in which the amniotic fluid is markedly decreased.

Oligospermia: Refers to a sperm count which is especially decreased.

Organic pathology: This refers to abnormal conditions in which are involved the formulation and integrity of the tissues themselves (as opposed to hormonal or endocrine pathology).

Os: Refers to an anatomic location that is at the opening, e.g., the external os of the cervix.

Ovarian wedge resection: This is a surgical procedure in which a pie-shaped wedge of tissue is removed from the enlarged ovary. This usually is performed in women who have polycystic ovaries and carries with it the best chance for them to have regular cycles, pregnancy and a return to more normal hormone patterns.

Ovulation cycle: This measures from ovulation in one cycle to the next ovulation in the next cycle.

Ovulation: This is the release of the ovum (egg) from the follicle.

P

Para: This refers to a woman who has carried a pregnancy beyond the 20th week.

Peak Day: This is the last day of the mucus that is clear, stretchy and/or lubricative.

Peak-type mucus: This is a mucus discharge that is either clear, stretchy and/or lubricative.

Perimenstrual: Refers to the days leading up to the onset of the menstrual flow and the first few days of the menstrual flow.

Perinatology: The study of high-risk pregnancies and is a subspecialty in obstetrics which specifically treats high-risk pregnancies.

Periovulatory: Refers to the days leading up to the time of ovulation and the few days following it.

Peritoneal fluid: This is fluid that accumulates within the peritoneal cavity (which is the abdominal cavity). The peritoneum is the lining tissue in the abdominal cavity. Some peritoneal fluid is normal, but there are abnormal conditions in which it can be excessive.

Peritubal cyst: This is a cyst which is usually located at the end of the fallopian tube. It usually is fairly small, but can grow to become 4 to 5 cm in size. These cysts are usually benign.

Pharmacology: This is the study of various medications.

Picture Dictionary: This is a teaching tool of the **CREIGHTON MODEL System** that allows for the descriptions to be recorded in an objective fashion.

Pituitary gland: This is the gland in the brain, sometimes referred to as the "master gland." It contains and releases both FSH and LH.

Placebo: This is a substance that has no pharmacologic activity. It usually is used in studies of a particular medication so that the effects of the medication can be compared to the effects of a placebo.

Placenta: The structure formed by the early developing fetus which attaches to the side wall of the uterus and provides a connection between the maternal circulation and the baby's circulation for growth and development.

Placenta previa: This refers to the placenta when it covers the internal opening of the cervix. Women who have placenta previa need to be delivered by Cesarean section.

Polycystic ovaries: These are ovaries that are generally enlarged, very smooth and have multiple small follicles within the ovary.

Post-coital test: This is a test of the interaction between the sperm and the cervical mucus. It is performed from two to six hours following intercourse. The woman comes into the doctor's office, a sample of mucus is taken from the cervix and examined under a microscope.

Posterior: In human anatomy, this refers to the back surface of the body. It is often used to indicate the position of one structure relative to another.

Postovulatory progesterone sum: This refers to a targeted progesterone evaluation in which each of the levels obtained on P+3, 5, 7, 9 and 11 are added up and a sum is identified.

Post-Peak phase of the cycle: This is the phase of the cycle from the first day following the Peak Day up through the last day prior to the beginning of menstruation.

Pregnancy Evaluation Form: This is a form that has been developed in the **CREIGHTON MODEL System** so that pregnancies can be properly evaluated and classified.

Pregnane: The parent compound to the formation of progesterone and several hormones of the adrenal gland.

Premature birth: This is the birth of any baby prior to 37 weeks gestation.

Premenstrual: Refers to those days leading up to the onset of menses.

Preovulatory: This refers to that phase of the cycle prior to ovulation.

Pre-Peak phase of the cycle: This is the portion of the cycle from day 1 of the cycle up to and including the Peak Day.

Progesterone: This is one of the main hormones produced following ovulation and it is produced in very large amounts during pregnancy.

Proliferative phase: This is the regenerating phase of the lining of the uterus following menstruation and prior to ovulation. It is usually under the control of estrogen.

Prophylaxis: Refers to the prevention of some condition which may be a disease or a process that can lead to disease.

Prospective: This refers to a looking forward as opposed to looking backward in the collection of study data.

Prostate gland: This is a gland in the man's body that is a primary source for the production of seminal fluid.

Proximal: Refers to an anatomic site nearest the point of its origin. An example would be the proximal portion of the fallopian tube, that portion of the fallopian tube that is nearest the uterus.

***P* value:** Refers to a number which is calculated using various statistical techniques. When the *P* value is equal to or less than 0.05, it indicates that there is a 95% chance or greater that the differences identified in two sets of data are there because of a specific difference in the data set as opposed to something that could happen simply because of a random selection.

R

Receptors: These are chemicals that are located either in the nucleus of the cell or in the material outside of the nucleus. For a hormone to be effective, it must link to a specific receptor.

Rectosigmoid colon: This is the portion of the colon which is descending down towards the rectum.

Reflex ovulation: This is an ovulation that occurs usually in response to copulation. The ovulation patterns of rabbits would be a good example of this form of ovulation pattern.

Relativism: A philosophical approach that sees truth in relation to the group or individual that proposes it. The important feature of relativism is that it sees no moral absolutes. Furthermore, it is not based in an objective judgment of what is morally right or wrong. An action might be considered morally wrong today, but through a subjective assessment, it might be considered morally right tomorrow.

Retroplacental hematoma: This is a blood clot that forms behind the placenta.

Retrospective: Refers to an evaluation of data which is collected after the fact and looking back at the data.

S

Secretory phase: This is the term describing the lining of the uterus following ovulation. The secretory cells develop as a result of the effect of progesterone.

Selective hysterosalpingography: This is an x-ray test of the lining of the uterus and both fallopian tubes. It allows for a catheter to be placed into the internal opening of the fallopian tube and each tube injected separately and thus studied separately.

Selective intercourse: This refers to the choices that couples who are using the **CREIGHTON MODEL System** make relative to the use of the system to either achieve or avoid pregnancy.

Serous cystadenoma: This refers to a histologically-benign tumor derived from glandular elements in which cystic accumulations of retained secretions are formed. When it is a mucinous cystadenoma, it usually collects a mucinous-like material within the cyst. This is a tumor which contains mucin (a secretion containing carbohydrate-rich glycoproteins). The fluid contained in a serous cystadenoma is serous in quality.

Spermatozoa: The cell of reproduction in the male.

SPICE: This refers to the multidimensional aspects of the human personality that are reflected in a cerebrocentric form of human sexuality. The acronym SPICE refers to the Spiritual, Physical, Intellectual, Creative and Emotional aspects of the individual man or woman.

Spontaneous abortion (SAB): Refers to a natural process in which a pregnancy is miscarried.

Spontaneous ovulation: This is a form of ovulation that is not affected by copulation. Human women are spontaneous ovulators.

Stamps: This refers to the various stamps that are used in charting the **CREIGHTON MODEL System**.

Standard curve: A statistical graph which has been developed usually by studying a group of normal patients. It then becomes a "normal" curve that other test results can be compared to.

Submucous: This usually refers, in gynecology, to the location of a fibroid tumor. In this case, it is just underneath the lining of the uterus and these tend to bleed more heavily and are more difficult to treat. Fibroid tumors can sometimes be located under the lining of the uterus and these are called submucous fibroids.

Suboptimal: This refers to blood levels which are less than desired and less than normal.

T

T_3: This refers to triiodothyronine, the active thyroid hormone which is formed on its own as well as due to a conversion from thyroxine (T_4).

Tailor-made: The learning of the **CREIGHTON MODEL System** is tailor-made to the individual couple in individual follow-up sessions that deal directly with the charting of their own fertility cycles.

Target organ dysfunction: This refers to an abnormal function of the target organ. As an example, this could refer to the lack of production of the cervical mucus from the cervix because of an inadequate amount of estrogen or its receptors.

Targeting the cycle: This refers to the measurement of hormones specific to the menstrual cycle and targeting it properly so that reliable results are obtained.

Teratogens: Refers to medications that have an outcome on the developing fetus which leads to a developmental abnormality.

Terbutaline: A drug that has the effect of quieting the pregnant uterus and is used specifically in the medical treatment of uterine contractions.

Terminal ileum: This is a portion of the small bowel which inserts into the cecum, the ascending colon.

Testicles: These are the glands in the male body that produce spermatozoa and also important hormones to reproduction.

Testosterone: This is the major male hormone produced in men.

Thermogenic: This refers to the increase in body temperature that is the result of the effect of progesterone.

Tocolytic therapy: This refers to therapy which is designed to stop or slow uterine contractions when a woman is in either early labor or labor. Tocolytic agents are those medicines used to provide tocolysis (the inhibition of uterine contractions).

Transcervical catheterization of the fallopian tubes: This is a situation in which the fallopian tube is catheterized with a floppy wire usually at the time of selective hysterosalpingography. This allows for some tubes to be unblocked, while other tubes can be more definitely identified as having an organic obstruction.

Trimester: Pregnancy is usually divided into three trimesters, roughly three months each in length, so there is the first, second and third trimester of pregnancy.

True family planning: This refers to a family planning system in which ovulation is not suppressed or fertility is not destroyed. In this system, the couple enjoys the capability to either choose to avoid a pregnancy or choose to achieve a pregnancy.

Truncated: Refers to an abbreviated function. In talking about a truncated menstrual cycle, for example, it refers to an abbreviated cycle or a shortened cycle. These cycles are usually not normal and are more common as women approach the menopause.

Tubal occlusion: This means a blockage in the fallopian tube at various positions along the tube. A proximal tubal occlusion occurs at the site of the insertion of the fallopian tube into the uterus. A distal tubal occlusion is a blockage with a tube at the very end of the fallopian tube.

Type E mucus: This refers to an estrogenic-type of mucus produced in the cervix around the time of ovulation. It facilitates the penetration of the sperm into the uterus.

Type G mucus: This is a form of mucus produced when the estrogen levels are extremely low or when progesterone is present. It forms a blocking type of mucus which closes the cervical canal to the entrance of the spermatozoa.

U

Ultrasound: This is a technology in which sound waves are beamed into a body cavity and the echo of those sound waves are heard by the transmitting instruments. Then, through sophisticated computer technology, this can be translated into an image. There is real-time ultrasound which is live-action, motion picture-type ultrasound and 3-D ultrasound which gives a three-dimensional appearance to its object. There is also 4-D ultrasound which is a combination of live-action and 3-D.

Urethra: This is the channel from the bladder to the outside of the body.

V

Vaginal Discharge Recording System: This is a unique recording system developed for the **CREIGHTON MODEL FertilityCare™ System**. It standardizes the observations, makes them objective and allows for the use of a common language so everybody can be speaking that same language.

Vaporization: This refers to the use of laser and its effects on tissue. It creates an environment where the tissue is changed to water vapor and cellular debris (the laser plume). Vaporization is usually referred to when talking about laser energy. It does produce surgical removal of the tissue.

Varicocele: This is a varicose vein of the testicle and sometimes is associated with abnormal sperm counts because it increases the heat within the testicle which is harmful to the sperm.

Vas deferens: This is the tube that runs from the epididymis and goes through the prostate gland into the male urethra. It is the channel in which the sperm migrate during sexual intercourse.

Index

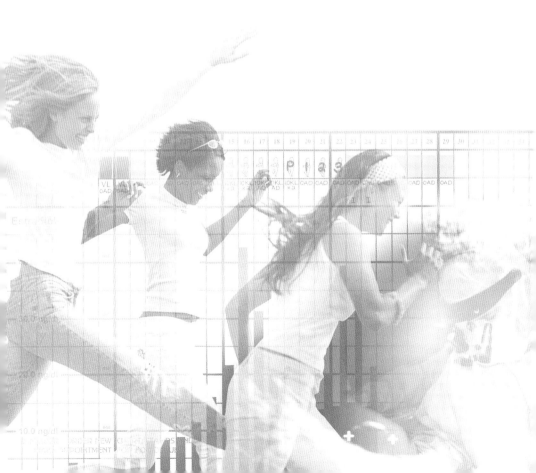

"Band-Aid" approach, 32, 37
"near-contact" laparoscopy, 161, 243
"per-woman" pregnancy rates, 219

A

Abandonment, 225, 383
Abortifacient, 22, 68, 403
Abortion
    increase in numbers, 16
    induced, 412
    selective reduction, 22
    spontaneous, 259ff
Abruption of the placenta, 140
Abnormal ovarian function, 115
Acquired immune deficiency syndrome
    (AIDS), 21, 403
    condom use, 21
Adenocarcinoma, 403
Adenomatous hyperplasia, 341, 403
Adenomyosis, 343, 403
Adherent placenta, 403
Adhesion prevention, 164
Adhesions, 172, 404
Adhesion-free surgery, 157ff
Adoption, family-building technique,
    234, 252
Allied Health Education Program, 38
Amenorrhea hormone profile, 238, 299,
    300, 404

Amenorrhea, 239ff
    hyperprolactinemia, 299
    hypothalamic, 244, 299
    polycystic ovaries, 299
    premature menopause, 299
American Academy of FertilityCare
    Professionals, 93
    Code of Ethics, 93
    in accreditation, 93
    in certification, 93
    in service programs of excellence, 93
American Academy of Natural Family
    Planning, 93
American Society of Reproductive
    Medicine (ASRM), xv
Ampicillin, 404
Anatomy, basic, 43
Androgenic, 404
Androstenedione, 404
Anorexia nervosa, 301
Anovulation, 404
ART, side-by-side comparison, 255
Artificial insemination, 211, 404
    intrauterine, 211, 307
    pregnancy rates, 211
Artificial reproductive technologies,
    212ff
Artimones, 127ff
    clinical effects, 136
    heteromolecular, (HMA), 131
    metabolic effects, 135

Association of Professors of Gynecology
and Obstetrics (APGO), xv
Azoospermia, 404

B

Bacterial vaginosis, 404
Basal body temperature (BBT), 404
systems, 60
Billings Ovulation Method, 9, 27
and infertility, 235
Billings, Dr. John, 27
Billings, Dr. Lyn, 27
Biological valve, 50, 51, 404
Biomarkers, 36, 237, 405
Birth control pill, 3, 131
androgenic activity, 133
health benefits, 393
irregular bleeding, 37
menstrual cramps, 37
most common progestins, 133
recurrent ovarian cysts, 37
Berman & Berman, 65
Bleeding, unusual, 331ff
Braxton Hicks contractions, 355
Breast cancer, 388
polycystic ovaries, 291
Bromocriptine, 302

C

Catheterization, fallopian tubes, 162
Cautionary note, xxi
Cerebrocentric sexuality, 405
Cervical canal, 45, 405
Cervical cancer, 20
invasive, 20
Cervical cerclage, 141, 364, 405
lengthening of cervix, 366
Cervical crypts, 45, 405
Cervical ectropion, 321, 407
Cervical eversion, 322
Cervical fluid, 49
Cervical infection, 326
Cervical inflammation
criteria for identifying, 321ff
hyfrecation of cervix, 325
identification of, 322
nabothian cysts, 323

Cervical mucus, 45, 405
leukocytes, 87
quantity, 87
sperm survival, 87
spinnbarkeit, 87
Type E, 420
Type G, 420
viscosity, 88
Cervix grading system, 322
Cervix, 45
Child abuse and neglect, 17
Childlessness, infertility, 19
Chlamydia, 19, 405
Chronic cervicitis, 336
Chronic discharge, green discharge,
326, 408
Chronic endometritis, 336
Civilization of love, 14
Clomiphene, 405
Cohen, Dr. M. R., 87
Comprehensive management review,
160, 237
Conception, 68, 405
estimated time of, 98
Condoms, development of AIDS, 21
Conscience, protection of, 391
Contraception, divorce rates, 16
Contraceptives, increase in use, 16
Cooperative approaches, 37
Corpus luteum, 48, 53, 58, 59
deficiency of, 117
Cost effectiveness, 377ff
quality of life outcomes, 384
Creighton Model FertilityCare™ System,
xvii, 11, 27, 43, 51, 60, 61, 64, 406
adenomatous hyperplasia, 341, 403
biological markers, 91
biomarkers, 36
calculating ETA, 98
case management, 74
causes of unusual bleeding, 336ff
cervical inflammation, 321ff
charting examples, 79ff
charting, 73ff
continuous discharge, 90, 321ff
cost of family planning, 377
criteria-driven system, 91
dating pregnancy, 97ff
descriptions, 79

effectiveness to avoid pregnancy, 69, 95
followup, 74
frequent "2W" observations, 326
implantation bleeding, 327
implantation mucus, 327
in achieving pregnancy, 90
in breast feeding, 89
in long cycles, 88
Introductory Session, 74, 412
legitimate choices, 36
locating a teacher, 95
male infertility success, 310ff
Medical Consultants, 73
NaproTracking, 92
non-Peak-type mucus, 77
ovarian cysts, 175ff
ovarian funtion, and, 116
Peak Day, 76
Peak-type mucus, 77
Picture Dictionary, 85
polycystic ovaries, 293
premenstrual syndrome, 181ff
professional infrastructure, 74
stamps, 78
standardization, 74
stress, and, 169
targeted hormone profiles, 106
teachers, 73
unusual bleeding, 331ff
use of pre-Peak yellow stamps, 328
Vaginal Discharge Recording System, 83
Creighton University School of Medicine, 9, 38
Crime rate, violent, 17
Cumulus oophorus, 406
Curse, the, 33
Cushing syndrome, 301
Cystic hyperplasia, 406

D

Daly, K. Diane, vii
Dalton, Dr. Katherina, 181
Davis, Dr. Kingsley, 62
Declaration of Geneva, 410
Depression, sexual activity, 18
Diethylstilbestrol (DES), 143

Discharges, 321ff
Dissent, 5
Divorce laws, 16
Divorce rate, 15
Divorce, sexual promiscuity, 22
Dodds, E. C., 131
Donor eggs, 213, 215
Donor embryos, 215
Donum Vitae, 233
Dostinex, 302
Double ovulation, 66, 407
Down syndrome, 33
Dry cycles, endometriosis, 281
Dry cycles, infertility, 236
Dysfunctional uterine bleeding (DUB), 333, 407
    polycystic ovaries, 291
Dysmenorrhea, 407

E

Ecologically-sensitive system, 45
Ectopic pregnancies, 19, 407
Ectropion, 407
Embryo cryopreservation, 215, 222
Embryo wastage, ART, 216
Encyclical letter, 5, 407
Endometrial biopsies, 341
Endometrial cancer rate, 20
Endometrial cancer, polycystic ovaries, 291
Endometrial hyperplasia, 341, 407
Endometrial polyp, 338, 408
Endometriosis, 275ff, 408
    20 years of "progress," 218
    development of, 278
    diagnosis, 278
    effects on fertility, 279, 283
    excision of endometrial implants, 283, 316
    laparoscopic photos, 280
    laparoscopy, 279
    laser vaporization, 316
    locations, 278
    mucus cycles, 281
    "near-contact" laparoscopy, 161, 243, 277
    treatment, 283
Endometritis, 336, 408

Enovid, 131
Estimated time of arrival (ETA), 98, 408
Estimated time of conception (ETC), 408
Estrogen, 49, 53, 57, 58, 408
    cooperative replacement, 106, 110
    effects, 129
    targeted evaluation, 103ff
Ethinyl estrodiol, 131
Evidence-based medicine, 70, 393, 408

F

Faith, 8
Fallopian tube, 49
    catheterization, 162
Familiaris Consortio, 62, 409
Family planning, 377
Family violence, increase, 23
Fecundity, impaired, 19
Fertility cycle, 409
Fertility pacemaker, 56
Fertility testing, timing of, 240
Fertility, combined, 45
Fertility, micromanagement, 222
FertilityCare™ Centres of Europe, 95
FertilityCare™ Centers International, 94
FertilityCare™ Centers of America, 94
FertilityCare™ Centers of Australasia, 95
FertilityCare™ Centers of Latin America, 95
FertilityCare™ Educator, 9, 409
FertilityCare™ Medical Consultant, 9, 409
FertilityCare™ Practitioner, 9, 38, 409
FertilityCare™ Supervisor, 9
Fertility-focused intercourse, 235
Fertilization, 68
Fetal age, 98
Fibroids, submucous, 339, 409
Fides et Ratio, 7
Fluoxitine, 409
Follicle development, dominance phase, 57
    recruitment phase, 56
    selection phase, 57

Follicle, 48, 54, 56, 409
    mature,48
Follicle stimulating hormone (FSH), 409
Follicular cysts, persistent, 176
Follicular phase deficiency, 121, 123, 409
Follicular phase, 57, 409
Follicular ultrasound series, 237
Folliculogenesis, abnormal, 229, 264
Follow-up, 410
Follow-up Form, 75, 409
Frequent "2W" observations, 326
FSH, 47, 53, 55, 56, 58
    pulsatile, 60

G

Gamete intrafallopian transfer (GIFT), 212
General Intake Form, 85
Genitocentric sexuality, 410
Gestational age, 97
Gestational carriers, 215
GIFT, 212
GnRH, pulsatile fashion, 55
Gonadotropin-releasing hormone (GnRH), 55, 410
Gore-Tex anti-adhesion barrier, 164
Green discharge, 326
Gynecological health, monitoring and maintaining, 91

H

Hart, Dr. R. D., 62
HCG,in short post-Peak phase, 267
    use in miscarriage, 269
Hilgers, Susan K., vii
Hilgers, Thomas W., vii
Hippocrates, 181
Hirsutism, polycystic ovaries, 291, 410
Hormonal dysfunction, 60
Hormone, 127, 410
Hormone, isomolecular (IMH), 132
Hormones, 127ff
    bioidentical, 132, 134, 135
    commonly used, 134
    delivery forms, 138
    dosing amounts and schedules, 138
    isomolecular preparations, 132ff
    ovarian, 117

Human chorionic gonadotropin (hCG),
58, 59, 110, 410
Human life, value and dignity, 36
Human papilloma virus, 20, 411
Human person, respect for, 36
total, 34
Human sexuality, the "inner soul" of,
62
Humanae Vitae, 5, 6, 7, 9, 411
Hyfrecation of cervix, 341, 411
Hyperprolactinemia, 299, 411
Hypospadias, 411
Hypothalamic amenorrhea, 239, 299
Hypothalamus, 55, 411
Hysterosalpingogram, 411
Hysteroscopy, 411

I

Ignorance, 61
Immature follicle, 120, 242
Implantation bleeding, 327
Implantation mucus, 327
in vitro fertilization, xi, 212ff, 412
cancellation rates, 214
dehumanizing process, 32
drop-out rates, 215
embryos wasted, 216
empty deficiencies, 221
first baby born, 4
ICSI, 212, 307
impersonal process, 32
live birth rates, 214
live birth rates, by age, 214
missing links, 223
multiple pregnancies, 217
outcome of pregnancies, 220
ovarian hyperstimulation syndrome
(OHSS), 217
Infant mortality rate, triplets, 19
Infertility treatment, history of, 32
Infertility, 37, 207ff, 227ff
approaches to treatment, 210
causes of, 209
current staircase approach, 210
definition of, 207, 235
endometriosis, 219
evaluation of, 208, 236
evaluation protocols, 236

female diagnosis, 244
fertility-focused intercourse (FFI), 311
incidence, 207
laparoscopic findings, 243
low multiple pregnancy rate, 246
male diagnosis, 244
male, 303ff
missing links, 223
multi-factorial aspects, 244
ovulation defects, 242
polycystic ovaries, 219
premenstrual symptoms, 241
primary, 207
regular menstrual cycles, 236
secondary, 207
staircase approach, 210, 234
The Missing Link, 228
treatment approaches, 210, 245
tubal factor, 220
ultrasound findings, 242
what "progress", 218
Insulin resistance, 238
polycystic ovaries, 292
Insults, 61
Insurance reform, 377ff
centers of excellence, 383
Intracytoplasmic sperm injection (ICSI),
323
Irregular bleeding, 37
Irregular cycles, 37
Irregular menses, polycystic ovaries,
293
IUD, 68

J

K

Kallmann syndrome, 300, 412
Knowledge, the power, 34
Kruger, Dr. T. F., 306
Kruger, strict criteria, 307

L

Laparoscopy review, 160
Laparoscopy, "near-contact", 161, 243

Laparoscopy, 411
  diagnostic, 243
  laser vaporization, 316
  operative, 158
  polycystic ovaries, 287
  variation in diagnostic skill, 315
Laparotomy, 412
Laser laparoscopy,
  subsequent hysterectomy, 317
Laser laparotomy,
  subsequent hysterectomy, 317
Laser uterosacral nerve ablation (LUNA),
  316ff
Laser vaporization, 316
Laser, 412
LH surge, 57, 58
LH test kits, 209, 242
LH, 47, 53, 55, 56, 57, 67
Libido, 412
  level of, 61
Limited mucus cycles, 241
  endometriosis, 281
  miscarriage, 260ff
L-norgestrel, relative potency, 132
Long cycles, 238ff
Long post-Peak phase, 237
Lubricants, vaginal, 310
Luteal cysts, persistent, 177
Luteal phase defects, 117ff
Luteal phase deficiency, 413
  type I, 117, 123
  type II, 117, 123
  type III, 117, 145
  type IV, 119
  type V, 119
Luteal phase deficiency, types, 117-119
Luteal phase, clinical estimates of,
  60, 413
  length of, 58
  short, 261
Luteinized Unruptured Follicle
  Syndrome, 242
Luteinizing hormone (LH), 413
Luteogenesis, abnormal, 229

M

Male infertility, fertility-focused
  intercourse, 311

medical treatment, 308
  success of clomiphene therapy, 309
  vaginal lubricants, 310
Marital bonding, 64
Marriage, the integrity of, 36
Masturbation, dehumanizing, 305
Medicine, the art of, xvii
Medicine, the science of, xvi
Medroxyprogesterone acetate, 413
  relative potency, 132
Men, fertility, 43
Menometrorrhagia, 333, 413
Menopause, premature onset of,
  299
Menorrhagia, 333, 413
Menotoxins, 65
Menses, excessively heavy, 334
Menstrual cramps, 313ff
  economic impact, 313
  incidence of severity, 313
  laser uterosacral nerve ablation, 316
Menstrual cycle hormone profile, 237
Menstrual cycle, 46, 54, 413
Menstrual cycle, truncated, 344
Menstrual fluid, toxicity of, 64
Menstruation, 48, 54, 55, 58, 413
  absence of, 299ff
  normal characteristics, 331
  normal, 331
  retrograde, 278
Metformin, 292
Methodological flaws,
  national IVF data, 215
Metrorrhagia, 333, 414
Michael, Professor R.T., 15
Micronized, 414
Miscarriage, antiphospholipid syndrome,
  274
  endometriosis, and, 264
  evaluation of, 267
  hormonal parameters, 263
  incidence of, 259
  length and variability of post-Peak
    phase, 263
  limited mucus cycle, 260ff
  luteal phase deficiencies, 266
  menstrual score, 260
  mucus cycle score, 260
  ovulation disorders, 264
  premenstrual symptoms, 264

recurrent, evaluation and treatment
    protocol, 267
recurrent, incidence of endometriosis,
    265
role of hCG, 267
role of progesterone, 265
short luteal phase, 261
short post-Peak phase, 261
subclinical infection, 269
Missing links, 223, 228
Morbidity, neonatal, 19
Morphology, 414
Mucus cycle score, 414
    endometriosis, 281
    normal fertility controls, 281
    polycystic ovaries, 293
Mucus cycle, 414
    classification of, 241
Mucus, 414
    type E, 50
    type G, 50
Mucus-enhancing agentsw, vitamin B6,
    245, 247
Multiple births, high order, 216, 246
Multiple pregnancy rate, 217
Multiple pregnancy, 19
Myths, 61

N

Nabothian cysts, 323, 414
Naltrexone, 414
    premenstrual syndrome, 189ff
NaProEducation Technology, 74, 414
NaProTECHNOLOGY,
    xvii, 9, 10, 24, 25, 61
    abnormal ovarian function, 115
    adoption, 252
    and family building, 253
    and hormone assessment, 229, 240
    and infertility, 227ff
    and laparoscopy, 243
    and selective hysterosalpingography,
        162
    assessment, 237
    biomarkers, 237
    breast cancer, 388
    child as gift, 233

comparative pregnancy rates to IVF,
    253
cooperative hormone replacement,
    106
cost effectiveness, 377ff
current research, 387ff
dysfunctional uterine bleeding, 105
education of the patient, 26
effectiveness in infertility, 248ff
Effectiveness Summary, 13
endometriosis, 250
fellowship, 39
goals of, 239
in recurrent miscarriage, 259ff
infertility and staircase approach,
    227ff
infertility evaluation protocols, 236
infertility, 105
infertility, cost effectiveness, 377ff
infertility treatment, 246
long and irregular cycles, 238
low multiple pregnancy rate, 246
male infertility, success, 308ff
multiple pregnancy rate, 217, 246
new insights, 387ff
osteoporosis, 390
ovarian cysts, 175ff
ovarian function, 118, 121
ovarian hyperstimulation syndrome
    (OHSS), 217
paradigm shift, 28
philosophy of, 232
polycystic ovaries, 251
postpartum depression (PPD), 199ff
prematurity prevention,
    cost effectiveness, 396
premenstrual syndrome (PMS),
    105, 181
preterm birth prevention, 105, 351ff
progesterone support during
    pregnancy, 137
progesterone support protocol, 150
protection of conscience, 391
quality of life outcomes, 384
recurrent miscarriage, 105
recurrent ovarian cysts, 105
side-by-side comparison, 255
spectrum of its application, 25
staircase approach, 234
success with endometriosis, 250

success with polycystic ovaries, 251
summary of costs, 381
surgical, 157
surgical, qualifications of the
    physician, 159
surgical, selection of patients, 159
targeted hormone evaluation, 103
term first used, 28
The Medical & Surgical Practice
    of, 12
therapeutic approaches, 26
timing of fertility tests, 240
underlying causes of infertility, 244
uterine cancer, 291
works cooperatively with, 37
Near adhesion-free surgery, 157
Neonatal morbidity, 19
Nihilism, 8
Non-Peak-type mucus, 77, 415
Norethindrone, relative potency, 132

O

Obstetrics, 415
Oligospermia, ideopathic, 308, 415
Operative laparoscopy, 158
Oral contraceptive, 3
Osteoporosis, 390
Ovarian cancer rate, 20
Ovarian cyst, assessment, 175ff
    recurrent, 175
Ovarian function, abnormal, 115
Ovarian hormone dysfunction, 241
Ovarian hormones, 117
Ovarian hyperstimulation syndrome
    (OHSS), 217
Ovarian wedge resection, 158, 296, 415
    hormonal changes, 290
Ovaries, congenital absence of, 301
Ovary, 53
Ovulation cycle, 47, 48, 54, 415
Ovulation defects, infertility, 242
Ovulation disorders,
    classification system, 120
    hormonal profiles, 125, 126
Ovulation test kits, 209, 242
Ovulation testing, current flaws, 242
Ovulation, 47, 48, 53, 57, 415
    abdominal pain, 57
    anatomic defects, 119

defective, 115, 120, 242
double, 66
LH detector kit, 209, 242
occurrence on day 14, 108
Ovulation, testing for, 115, 120
Ovulation, ultrasound assessment,
    116, 167, 242
Ovulatory events, 242

P

Patient abandonment, 29
Peak Day, 53, 76, 100, 415
Peak-type mucus, 77, 415
Pelvic pain scale, 314
Pelvic pain, 313ff
    causes of, 316
    premenstrual syndrome, 319
perinatology, abortion, 33
Perinatology, xii, 416
Periodic abstinence 63
Persistent follicular cysts, 176
Persistent luteal cysts, 177
Philosophy of Nothingness, 8, 223
Physiology, basic, 43
Picture Dictionary, 75, 85, 416
Pituitary gland, 53, 416
Placebo, 416
Placenta, adherent, 416
Planned Parenthood, 18
Polycystic ovarian disease,
    285ff
    ovarian wedge resection, 294
    use of progesterone, 294
Polycystic ovaries, 416
    50 years of "progress," 218
    and breast cancer, 291
    and endometrial cancer, 291
    and endometriosis, 245, 290
    cycle length, 238, 299
    diagnosis, 287
    dysfunctional uterine bleeding,
        291, 341
    endometriosis, 290
    hirsutism, 291
    hormonal correlates, 289
    hypertension, 291
    infertility, 294
    insulin resistance, 238, 292

irregular menses, 291
laparoscopic photos, 288
laparoscopy, 295
long-term medical impact, 290
mucus cycle score, 293
post-Peak phase, 293
progesterone prophylaxis, 294
risk factors, 290ff
ultrasound photos, 288, 289
wedge resection, 296
Polycystic ovary syndrome, 286
Pope John Paul II, 7, 8, 62, 63
Pope Paul VI, 5, 6, 9
Pope Paul VI Institute, 39, 67
development of
NaProTECHNOLOGY, 91
progesterone protocol, 137ff
protocol for progesterone support,
137ff
ultrasound of ovulation, 116
web site, 39
Pornographic literature, 21
Postcoital test, 240, 416
Post menstrual brown bleeding, 333
Postovulatory phase, 46, 58
Postpartum depression, 199ff
cause, 200
Phase I study, 202
Phase II study, 203
treatment protocol, 205
usual approaches to treatment, 201
Postpartum psychosis, 199
Post-Peak phase, 60, 417
long, 177
short, 261
unstable, 263
Practitioner, FertilityCare™, 38
Practitioner, natural family planning,
38
Prebil, Ann M., vii
Pre-embryo, definition, 222
Pregnancy evaluation form, 75, 417
Pregnancy rates, "per woman" in IVF,
219
Pregnancy, ectopic, 19, 407
Pregnancy, out-of-wedlock, 17
Pregnancy-induced hypertension, 143
Pregnanediol, 142
Premature birth, definition, 417

Premature rupture of membranes,
33, 140
Prematurity prevention program,
351ff
Prematurity prevention,
twin pregnancies, 367
Prematurity rate, 18, 351
Premenstrual bleeding, 338
Premenstrual Dysphoric Disorder,
183ff
Premenstrual spotting, 237, 337
Premenstrual syndrome (PMS), 181ff
APGO, and, 183, 184
beta-endorphin levels, 189ff
common symptoms, 190
cost effectiveness, 378
fluoxetine hydrochloride, 192
incidence of symptoms, 191
infertility, 241
naltrexone, 189
NaProTECHNOLOGY diagnosis,
190
non-pharmacologic approaches, 184
pelvic pain, 319
pharmacologic therapy, 185
progesterone treatment, 186ff
spontaneous abortion, 193
Preovulatory phase, 46, 57
Pre-Peak phase of the cycle, 419
Preterm birth, 351ff
antibiotic therapy, 361
case reports, 368ff
cost of, 378
delivery rates, Pope Paul VI Institute
Protocol, 353, 367
fetal fibronectin, 354
medical and developmental problems,
352
obstetrical health maintenance, 358
Office Assessment Form, 351
prematurity prevention program, 353
prematurity rate, 351
short cervix, 364
tocolytic therapy, 360
use of antibiotics, 361
use of cervical cerclage, 364
use of progesterone, 357
Preterm delivery, 145
Preventing adhesions, 164

Progesterone changes in pregnancy, 147
Progesterone in pregnancy, luteal phase deficiencies, 115ff
Progesterone support during pregnancy, 137ff
  protocol, 150
Progesterone treatment, non-targeted therapy, 187
Progesterone treatment, PMS, 186
Progesterone treatment, targeted therapy, 188
Progesterone use, multiple pregnancies, 140
Progesterone, 49, 53, 58, 59, 127ff, 417
  absorption patterns, 134ff
  assessment in pregnancy, 141
  concentrations, 135, 151
  cooperative replacement 106
  day 22 levels, 104
  effects, 128
  human-identical in pregnancy, 131
  important functions, 138
  in pregnancy, 139
  injections, 109
  isomolecular, 131
  levels in miscarriage, 265ff
  lozenges (troches), 134
  micronized, 109
  normogram, 151
  oral micronized, 109
  potency, 132
  pregnancy uses, 139
  production in pregnancy, 138
  regulation of cycle, 110
  safety in pregnancy, 143ff
  support in pregnancy, 137
  targeted evaluation, 103ff
  thermogenic action, 54
  types of support, 108
  vaginal capsules, 109
  zones, 152
Progestin, C-21, 146
Proliferative phase, 48, 54, 57, 417
Prospective data collection, 36, 417
Prostate gland, 44, 417
Protection of conscience, 391

Q

Quality-adjusted life year (QALY), 384
Quality life outcomes, 384

R

Randomized controlled trials, 394
Receptor, estrogen, 59
Receptors, 59, 418
  cytoplasmic, 60
  intranuclear, 60
  steroid, 60
Reconstructive pelvic surgery, 157ff
Recruitment phase, 56
Recurrent miscarriage, 259ff
Recurrent ovarian cysts, 37
Reflex ovulators, 66, 418
Relativism, 418
Reproductive health, monitoring and maintaining, 91
Reproductive medicine, history of, 36
  two approaches, 31
Reproductive system, mission control, 56
Reproductive technologies, empty deficiencies, 221
Research, 12
Retrograde menstruation, 278
Retrospective, 418
Roe v. Wade, 4, 16, 391
Roman Catholic Church, 5

S

SART, 213
Secretory endometrium, 58
Secretory phase, 48, 54, 57, 58, 418
Selective hysterosalpingogram, 162, 234, 418
Selective intercourse, 63, 418
Selective reduction, 22, 33
Semen analysis, World Health Organization reference, 307
Seminal collection device, perforated, 305

Seminal fluid analysis, 304
  standards of adequacy, 306
  strict Kruger criteria, 306
Sexual abuse, 14
Sexual activity, depression, 18
  use of alcohol, 18
Sexual freedom, authentic,
  sexual license, 35
Sexual license, sexual freedom, 35
Sexual retardation, 21
Sexual revolution, 21, 35
Sexuality, cerebrocentric, 64, 405
  dehumanization, 64
  depersonalization, 64
  genitocentric, 64, 410
Sexually-transmitted disease, pregnancy,
  34
Sexually-transmitted diseases, 19, 23
Short post-Peak phase, 261
  use of hCG, 267
Sims-Huhner test, 240, 416
Society for Assisted Reproductive
  Technology (SART), xv, 213
Society of Reproductive Surgeons, 158
Sociologic and medical trends, 24
Sperm (spermatozoa), 43, 419
Sperm survival, 49
SPICE, 64, 419
Spontaneity, 61
Spontaneous abortion, history of 140,
  419
  premenstrual syndrome, 193
Spontaneous ovulators, 66, 419
St. Louis University School of
  Medicine, 9
St. Thomas Aquinas, 8
Standard of care, 28, 29
Standardization, 11, 74
Stein and Leventhal, Drs., 286
Stein-Leventhal Syndrome, 286
Stillbirth, 145
Stress, 169ff
  acute, 169
  chronic, 169
  emotional, 169
  physical, 169
Suicide rates, 17
Super-ovulation strategies, 210
Surgical NaProTECHNOLOGY, 157ff

T

Tail-end brown bleeding, 237
Targeted hormone evaluation, 103ff, 240
Targeting the cycle, 419
Testes, 43
Testicles, 43, 419
The American College of Obstetricians
  and Gynecologists (ACOG), xiii
  Code of Professional Ethics, 28
  committee opinions, 29
Thyroid dysfunction, 341
Tietze, Christopher, 207
Toxemia of pregnancy, 140
Trends, sociologic and medical, 24
True family planning, 420
Truncated, 420
Tubal factor infertility,
  23 years of "progress," 227
Tubal occlusion, 420
Type E mucus, 420
Type G mucus, 420

U

Ultrasound, 421
  evaluation of ovulation, 119
  study of ovulation, 67
Understanding, the power, 34
Unusual bleeding, 331ff
  adenomyosis, 343
  causes of, 336
  characteristics of, 332
  classifications of, 120
  organic causes, 336
  thyroid dysfunction, 341
Urethra, 44
Uterine cancer, 387
Uterine contractions, self-monitoring,
  354
  symptoms of in pregnancy, 355
Uterine fibroids, 339, 409

V

Vaginal Discharge Recording System
  (VDRS), 75, 83, 241, 421
Vaginal discharges, chronic, 321ff
Van Leeuwenhoek, Antoine, 303

Vaporization, 421
Varicocele, 304, 421
Vas deferens, 44
    obstruction of, 304, 421
Vitamin B6, mucus-enhancing agent,
    247

W

Web site, FertilityCare™ Centers of
    America, 39
Women, fertility, 44
    the dignity of, 36

Z

Zygote intrafollopian transfer (ZIFT),
    213